T0230601

Breast Cancer

Translational Medicine Series

Breast Cancer

Translational Therapeutic Strategies

Edited by

Gary H. Lyman

University of Rochester School of Medicine and Dentistry
and James P. Wilmot Cancer Center
University of Rochester Medical Center–
Strong Memorial Hospital
Rochester, New York, U.S.A.

Harold J. Burstein

Dana-Farber Cancer Institute
Harvard Medical School
Boston, Massachusetts, U.S.A.

informa
healthcare

New York London

First published in 2007 by Informa Healthcare, Telephone House, 69-77 Paul Street, London EC2A 4LQ, UK.

Simultaneously published in the USA by Informa Healthcare, 52 Vanderbilt Avenue, 7th Floor, New York, NY 10017, USA.

Informa Healthcare is a trading division of Informa UK Ltd. Registered Office: 37–41 Mortimer Street, London W1T 3JH, UK. Registered in England and Wales number 1072954.

A CIP record for this book is available from the British Library.

Library of Congress Cataloging-in-Publication Data available on application

ISBN-13: 978-0-8493-7416-6

Orders may be sent to: Informa Healthcare, Sheepen Place, Colchester, Essex CO3 3LP, UK
Telephone: +44 (0)20 7017 5540
Email: CSDhealthcarebooks@informa.com
Website: http://informahealthcarebooks.com/

For corporate sales please contact: CorporateBooksIHC@informa.com
For foreign rights please contact: RightsIHC@informa.com
For reprint permissions please contact: PermissionsIHC@informa.com

Printed and bound by CPI Group (UK) Ltd, Croydon, CR0 4YY

Transferred to Digital Print 2012

To my wife, Nicole, and my sons, Stephen and Christopher.
—G. H. L.

To Mary.
—H. J. B.

Foreword

The past 30 years have seen considerable progress in the detection, diagnosis, treatment and prevention of breast cancer. Such progress followed developments on two parallel tracks: empirical observations and, increasingly, translational research. Empirical observations have been at the heart of medical progress for millennia and, until the middle of the 19th century, were largely responsible for all progress in medicine. The emerging fields of biology and genetics have achieved increasing importance, and over the past 30 years the explosion of knowledge about the process of malignant transformation has been dramatic. We now understand that all cancers, including all breast cancers, are ultimately the result of one or more molecular genetic anomalies that result in the loss of customary control processes for cell growth and communal organization. These molecular genetic anomalies can result from a variety of inherited conditions, or external or internal influences. Certainly exposure to environmental carcinogens is one obvious mechanism, but dysregulation of physiologic processes is another common pathway. Research in this area has revealed the central importance of steroid hormone physiology and, in its diseased state, pathophysiology in the development of premalignant and malignant changes of breast tissue. Further research has identified other critical growth hormone and receptor systems, including the type I tyrosine kinase receptor family. Other growth hormone families and the intricate network of intracellular signaling steps that govern cellular behavior and survival have acquired more prominent roles in our global understanding of breast cancer. All these pieces of the puzzle also serve to open opportunities for identifying therapeutic targets and lead to the development of molecularly targeted therapies. The past few years have witnessed the coming together of these various discoveries and led to a substantive paradigm change in our approach to breast cancer. Tamoxifen, as a targeted approach to the estrogen receptor signaling network, and trastuzumab, as a molecular modulator of HER2 signaling, became the prototypes of what many of us hope will be an increasing stream of smart drugs that will approach breast cancer treatment by identifying specific molecular targets that are critical to the survival of the malignant cell and cutting that lifeline.

Recent years have also witnessed our increased understanding of the critical importance of stroma in the development and prospering of cancer cell colonies, whether primary or metastatic. Stromal cells mediate the progression from in situ to invasive breast cancer; normal vascular cells are the precursors of tumor neovascularity in an incestuous relationship with malignant cells. Stromal cells signal to malignant cells and provide the complement of growth factors and cytokines needed for tissue homing, invasion, and metastasis. Such developments opened avenues for entirely novel therapeutic strategies already shown to be clinically effective and relevant.

It is important to understand that this process of discovery to clinical application is delicate, frail, and can be derailed by a variety of external influences.

Our understanding of basic biology, while markedly expanded compared to a few decades ago, is still woefully incomplete. The path from discovery of a potentially active compound in an in vitro system to a drug candidate depends on a series of economically motivated, and sometimes politically charged, influences within pharmaceutical companies, and on the uncertainties of peer-reviewed research support and the vagaries of health care reimbursement in academic centers. Strong credentials and sometimes luck are helpful for new drugs to succeed. A persistent champion that pushed the candidate drug through the existing system is often largely responsible for success or failure.

The process of translating laboratory-based discoveries into practical clinical tools is convoluted and full of obstacles. Basic scientists are ill equipped to travel this road, and most clinical investigators are unskilled to initiate the process. The necessary bridge to make this process succeed is that rare breed of physician scientists labeled "translational investigators." Few centers are equipped to train such individuals, and even fewer provide the support and career opportunities to ensure their success. Clinicians look at translational investigators as incomplete physicians, while basic scientists might consider them intruders with inadequate credentials. They compete, on a part-time basis, with full-time scientists of clinical investigators, and they are expected to not only succeed, but also to drag their skeptical colleagues to follow their lead. And yet, if we don't foster the development of well-trained, biologically oriented translational investigators, basic science discoveries, as critical as they might be, will languish in someone's desk drawer for lack of an effective "translator."

This volume brings together scientists and clinicians, laboratory investigators and clinical trialists. Ably led by the two editors, accomplished translational investigators themselves, it brings to light the accomplishments and challenges of the paradigm shift mentioned previously. While our accomplishments to date are solidly anchored on the increased acceptance and use of the randomized clinical trial, it is clear that many of our new therapeutics will need novel clinical trial approaches for optimal effectiveness and to minimize the possibility of discarding new drugs with biological effects different from traditionally understood cytotoxicity. The development of high-throughput analytical methods have enhanced manifold our ability to analyze the genome, proteome, and metabolome, but also led to new challenges in the interpretation and analysis of massive amounts of data, often obtained from limited numbers of samples. Minimizing the probability of false discovery has become a major task of our statisticians, and maintaining a balance between discovery-led investigations and hypothesis-based research has become an important objective in itself. Technological advances now permit testing not only for overt molecular genetic abnormalities, but also for genetic polymorphisms that are considered to be normal variants. This field will expand substantially in years to come, since it might explain the substantial variability in pharmacokinetics and, more importantly, pharmacodynamics of most drugs, and especially those that require metabolic activation or catabolism. This might lead to improved dosification of all our therapeutics, and perhaps a marked increase in the therapeutic ration of potentially toxic drugs. Clinical and biochemical markers of prognosis have emerged over the past few decades. Most provide reasonably accurate prognostic information for groups of patients but are seldom useful for prognostication of individuals. New molecular markers might provide individually accurate markers of prognosis or predictors of response or resistance to therapy. It is also possible that combinations of multiple markers, as in gene expression profiles, might provide the best prognostic models. The volume also summarizes evolving knowledge about multiple molecularly targeted therapeutic strategies and points out directions for future research.

These are exciting times to be involved in oncology. The pace of discovery, the opportunities to improve our care for patients with breast cancer, and the increasing possibility of developing effective and nontoxic prevention strategies make this an invigorating and intellectually challenging field. How rapidly conceptual advances translate into applicable clinical tools will depend on the process of translation and the dedication and skills of our translational investigators, as well as the increasing involvement of the oncology community at large to effect the clinical validation of novel scientific concepts. I invite you to enjoy this excellent primer and hope it will provide useful, practical information and further provoke your intellectual curiosity.

Gabriel N. Hortobagyi, MD, FACP
Professor and Chair, Department of Breast Medical Oncology, and
Nellie B. Connally Chair in Breast Cancer,
The University of Texas M. D. Anderson Cancer Center
Houston, Texas, U.S.A.

Preface

> Full fathom five thy father lies;
> Of his bones are coral made;
> Those are pearls that were his eyes:
> Nothing of him that doth fade
> But doth suffer a sea-change
> Into something rich and strange.
>
> —William Shakespeare, *The Tempest*

We are living amidst a sea-change in our treatment of breast cancer. As Shakespeare imagined the sailor under the sea, so this medical transformation is both rich and strange. It was this richness, and a desire to make it less strange, that prompted this book, *Breast Cancer: Translational Therapeutic Strategies*.

While the processes of the ocean are timeless, it is worth asking why the sea-change in breast cancer medicine is happening now. There are several major contributors to this transformation. The first has been the recent availability of novel targeted drugs. Breast cancer medicine had for decades depended on two systemic treatment options—chemotherapy and endocrine therapy; the latter representing the earliest successful effort to target therapies based on an improved understanding of tumor biology and biomarker testing. The emergence of anti-HER2 targeted therapy with the humanized monoclonal antibody trastuzumab in the 1990s heralded a major new class of therapeutic modalities. Laboratory and clinical evidence indicated that trastuzumab would be effective only in tumors that were markedly HER2 overexpressing. This created a pressing need for diagnostic tests for HER2 overexpression so that tumors, and thus patients, could be appropriately selected for therapy. The impact of trastuzumab on HER2-positive metastatic breast cancer revised treatment algorithms such that therapy depended entirely on tumor HER2 status. In 2005, reports from several major adjuvant trials of trastuzumab demonstrated that this therapeutic impact extended into early stage breast cancer management as well.

In addition to the apparent clinical benefits of targeted therapy, the focus on HER2 testing and targeted treatment fueled research into the second major transforming event in breast cancer medicine—the characterization of clinical subsets of breast cancer. It became obvious that not all breast cancers were the same. Indeed, several major clinical types of breast cancer could be characterized by marker analysis: estrogen receptor and/or progesterone receptor positive, HER2 positive, and "triple negative" (lacking estrogen receptor and/or progesterone receptor and HER2 expression) subsets. These subsets had immediate practical clinical implications in terms of selecting therapy for both early- and late-stage breast cancers.

Biotechnology advances that facilitated the development of new therapeutics like trastuzumab were accompanied by a further explosion of interest in the large-scale study of gene expression patterns. When genomic tools were applied to breast cancer, the tumor subsets defined by treatment options (hormone receptor subsets, HER2 subsets) were immediately rediscovered, as these tumors all possessed strikingly different patterns of gene expression for one another. In fact, the use of gene expression profiling to characterize breast cancers further deepened the appreciation of breast cancer subsets, as it was found that differences between tumors are not merely "skin deep" and limited to small numbers of growth factors. Rather, the differences between subsets were profound and affected expression of literally hundreds of genes throughout the tumor cell genome. With these observations, the field quickly shifted from the question, "Are there important subsets of breast cancer?" to the questions, "Since there are important subsets, how much pathobiological information do we need to characterize these subsets, and how best should such characterization be done?"

The final major contribution to the transformation of breast cancer treatment has not been a technical or pharmacological revolution, but rather a transformation in the way we think about the disease and its treatment. Namely, clinical researchers and clinicians have become increasingly willing to accept the scientific observations on breast cancer heterogeneity and novel breast cancer therapeutics, and clearly show a willingness to incorporate this new understanding into day-to-day clinical practice. This final step may yet prove to be the most critical. Paradigms of breast cancer treatment that developed from the 1960s through the 1990s were more or less premised on the concepts that all breast tumors were fundamentally similar and should be treated with similar techniques. Thus, seminal trials of breast cancer surgery, radiation therapy, and chemotherapy accrued patients irrespective of tumor biology. As a result, treatment principles learned in these trials were held as true for all types of breast cancer. Lacking better tools to characterize breast cancer variation, investigators did the best they could.

The tools to describe this heterogeneity among breast cancers, however, now exist. Fortunately, the clinical community has been receptive to using these tools both to describe and explain, and ultimately to treat, breast cancers in different and individually tailored fashions based on the biology of the underlying tumor. In fact, few recent trends in oncology better highlight that oft-cited cliché of "bench to bedside" than the evolution in breast cancer treatment in recent years. Truly, this is the exemplar par excellence of translational therapy, where research discoveries in the lab and the clinic have become integrated into ordinary medical care. The rapid incorporation of new discoveries into standard practice is one of the marvels of both the scientific enterprise and clinical care.

This book, assembled with the help of some of the finest clinical investigators in breast cancer medicine today, is designed to highlight the sea-change in breast cancer treatment that has and continues to occur. The book is divided into three major sections. The first section addresses methodological issues for translational medicine and research in oncology. Despite exciting new diagnostic and treatment tools, traditional challenges persist. These include the proper design and analysis of clinical trials, probably nowhere better illustrated than in studies involving high throughput microarrays, which are all the more critical when coping with myriad clinical subsets of tumors, and the limitless quantity of bioinformation entering databases make proper analyses essential. There is a need to explore novel treatment approaches in the geriatric patient population, a demographic group that comprises the largest number of breast cancer patients but which continues to be underrepresented in clinical and scientific studies of breast cancer. Finally, there is a discussion of neoadjuvant breast cancer treatment, a strategy that is increasingly being looked to for early insights into tumor biology and treatment effects.

The second section of the book explores the molecular and cellular heterogeneity of breast cancer. New techniques have emerged to characterize breast cancers into pathobiological subtypes and to detect microscopic foci of cancer. The clinical implications of these new technologies are rapidly emerging and promise to redefine the fundamental nature of our understanding of breast tumors, the traditional methods of determining breast cancer prognosis and selection of therapy, and the monitoring of treatment efficacy.

Finally, the volume closes with a section on novel treatments for breast cancer. This portion of the book includes updates on important tailored therapies, including new endocrine options for ER-positive breast cancer. There are chapters discussing the state of the art for targeted treatments for HER2-positive breast cancer, which are already entering the "next generation" of trials, and other targeted small molecule growth factor inhibitors. In addition, this section highlights the development of new antiangiogenic agents as breast cancer treatments, an entire new avenue of targeted therapy now entering clinical practice. Finally, there is an update on emerging chemotherapeutics, which retain a critical role in breast cancer treatment. It is interesting to note that despite the understandable excitement and enthusiasm for novel targeted drugs, chemotherapy continues to be the backbone upon which most of these treatments have proven their worth. In fact, the ability of chemotherapy to potentiate the effects of newer biological agents means that chemotherapy advances are more relevant to clinical practice than ever.

We believe strongly that *Breast Cancer: Translational Therapeutic Strategies* is arriving at a most timely moment. The confluence of science, technology, and clinical thinking is reshaping the discourse of breast cancer care just as it promises to improve results for breast cancer patients. We hope that this volume continues the transformation of our approaches to breast cancer into future progress that is even richer, and undoubtedly no less strange.

Gary H. Lyman
Harold J. Burstein

Contents

Contributors

Douglas G. Altman   Centre for Statistics in Medicine, University of Oxford, Oxford, U.K.

Karen S. Anderson   Cancer Vaccine Center, Dana-Farber Cancer Institute, Harvard Medical School, Boston, Massachusetts, U.S.A.

Doris Auer   Department of Obstetrics and Gynecology, Innsbruck Medical University, Innsbruck, Austria

Lodovico Balducci   Senior Adult Oncology Program, H. Lee Moffitt Cancer Center and Research Institute, Tampa, Florida, U.S.A.

Mansoina Baweja   Mayo Clinic, Jacksonville, Florida, U.S.A.

Kimberly Blackwell   Departments of Medicine and Radiation Oncology, Duke University Medical Center, Durham, North Carolina, U.S.A.

Joanne L. Blum   Baylor-Charles A. Sammons Cancer Center, Texas Oncology, P.A. and U.S. Oncology, Dallas, Texas, U.S.A.

Stephan Braun   Department of Obstetrics and Gynecology, Innsbruck Medical University, Innsbruck, Austria

Craig A. Bunnell   Dana-Farber Cancer Institute, Harvard Medical School, Boston, Massachusetts, U.S.A.

Harold J. Burstein   Dana-Farber Cancer Institute, Harvard Medical School, Boston, Massachusetts, U.S.A.

Susana M. Campos   Department of Breast and Gynecology, Dana-Farber Cancer Institute, Harvard University, Boston, Massachusetts, U.S.A.

Lisa A. Carey   University of North Carolina, Chapel Hill, North Carolina, U.S.A.

Steven E. Come   Breast Cancer Program, Beth Israel Deaconess Medical Center and Harvard Medical School, Boston, Massachusetts, U.S.A.

Leon E. Cosler   Department of Pharmacy Practice, Albany College of Pharmacy, Albany, New York, U.S.A.

Nancy E. Davidson   Department of Oncology, Johns Hopkins University, Baltimore, Maryland, U.S.A.

Shaheenah Dawood   Department of Oncology, Dubai Hospital, Dubai, United Arab Emirates

Christine Desmedt   Department of Medical Oncology, Jules Bordet Institute, Brussels, Belgium

Amylou Dueck Division of Biostatistics, Mayo Clinic, Rochester, Minnesota, U.S.A.

Daniel F. Hayes Department of Internal Medicine, University of Michigan, Ann Arbor, Michigan, U.S.A.

Nicole M. Kuderer Department of Medicine, University of Rochester School of Medicine and Dentistry and the James P. Wilmot Cancer Center, Rochester, New York, U.S.A.

Brian Leyland-Jones Departments of Oncology and Medicine, McGill University, Montreal, Quebec, Canada

Tianhong Li Department of Oncology, Montefiore Medical Center, Albert Einstein Cancer Center, New York, New York, U.S.A.

Gary H. Lyman Department of Medicine, University of Rochester School of Medicine and Dentistry and the James P. Wilmot Cancer Center, University of Rochester Medical Center–Strong Memorial Hospital, Rochester, New York, U.S.A.

Christian Marth Department of Obstetrics and Gynecology, Innsbruck Medical University, Innsbruck, Austria

Erica L. Mayer Dana-Farber Cancer Institute, Harvard Medical School, Boston, Massachusetts, U.S.A.

Rebecca A. Miksad Division of Hematology–Oncology, Beth Israel Deaconess Medical Center and Harvard Medical School, Boston, Massachusetts, U.S.A.

Kathy D. Miller Division of Hematology/Oncology, Indiana University, Indianapolis, Indiana, U.S.A.

Jeffrey Peppercorn University of North Carolina, Chapel Hill, North Carolina, U.S.A.

Edith A. Perez Mayo Clinic, Jacksonville, Florida, U.S.A.

Charles M. Perou University of North Carolina, Chapel Hill, North Carolina, U.S.A.

Martine J. Piccart-Gebhart Department of Medical Oncology, Jules Bordet Institute, Brussels, Belgium

John T. Salter Division of Hematology/Oncology, Indiana University, Indianapolis, Indiana, U.S.A.

Daniel J. Sargent Division of Biostatistics, Mayo Clinic, Rochester, Minnesota, U.S.A.

Richard Simon Biometric Research Branch, Division of Cancer Treatment and Diagnosis, National Cancer Institute, Bethesda, Maryland, U.S.A.

Jeffrey B. Smerage Department of Internal Medicine, University of Michigan, Ann Arbor, Michigan, U.S.A.

Christos Sotiriou Department of Medical Oncology, Jules Bordet Institute, Brussels, Belgium

Joseph A. Sparano   Department of Oncology, Montefiore Medical Center, Albert Einstein Cancer Center, New York, New York, U.S.A.

Vered Stearns   Department of Oncology, Johns Hopkins University, Baltimore, Maryland, U.S.A.

Vera J. Suman   Division of Biostatistics, Mayo Clinic, Rochester, Minnesota, U.S.A.

Carmel S. Verrier   Departments of Medicine and Radiation Oncology, Duke University Medical Center, Durham, Noth Carolina, U.S.A.

Donald L. Weaver   Department of Pathology, University of Vermont College of Medicine, Burlington, Vermont, U.S.A.

Eric P. Winer   Dana-Farber Cancer Institute, Harvard Medical School, Boston, Massachusetts, U.S.A.

Qun Zhou   Department of Oncology, Johns Hopkins University, Baltimore, Maryland, U.S.A.

1   Clinical Trials of Novel and Targeted Therapies: Endpoints, Trial Design, and Analysis

Vera J. Suman, Amylou Dueck, and Daniel J. Sargent
Division of Biostatistics, Mayo Clinic, Rochester, Minnesota, U.S.A.

INTRODUCTION

With the growth in knowledge of tumorigenesis, the development of agents to combat cancer has evolved from examining the ability of a compound to destroy more tumor cells than healthy cells without imparting excessive toxicity to developing agents that target aberrant antiproliferation signaling, tumor angiogenesis and invasion, resistance to apoptosis, cell immortalization, and/or capacity to metastasize (1). This evolution in cancer drug development has led to modifications in traditional cancer clinical trial designs. This chapter discusses some of these modifications, both proposed and in current use, to traditional phase I, II, and III cancer clinical trial designs for the identification and evaluation of promising targeted agents.

PHASE I DESIGNS

The clinical trial paradigm was developed in the setting of evaluating cytotoxic agents or combinations of cytotoxic agents. The first step in assessing a cytotoxic agent in humans, a phase I clinical trial, is to determine its safety profile, pharmacokinetic characteristics, and a schedule for its administration. Trial designs were developed under the assumption that as the amount of the agent administered increases, the number of tumor cells destroyed increases, and the patient's ability to tolerate the agent decreases. The traditional goal of a phase I trial is to find the maximum amount of the agent that can be administered without inducing intolerable toxicity [maximum tolerated dose (MTD)]. The intent is one of estimation, not hypothesis testing. As the focus is tolerability not clinical benefit, the size of phase I trials is kept small (three to six patients per dose level), intrapatient dose escalation is not usually seen, and enrollment is open to patients of any tumor type, who have exhausted standard treatment options.

The traditional phase I clinical trial design begins enrollment at a dose based on findings from animal studies—for example, one-tenth of the murine equivalent LD10 (the dose that is lethal in approximately 10% of mice it is administered to). The dose escalation scheme is based upon the modified Fibonacci series (e.g., increase by 100%, 65%, 50%, 40%, and then 33% for all subsequent dose levels) as well as a threshold for declaring when excessive toxicity has been encountered (e.g., 33% of the patients treated at the dose will develop an unacceptable degree of toxicity). The toxicities associated with an experimental agent may be anticipated from the toxicities observed in animal or other human studies or the toxicity profile of agents in the same class of drugs. A set of toxicities and the degree of their severity [called dose-limiting toxicities (DLTs)] is defined, which halts dose escalation at the present dose level if an unacceptable proportion of patients treated at that dose level develop a DLT. This event leads to the conclusion that the dose level currently being examined induces unacceptable levels of toxicity and the next lower dose level is declared to be the MTD. See Geller (2) for more details on traditional phase I clinical trial design.

Alternatives to the traditional design have been proposed to reduce the number of patients, who are exposed to dose levels that may not be therapeutic or too toxic and to shorten trial duration. Storer (3) considered a dose escalation scheme in which one patient per dose level is enrolled until a DLT is observed, and then a traditional dose escalation scheme is initiated starting at the dose just prior to the dose producing the DLT. This approach was regarded by some to be too aggressive in the pace at which doses were escalated. Korn et al. (4) offered an alternative to counter this concern in the setting in which the DLT is a severe [National Cancer Institute Common Terminology Criteria for Adverse Events (NCI-CTCAE) Grade 3] or life-threatening toxicity (NCI-CTCAE Grade 4). They suggested that two patients per dose level be enrolled until a DLT is observed or until the second instance of a moderate (NCI-CTC Grade 2) toxicity is reported, then enrollment continues using a traditional dose escalation scheme (4,5).

Ivanova et al. (6) examined the properties of several up-and-down rules for sequentially assigning patients to a dose level. One rule proposed by Gezmu (7) suggests entering as many as k patients per dose level, where ρ is the target probability of developing a DLT at the MTD and k is the value that satisfies the equation $\rho = 1 - (0.5)^{1/k}$. The rules for dose escalation are as follows: If the last patient entered on trial was enrolled onto the dth dose level and developed a DLT, then the next patient enters onto the $(d-1)$th dose level. If the last patient entered was enrolled onto the dth dose level and did not develop a DLT and the previous $k-1$ patients entered were enrolled on the dth dose level and did not develop a DLT, then the next patient enrolled is entered onto the $(d+1)$th dose level. If the last patient entered was enrolled onto the dth dose level and did not develop a DLT and the previous j patients entered were enrolled onto the dth dose level and did not develop a DLT but $j < k-1$, then the next patient enrolled is entered onto the dth dose level.

Another variation of an up-and-down rule was proposed by Narayana (8) in which the criteria for assigning the $(s+1)$th patient to a dose level is based on the proportion of patients, who develop a DLT among those enrolled on the jth dose level up to that time point, p_{js}. Ivanova et al. (6) found that these designs perform well in terms of assigning patients to doses close to the MTD.

The up-and-down designs of Narayana (8) and Ivanova et al. (6) use dose escalation schemes in which the toxicity data from patients treated at the current dose level are used to determine the dose level to assign to the next patient enrolled. The Bayesian approach does not restrict its dose escalation criteria to the toxicity data from the current dose level, but uses all the toxicity data up to that point. The Bayesian approach not only requires specifying the set of toxicities to be considered DLTs, the target probability for developing a DLT at the MTD, and the dose levels of interest, but requires the investigators to specify a functional form for the dose–toxicity relationship (e.g., a logit or probit model) and a probability distribution function for the unknown parameters of the dose–toxicity relationship (e.g., the uniform or beta distributions). Based on these initial specifications, O'Quigley et al. (9) proposed that the dose with the estimated probability of inducing a DLT nearest to the target probability be given to the first patient enrolled. After each patient is entered onto the trial and her toxicity results are ascertained, the probability distribution function for the unknown parameters of the dose–toxicity relationship is updated using Bayes theorem. The expected values of the unknown parameters are used to update the dose–toxicity function and the dose with the estimated probability of inducing a DLT nearest to the target probability is assigned to the next patient enrolled. This approach is referred to as the continual reassessment method (CRM) (9,10). Several recommendations have been made as to when to end enrollment such as after a prespecified number of patients have entered, when a prespecified number of patients have been treated at the nominal MTD, or when the estimate of the MTD is within 10% of its previous estimate.

CRM has been criticized for many reasons including the time required to complete such a trial since the jth patient's outcome must be known before the $(j+1)$th patient can be enrolled, the appropriateness of the initial guess as to the dose–toxicity relationship, the possibility of a sizeable increases in the dose, and the possibility of enrolling patients at too toxic a dose level. Goodman et al. (11) demonstrated that restricting dose escalation to one dose level (de-escalations can be any number of dose levels), starting at the lowest dose level, assigning two to three patients per dose level, and terminating enrollment at a prespecified number of patients can shorten trial duration and incidence of DLTs.

Moller (12) suggested a blending of the standard and CRM designs to estimate the MTD. Patients are enrolled onto the trial using the standard trial design until the first DLT is observed. The data from this first stage of the trial are used to find an initial estimate for the dose–response relationship. The second stage of the trial is then carried out using the CRM dose escalation.

The growing body of knowledge in the area of tumor biology and cancer genetics has led to the development of agents that target errant signaling molecules, cell cycle checkpoint control, tumor differentiation, tumor suppressor oncogenes, angiogenesis, apoptosis, and immune intolerance. These agents seek to alter a critical mechanism of action driving the malignant process. Their effect may not result in the tumor shrinking, but in arresting its progression. In addition, the targets of these agents may be expressed differently in tumor cells compared to normal cells, and the mechanism by which a biological effect is gained may be different than the mechanism that induces severe or life-threatening toxicities. Thus, the relationship between the dose administered and the biological effect of the targeting agent may not follow the behavior associated with a dose–toxicity relationship. The dose where maximum modulation of the target occurs may not correspond to the MTD. As such, the goal of a phase I trial of a targeted agent (that does not shrink the tumor in a dose-dependent manner) becomes one of finding the dose that corresponds to the maximum modulation of the target while maintaining the toxicity rate within an acceptance range. Korn et al. (13) pointed out that finding the dose that provides maximum modulation of the target requires more patients than the number traditionally enrolled in phase I trials.

Enrollment to these trials is often limited to patients of a single tumor type whose tumors have the target under investigation. The starting dose is based on the results of animal models. Difficulties arise in defining what is considered a biologically meaningful effect, the minimum proportion of patients for whom the effect should be observed, and how aggressively doses can be escalated. Requisite to designing trials to evaluate biological parameter is the ability to obtain a measure of biological effect, such as through serial biopsies or noninvasive techniques that yield a surrogate for the biological effect of the agent (e.g., serum levels of the target, imaging parameters from PET or MRI scans). Presence of such a marker is not sufficient; the marker must also be able to be measured in a valid, reliable, and repeatable manner, and supported by evidence that modulation of the target correlates with clinical benefit (14–18).

Hunsberger et al. (19) suggested that a biologically adequate dose be sought where the dose yields a prespecified level of effect or lies in the plateau of the dose–response curve where neighboring dose levels yield effect levels within 10% of each other. They examined dose finding trial designs where the targeted agent does not induce excessive toxicity so that the dose escalation scheme is solely based on the dose–response curve. When the response rate is thought to increase with increasing doses of the agent, a modification of the standard dose escalation scheme is suggested based on the maximum response rate considered too low to be of clinical benefit and the minimum response rate considered to be of potential clinical benefit. When the dose–response curve is thought to plateau, the dose escalation scheme is based on the slope of the regression line through the last highest three to four dose levels. When the estimated slope of this regression line is near or below zero and at least one response rate is seen among these three to four highest dose levels, dose escalation stops. The recommended dose is the one with the highest proportion of responses.

Thall et al. (20) proposed a Bayesian dose-finding strategy where the "best" dose for the next cohort of patients depends upon the prespecified values for the minimum probability of a biological effect and the maximum probability of a DLT, as well as the toxicity and biological effects seen among all of the patients previously enrolled into the trial. This approach assumes that at a given dose level, the patient either develops a DLT, has documented tumor response, or neither. The number of patients to be treated per dose level is small, usually one, two, or three patients. At any step in the dose escalation process, if the estimated tumor response is similar for two or more doses (within say 5% of each other), they suggest that the dose with the lowest estimated probability of developing a DLT be chosen for the next cohort of patients to be enrolled. In terms of determining the maximum number of patients to be enrolled, Thall et al. (20) recommend that this be determined from the results of the simulations with clinically plausible dose–response scenarios. Thall and Cook (21) and Zhang et al. (22) presented alternative methods based on a similar approach of modeling both toxicity and efficacy in the phase I trial, extending the methodology to allow for a non-monotone dose–efficacy relationship.

PHASE II DESIGNS

A phase II clinical trial of a cytotoxic agent is conducted to assess its antitumor activity and to further describe its safety profile in a well-specified patient population of a given tumor type. Evidence of antitumor activity is usually based on the proportion of patients whose tumors significantly shrink (response rate) without the patients experiencing extensive toxicity. As such, enrollment is limited to patients whose lesions can be accurately measured on physical examination or imaging studies. The underlying assumption in this approach is that shrinking the tumor leads to longer progression-free or overall survival time.

A typical phase II trial of a cytotoxic agent is designed to test whether the proportion of patients whose tumors respond to treatment is so small that the agent is considered to have insufficient antitumor activity to further pursue in this patient population, against the alternative that the proportion of patients whose tumors respond to treatment is large enough to consider further testing of the agent in this population. The "too little" and "large enough" thresholds are chosen based upon published response rates with other agents in a similar patient population. Secondary endpoints may include progression-free or overall survival time.

Having specified the upper and lower thresholds for response and the size of the type I and type II errors, a trial can be designed to enroll patients in a single stage or multiple stage design. Multi-stage trials allow discontinuation of accrual after a prespecified number of patients if there is insufficient evidence of antitumor activity or overwhelming evidence of antitumor activity (23,24). These trial designs have been extended to include an endpoint composed of both tumor response and progression-free survival rates (25,26).

Some targeted agents may be cytotoxic and as such, tumor response would be an appropriate means to assess clinical benefit. Other targeted agents may slow or block further growth of the tumor, but not shrink the tumor. The progression-free survival rate and growth modulation index have been proposed as endpoints when assessing cytostatic agents (13).

Progression-free survival at say six months or one year captures clinical benefit associated with stable disease. However, in a two-stage design, accrual must be halted for six months or one year for patients to become evaluable. Accrual to the second stage can be hindered following a long break. Additionally, the progression-free survival rate is not a clear indication of clinical activity. In other words, some patients on study would have been progression-free after six months even had they not received the experimental treatment (whereas tumor response is a clear indication of treatment activity such that tumors rarely shrink in the absence of treatment). Lastly, in many cases it is difficult to select the appropriate control progression-free survival rate if historical data are unavailable.

The growth modulation index (27) is an alternative endpoint which is intended to measure whether an agent changes the natural course of the disease using each patient as her own control. This endpoint avoids the issue of selecting a historical control as is often problematic when using six-month progression-free survival. If a patient's time to progression on the experimental regimen is substantially longer (say by 33%) than the patient's time to progression on her prior therapy, then the experimental regimen is likely to have had an effect on the natural history of the patient's tumor. Though intuitively appealing, this endpoint may suffer from selection bias (enrollment of patients who progressed on first-line therapy) as well as bias from investigators prematurely classifying progression in a first-line setting in order to treat patients with the second-line experimental cytostatic agent. Other potential phase II endpoints for cytostatic agents are discussed by Korn et al. (13).

Randomized Phase II Designs

Evaluating the promise of a new agent/regimen to become the experimental arm for a phase III clinical trial from among those evaluated in a series of single-arm phase II trials is difficult given the variability among studies in terms of patient eligibility, dosing schedules, disease evaluations, and endpoint definitions. The randomized phase II design has been suggested as a means to overcome these sources of variability.

In randomized phase II designs, patients are randomized to one of k regimens where one of the regimens may be the standard treatment for the disease.

A common randomized phase II trial design is to conduct concurrently a stand-alone standard phase II clinical trial for each regimen under consideration using the same patient eligibility criteria, but randomizing eligible patients among the independent trials [e.g., see (28,29)]. In the event that two or more experimental regimens are deemed promising, but only a single experimental regimen may be moved forward to the phase III trial, the decision to move one experimental regimen to a phase III over another is not based on a formal comparison of the primary endpoint. The decision is based on consideration of efficacy, adverse event profiles, costs, quality of life, feasibility, etc.

Although these trials are not of a sufficient size to formally compare experimental regimens with a standard regimen, Herson and Carter (30) noted that there is potential value in randomizing to experimental and standard regimens within a phase II trial. Particularly, if a substantially smaller than anticipated success rate with the standard regimen is observed, then a small success rate with the experimental regimen may not indicate lack of efficacy of the experimental regimen. Similarly, a substantially larger than anticipated success rate with the standard regimen would lead to distrust of a high success rate with the experimental regimen.

Rubinstein et al. (31) suggested powering a randomized phase II trial for a formal (though not definitive) comparison between experimental and standard regimens. In order to reduce the sample size of such a comparison, Rubinstein et al. (31) suggested using a binary endpoint such as progression-free or overall survival at a fixed time point (e.g., six-month progression-free survival), as well as relaxing the type I and II error rates to 10% or 20%. The sample size is both the advantage and the disadvantage of this design. It is the advantage in that this design does not require substantially more patients than a pair of simultaneous single-arm phase II trials while still allowing a formal comparison between regimens of the primary endpoint. It is the disadvantage in that it still requires roughly twice as many patients as a single-arm phase II trial. Rubinstein et al. (31) ultimately concluded that this design is most appropriate as a preliminary test of a regimen in which a new agent is added to a standard regimen.

In a randomized phase II screening design, patients are again randomized to two or more experimental regimens and the regimen which exhibits the highest success rate is selected for further study (32). The sample size is determined to assure a high probability (such as 90%) of selecting the best experimental regimen if the success rate of that regimen is higher than the success rate of the other experimental regimens by some prespecified margin (such as 15%). An alternative to this design was proposed by Sargent and Goldberg (33) to allow additional factors to enter into the selection among experimental regimens for phase III testing when the outcome on the primary endpoint is not clear-cut.

Thall et al. (34) proposed a sequential randomized phase II design approach in which patients are randomized to two or more experimental regimens in the first stage, and then the most active experimental regimen identified in the first stage is compared in a randomized phase II fashion with a control regimen in the second stage. Another sequential randomized design discussed by Strauss and Simon (35) randomizes patients to one of two or more experimental regimens in the first stage and then the most active experimental regimen of the first stage becomes the control regimen in subsequent stages. Ma et al. (16) indicate that sequential designs are most useful when activity among experimental regimens and the control regimen is not substantially different.

An enrichment or discontinuation design is a sequential randomized phase II design which attempts to "enrich" the study cohort by selecting patients, who have a higher chance of responding to a targeted agent [e.g., see (36)]. Freidlin and Simon (37) indicate that this design may be informative when the assay for the target is not readily available or a molecular target has not been identified. In the first stage of this design, all patients are treated with the experimental regimen for a fixed duration of time. At the end of this phase, those with partial or complete tumor responses continue on active treatment whereas patients with stable disease are randomized to either active treatment or a placebo. Patients are taken off study at time of progression throughout the design.

Randomized phase II trials should not be viewed as substitutes for phase III trials (38). Randomized phase II trials are powered for selecting experimental regimens for a phase III trial as opposed to detecting definitive superiority or equivalence among experimental and/or standard regimens. Though randomized phase II trials allow for unbiased comparisons of typical phase III endpoints such as progression-free and overall survival, these secondary analyses suffer from multiplicity when many secondary endpoints are considered and should only be reported as exploratory (38). Additionally, a two-arm randomized phase II trial requires two to four times more patients than a single-arm phase II trial. A randomized phase II trial may be useful for selecting one of two novel agents for a phase III trial or selecting one of two dosing schedules of a novel agent (i.e., a two-arm randomized phase II trial requires roughly the same number of patients as two single-arm phase II trials). One must carefully consider, however, whether the benefit of including a control arm in a randomized phase II trial outweighs the delay of a definitive phase III trial.

PHASE III DESIGNS

The most common targeted design in the phase III setting is a trial in which the only patients randomized are those who are most likely to respond to the experimental agent, such as those patients who overexpress or dysregulate the novel agent's molecular target. Several authors have suggested that such a targeted phase III design is more efficient for determining the efficacy of novel agents (16,39,40). The targeted design assumes that a subpopulation likely to benefit has been identified and an assay is available for practical use for selecting such patients within the definitive phase III trial (41). Loi et al. (41) cite trastuzumab in breast cancer as a success story in terms of a targeted phase III design and gefitinib in nonsmall cell lung cancer as a failure. In several phase III trials of trastuzumab (42,43), a monoclonal antibody against HER2, only patients identified to be HER2+ were randomized and the benefit of trastuzumab was clearly identified. In an untargeted fashion, gefitinib [an antiepidermal growth factor receptor (EGFR) tyrosine kinase inhibitor] was tested in two phase III trials in widely heterogeneous populations (44,45). Subgroup analyses identified some subpopulations that may have benefited. Additional work in pharamacogenetics identified that somatic mutations of the tyrosine kinase domain of the EGFR were associated with sensitivity to gefitinib (46), which are typically present in many of the patients in the subgroups identified to have benefited from gefitinib in the phase III trials. Loi et al. (41) speculated that a targeted phase III trial of gefitinib may have identified it as successful within patients with somatic mutations of the tyrosine kinase domain of the EGFR similar to trastuzumab being identified as successful within patients with HER2+ breast cancer.

Simon and Maitournam investigated the relative efficiency of a targeted phase III design relative to an untargeted design with a binary endpoint (39) or a continuous response distribution-free endpoint (40). The authors speculated that their results most likely extend to right-censored survival data, but they have not extended the work thus far. This phase III design applies to restricting eligibility to patients predicted to be responsive to the drug as opposed to broader eligibility criteria. In the targeted design, patients are screened in order to identify patients with the required molecular target. An equal number of patients with the required molecular target are then randomized to the regimen containing the novel agent versus the control regimen. The authors found that when the treatment effect is limited to the targeted population and the sensitivity/specificity of the assay used for identifying patients likely to respond are high, the targeted design is far more efficient in the number needed for randomization and number needed for screening than the number needed for randomization in the untargeted design.

In many cases, however, the mechanism of action of an agent may be less well understood, and a targeted trial strategy may miss a true effect. Consider the monoclonal antibody cetuximab, which specifically targets EGFR. Initial trials with this agent restricted eligibility to those found to express EGFR (47), and as such, the initial FDA labeling for cetuximab only specified use for patients with EGFR positive tumors. Subsequent testing has demonstrated similar activity of cetuximab in both EGFR positive and negative tumors (48,49). Thus, depending on the knowledge base from which a drug development platform is mounted, a strategy of targeted trials may have positive or negative consequences. If an untargeted approach is proposed, prospective formal consideration of a subgroup analysis in patients expressing the target of interest is recommended. Sargent et al. (50) present additional statistical considerations for phase III trial designs to validate putative predictive markers.

CONCLUDING REMARKS

Targeted therapies require clinical investigators to reconsider all aspects of clinical development. Agents with limited toxicity require new phase I designs, agents with limited or no cytotoxic effect require new phase II designs, and agents whose activity is limited to biologically defined subsets alter phase III testing strategies. However, for each new agent that follows the prototypical pathway of a targeted therapy (such as imatinib), it seems another is developed that shares at least some similarities with standard cytotoxic agents (such as erlotinib). Trialists would be advised to use multiple approaches in early clinical trials, exploring several endpoints and avoiding a rush to phase III trials, which can result in large-scale disappointment [such as PTK-787 in colorectal cancer (51)]. The field remains ripe for further innovation.

REFERENCES

1. Hanahan D, Weinberg R. The hallmarks of cancer. Cell 2000; 100(1):57–70.
2. Geller N. Design of phase I and phase II clinical trials in cancer: a statistician's view. Cancer Invest 1984; 2:483–491.
3. Storer BE. Design and analysis of phase I clinical trials. Biometrics 1989; 45(3):925–937.
4. Korn EL, Midthune D, Chen TT, Rubinstein LV, Simon RM. A comparison of two phase I trial designs. Stat Med 1994; 13(18):1799–1806.

5. Simon R, Freidlin B, Rubinstein L, Arbuck SG, Collin J, Christian MC. Accelerated titration designs for phase I clinical trials in oncology. JNCI 1997; 89(15):1138–1147.
6. Ivanova A, Montazer-Haghighi A, Mohanty SG, Durham SD. Improved up-and-down designs for phase I trials. Stat Med 2003; 22:69–82.
7. Gezmu M. The Geometric Up-and-Down Design for Allocating Dosage Levels. Dissertation, American University, 1996.
8. Narayana TV. Sequential Procedures in the Probit Analysis. Dissertation, University of North Carolina, Chapel Hill, 1953.
9. O'Quigley J, Pepe M, Fisher L. Continual reassessment method: a practical design for phase I clinical trials in cancer. Biometrics 1990; 45:33–48.
10. Chevret S. The continual reassessment method in cancer phase I clinical trials: a simulation study. Stat Med 1993; 12:1093–1108.
11. Goodman SN, Zahurak ML, Piantadosi S. Some practical improvements in the continual reassessment method for phase I studies. Stat Med 1995; 14:1149–1161.
12. Moller S. An extension of the continual reassessment methods using a preliminary up-and-down design in a dose-finding study in cancer patients, in order to investigate a greater range of doses. Stat Med 1995; 14:911–922.
13. Korn EL, Arbuck SG, Pluda JM, Simon R, Kaplan RS, Christian MC. Clinical trial designs for cytostatic agents: are new approaches needed? J Clin Onc 2001; 19(1): 265–272.
14. Parulekar WR, Eisenhauer EA. Phase I trial design for solid tumor studies of targeted, non-cytotoxic agents: theory and practice. JNCI 2004; 96(13):990–997.
15. Ranson M, Jayson G. Targeted antitumor therapy-future perspective. British Journal of Cancer 2005; 92(suppl 1):S28–S31.
16. Ma BB, Britten CD, Siu LL. Clinical trial designs for targeted agents. Hematol Oncol Clin North Am 2002; 16(5):1287–1305.
17. Rowinsky E. The pursuit of optimal outcomes in cancer therapy in a new age of rationally designed target-based anti-cancer agents. Drugs 2000; 60(suppl 1):1–14.
18. Gelmon KA, Eisenhauer EA, Harris AL, Ratain M, Workman P. Anticancer agents targeting signaling molecules and cancer cell development: challenges for drug development? JNCI 1999; 91(15):1281–1287.
19. Hunsberger S, Rubinstein LV, Dancey J, Korn EL. Dose escalation trial designs based on molecularly targeted endpoint. Stat Med 2005; 24:2171–2181.
20. Thall PF, Estey E, Sung H. A new statistical method for dose-finding based on efficacy and toxicity in early phase clinical trial. Invest New Drugs 1999; 17:155–167.
21. Thall PF, Cook JD. Dose-finding based on efficacy-toxicity trade-offs. Biometrics 2004; 60(3):684–693.
22. Zhang W, Sargent DJ, Mandrekar S. An adaptive dose-finding design incorporating both toxicity and efficacy. Stat Med 2005; 25(14):2365–2383.
23. Simon R. Optimal two-stage designs for phase II clinical trials. Control Clin Trials 1989; 10:1–10.
24. Fleming TR. One-sample multiple testing procedure for phase II clinical trials. Biometrics 1982; 38(1):143–151.
25. Dent S, Zee B, Dancey J, Hanauske A, Wanders J, Eisenhauer E. Application of a new multinomial phase II stopping rule using response and early progression. J Clin Oncol 2001; 19(3):785–791.
26. Zee B, Melnychuk D, Dancey J, Eisenhauer E. Multinomial phase II cancer trials incorporating response and early progression. J Biopharm Stat 1999; 9(2):351–363.
27. Von Hoff DD. There are no bad anticancer agents, only bad clinical trial designs— twenty-first Richard and Hinda Rosenthal Foundation Award Lecture. Clin Cancer Res 1998; 4(5):1079–1086.
28. Chan S, Scheulen ME, Johnston S, et al. Phase II study of temsirolimus (CCI-779), a novel inhibitor of mTOR, in heavily pretreated patients with locally advanced or metastatic breast cancer. J Clin Oncol 2005; 23(23):5314–5322.
29. Perez EA, Geeraerts L, Suman VJ, et al. A randomized phase II study of sequential docetaxel and doxorubicin/cyclophosphamide in patients with metastatic breast cancer. Ann Oncol 2002; 13(8):1225–1235.
30. Herson J, Carter SK. Calibrated phase II clinical trials in oncology. Stat Med 1986; 5(5):441–447.

31. Rubinstein LV, Korn EL, Freidlin B, Hunsberger S, Ivy SP, Smith MA. Design issues of randomized phase II trials and a proposal for phase II screening trials. J Clin Oncol 2005; 23(28):7199–7206.

32. Simon R, Wittes RE, Ellenberg SS. Randomized phase II clinical trials. Cancer Treat Rep 1985; 69(12):1375–1381.

33. Sargent DJ, Goldberg RM. A flexible design for multiple armed screening trials. Stat Med 2001; 20(7):1051–1060.

34. Thall PF, Simon R, Ellenberg SS. A two-stage design for choosing among several experimental treatments and a control in clinical trials. Biometrics 1989; 45(2):537–547.

35. Strauss N, Simon R. Investigating a sequence of randomized phase II trials to discover promising treatments. Stat Med 1995; 14:1479–1489.

36. Stadler WM, Rosner G, Small E, et al. Successful implementation of the randomized discontinuation trial design: an application to the study of the putative antiangiogenic agent carboxyaminoimidazole in renal cell carcinoma—CALGB 69901. J Clin Oncol 2005; 23(16):3726–3732.

37. Freidlin B, Simon R. Evaluation of randomized discontinuation design. J Clin Oncol 2005; 23(22):5094–5098.

38. Wieand HS. Randomized phase II trials: what does randomization gain? J Clin Oncol 2005; 23(9):1794–1795.

39. Simon R, Maitournam A. Evaluating the efficiency of targeted designs for randomized clinical trials. Clin Cancer Res 2004; 10(20):6759–6763.

40. Maitournam A, Simon R. On the efficiency of targeted clinical trials. Stat Med 2005; 24(3):329–339.

41. Loi S, Buyse M, Sotiriou C, Cardoso F. Challenges in breast cancer clinical trial design in the postgenomic era. Curr Opin Oncol 2004; 16:536–541.

42. Slamon DJ, Leyland-Jones B, Shak S, et al. Use of chemotherapy plus a monoclonal antibody against HER2 for metastatic breast cancer that overexpresses HER2. N Engl J Med 2001; 344(11):783–792.

43. Romond EH, Perez EA, Bryant J, et al. Trastuzumab plus adjuvant chemotherapy for operable HER2-positive breast cancer. N Engl J Med 2005; 353(16):1673–1684.

44. Herbst RS, Giaccone G, Schiller JH, et al. Gefitinib in combination with paclitaxel and carboplatin in advanced non-small-cell lung cancer: a phase III trial–INTACT 2. J Clin Oncol 2004; 22(5):785–794.

45. Giaccone G, Herbst RS, Manegold C, et al. Gefitinib in combination with gemcitabine and cisplatin in advanced non-small-cell lung cancer: a phase III trial–INTACT 1. J Clin Oncol 2004; 22(5):777–784.

46. Lynch TJ, Bell DW, Sordella R, et al. Activating mutations in the epidermal growth factor receptor underlying responsiveness of non-small-cell lung cancer to gefitinib. N Engl J Med 2004; 350(21):2129–2139.

47. Cunningham D, Humblet Y, Siena S, et al. Cetuximab monotherapy and cetuximab plus irinotecan in irinotecan-refractory metastatic colorectal cancer. N Engl J Med 2004; 351(4):337–345.

48. Chung KY, Shia J, Kemeny NE, et al. Cetuximab shows activity in colorectal cancer patients with tumors that do not express the epidermal growth factor receptor by immunohistochemistry. J Clin Oncol 2005; 23(9):1803–1810.

49. Saltz LB. Can the addition of cetuximab to irinotecan improve outcome in colorectal cancer? Nat Clin Pract Oncol 2005; 2(1):20–21.

50. Sargent DJ, Conley BA, Allegra C, Collette L. Clinical trial designs for predictive marker validation in cancer treatment trials. J Clin Oncol 2005; 23(9):2020–2027.

51. Hecht JR, Trarbach T, Jaeger E, et al. A randomized, double-blind, placebo-controlled, phase III study in patients (pts) with metastatic adenocarcinoma of the colon or rectum receiving first-line chemotherapy with oxaliplatin/5-fluorouracil/leucovorin and PTK787/ZK 222584 or placebo (CONFIRM-1). J Clin Oncol, 2005 ASCO Annual Meeting Proceedings, 2005; 23(16S):3.

2 Prognostic Models: A Methodological Framework and Review of Models for Breast Cancer

Douglas G. Altman

Centre for Statistics in Medicine, University of Oxford, Oxford, U.K.

INTRODUCTION

Prognostic models are widely used in cancer for investigating patient outcome in relation to multiple patient and disease characteristics. Such a model may allow the (reasonably) reliable classification of patients into two or more groups with different prognoses. It may be of particular interest to identify patients with a good prognosis that adjuvant therapy would not be (cost-)beneficial, or a group with a poor prognosis that more aggressive adjuvant therapy would not be justified (1).

We can define a prognostic model as a combination of at least two separate variables to predict patient outcome. In this chapter, I describe a review of published prognostic models that have been developed to predict the outcome of future breast cancer patients. Studies were considered where the specific aim was either to develop a new prognostic model or to attempt to validate an existing model for newly diagnosed patients, and where at least one of the endpoints of death, cancer death, or recurrence of disease was studied. A full account is available elsewhere (2).

It is clear that a prognostic model will have no clinical value unless it can be shown to predict outcome with some success; unless the model is shown to be useful it will be quickly forgotten (3). Thus, there is a particular interest in identifying prognostic models for which there has been an evaluation of how successful the models have been when used in a different setting, that is, models which have been validated externally (1,4,5).

DEVELOPING RELIABLE PROGNOSTIC MODELS

Although prognostic models can be of great clinical assistance, few prognostic models are in common use (not just in cancer) (6). As Wyatt and Altman (3) observed: "However accurate a model is in statistical terms, doctors will be reluctant to use it to inform their patient management decisions unless they believe in the model and its predictions." They suggested the following conditions for clinical credibility: (*i*) All clinically relevant patient data should have been tested for inclusion in the model; (*ii*) it should be simple for doctors to obtain all the patient data required, reliably and without expending undue resources, in time to generate the prediction and guide decisions; (*iii*) model builders should try to avoid arbitrary thresholds for continuous variables; (*iv*) the model's structure should be apparent and its predictions should make sense to the doctors who will rely on them; and (*v*) it should be simple for doctors to calculate the model's prediction for a patient. The difficulties of developing reliable multiple regression models have been much discussed (7–10). Both clinical and statistical aspects are critical.

Study Design

Important considerations for the design of studies to develop a prognostic model include the advantages of a prospective study, the need for patients to be followed-up from a common event (such as surgery or diagnosis), and the quality of measurements. In prospective studies, eligible patients are enrolled, complete baseline measurements are made in a standardized way, and they are followed for an adequate length of time to allow a comparison of survival experience in relation to baseline variables including tumor marker values. Some randomized trials sensibly incorporate the collection of tumor markers for prognostic studies; otherwise, prospective studies are rare. Most prognostic studies in cancer use existing clinical data, however. These studies have the considerable advantage of the ready availability of a cohort with a long enough follow-up for assessment of a substantial number of outcome events (e.g., deaths or recurrences). But the cohort may not be complete, measurements may not be standardized, and some baseline data may be missing. Also, treatments given to patients will usually vary, with the choice of treatment partly related to prognostic information.

Patient Sample

A reliable prognostic study ideally requires a well-defined "inception" cohort of patients at the same stage of their disease, commonly at the time of first diagnosis of cancer. Apart from the stage of cancer, there may be additional selection criteria such as age, whereas exclusion criteria might include prior cancer or non-standard treatment. Eligible patients should not be excluded because of missing data or loss to follow-up. Only unselected cases or random samples from a given population will produce unbiased survival estimates.

Sample Size

Several authors have addressed the issue of sample size for prognostic studies (11,12). It is important to recognize that the power of a study depends on the number of observed events and not the number of patients. Thus, a small sample with long follow-up may yield better information than a large study with short follow-up. It follows that a study will have less power to investigate rarer endpoints; in the present context, there is more power to investigate recurrence than death.

For studies that aim to develop a prognostic model, the sample size needs to be large enough to override the problems of multiple comparisons in the selection of variables and the comparison of models. Various authors have suggested that the number of events should be at least 10 times the number of potential prognostic variables investigated, a value supported by a simulation study (10,13–15), a level most published studies fail to achieve. Small sample size is likely to be a major source of unreliability, especially when authors have used some stepwise algorithm for selecting the model (as most researchers do). If continuous markers are dichotomized (see below), the effective sample size is reduced by 30% or more, so that considerably more patients would be needed to achieve the same statistical power. Any investigation of interactions between prognostic factors and consideration of multiple cutpoints will further increase the sample size required. Altman and Lyman (9) suggested that such studies should be based on at least 250 to 500 events. Although a large sample size can improve precision, it cannot compensate for other weaknesses of a study.

Missing Data

Incomplete data is a common and often serious problem for studies developing prognostic models. Although the sample size may be large, patients missing one or more variables are generally excluded from a modeling exercise. The obvious effect will be to reduce power, but a much more serious possibility is the risk of introducing bias. Notably, banked tumor material is likely to be unavailable after some while in subjects with small initial tumor size (16) and its absence may be associated with other prognostic factors (17). Such selection bias cannot be discerned by readers unless published articles report on the selection of individuals for inclusion in a study and provide a comparison of the characteristics of those with and without available tumor material. Recent developments in imputation of missing data have as yet found little uptake in this field.

The completeness of the data should be reported, both by variable and overall (18). Some authors include data completeness as an inclusion criterion, making it impossible for the reader to know how representative the sample was. This practice is not recommended.

Statistical Analysis

Continuous Variables

A particularly important aspect of modeling is the handling of continuous variables. The choice is primarily between keeping such variables continuous, usually leading to the specification of a linear relation between the variable and the log hazard, or creating categories and thus largely avoiding the problem of model specification. There are considerable advantages in keeping variables continuous (19–21). However, categorization is extremely common in oncology— indeed splitting into two groups (dichotomization) is the norm.

Categorizing patients into high- and low-risk groups based on a marker cutpoint effectively assumes a constant risk up to the threshold and then a different constant risk for all values beyond the threshold. Such dichotomization is artificial and often unnecessary. Further, it discards potentially important quantitative information, thus reducing the power to detect a real association with survival (21,22). A continuous, if not linear, relationship between the value of marker and prognosis is far more plausible than a jump in risk at some (unknown) value of the marker.

Patients are often divided into two equal groups by splitting at the median value. Although this approach will be unbiased, there is no a priori reason to suppose that half of the patients are at higher risk. Some investigators compute the statistical significance level for all possible cutpoints and then select the cutpoint giving the smallest *P*-value. There are several serious problems associated with this so-called "optimal cutpoint" approach and it should never be used (23,24).

Models

The most common analytical technique in prognostic studies in cancer is the Cox proportional hazards (PH) model, which describes the relationship between the event incidence, as expressed by the hazard function, and a set of covariates (10,25). Under the model, the covariates act multiplicatively on the hazard at any point in time, and this provides us with the key assumption that the hazard of the event in any group is a constant multiple of the hazard in any other. A covariate with a hazard ratio greater than one (equivalent to a regression coefficient greater than zero) indicates that as the covariate increases the event hazard increases and thus the length of survival decreases. This proportionality assumption is often appropriate for survival time data but ought to be verified for each data set.

Rather than just fit all the possible (candidate) variables in a prognostic model, many studies seek parsimonious prediction models by retaining only the most important prognostic factors. It is common to include all variables significant at an arbitrary level of significance of 0.05 in the final model. Unfortunately, the results of stepwise regression analyses may be misleading (8,9). With a small sample there will be an increased risk of selecting unimportant variables and failing to include important ones. Also, the classification of certain variables as important (and others as not important) misrepresents the fact that models based on very different sets of variables may predict equally well. The wide use of such methods supports the need to carry out a validation study before claiming that a model is useful. Recognized prognostic factors should generally not be subjected to the selection process. It will often be sensible to force known important variables into the model and use selection for the remainder, but such practice is rare.

Parametric PH models work in broadly the same way as Cox models but the underlying hazard function is estimated by means of assuming a particular distribution for the survival times (such as the exponential or Weibull) (25–27). Other approaches occasionally used in studies exploring multiple factors simultaneously are classification trees and artificial neural networks (10,12). There is no good evidence that they tend to improve on Cox regression.

Creation of Risk Groups

Regardless of whether specific prognostic variables are kept as continuous or categorized when developing a model, the predicted outcomes will often need to be grouped in some way to apply that model. With a model containing just binary or categorical predictors, risk groups may be created by collapsing a multi-way categorization. With one or more continuous variables it is usually necessary to calculate a prognostic index (PI) and divide the range of values into bands representing different levels of risk. Kaplan–Meier survival curves are a good way to illustrate the degree of prognostic separation achieved by the classification.

The PI is the weighted combination of the variables in the model with the regression coefficients as weights. There is no consensus on how many groups should be created, nor on how to choose the cutpoints (19). Equally spaced intervals will tend to give extreme groups with rather few patients, so some researchers choose groups with similar number of patients, at the expense of some reduction in the separation of the survival curves. Although the separation between groups will generally increase with more groups, the clinical use of such a classification needs to be kept in mind. Elston and Ellis (28) observed that because prognosis needs to be considered in relationship to the available treatment options, there was little value in having more than three risk groups for categorizing breast cancer patients.

Validation of a Model

The idea of validating a prognostic or diagnostic model is generally taken to mean establishing that it works satisfactorily for patients other than those from whose data the model was derived (4). Strictly, a model would be described as validated only when that evaluation gave results deemed satisfactory in some sense.

The performance of a model will tend to be poorer in new data than in the data set on which the model was derived. One main reason is the data-dependent choice of a model that is in some sense "best" among many alternative models, but differences in the patients and settings in the two data sets may be important. A validation exercise may be carried out on additional patients in the same center(s) as the original data or elsewhere. The latter is a harder, and more valuable, test of a model, as it mimics the reality of taking a model and applying it in clinical practice in different settings (4).

It does not matter if performance of a model is less good in a different context if that performance remains clinically useful. Arguably, the best indicator of usefulness is the separation between risk groups in a plot showing Kaplan–Meier survival curves, which can be quantified using the D-statistic (29). The method can be used regardless of whether groups are created, or how many there are.

REVIEW OF PUBLISHED PROGNOSTIC MODELS IN BREAST CANCER
Methodology

Papers were sought that presented new prognostic models for patients with operable breast cancer, or which evaluated a previously published model (validation study), or both of these. Medline®, Embase®, CancerLit®, and other databases were searched late in 2001 (2). Some additional articles were identified after the main searches.

Of the 78 identified articles 17 were excluded as ineligible. The findings that follow are thus based on analysis of data from 61 studies published between 1982 and 2001: 54 presented one or more new prognostic models and 19 included model validation. Table 1 gives characteristics of the studies and the included patients, and Table 2 shows methodological details. Full details of the findings are available elsewhere (2).

Study Design

Descriptions of key aspects of study design were very poor. No paper gave a justification for the sample size for the study. It was very hard to identify which studies were prospective, in the sense that there was a clear a priori intent to collect data with the specific aim of generating a prognostic model.

It was rarely possible to derive the number of eligible patients, the number included in univariate analyses, and, in particular, the number contributing data to the generation of the prognostic model. Thus, the number of patients with complete data was often not stated, yet missing data can lead to a substantial reduction in overall sample size. The number of events per variable could be calculated for only about half of the studies, many of which had fewer than 10 events per candidate variable.

Patient Characteristics

Patient characteristics were poorly reported. Stage of breast cancer was rarely reported explicitly, but all studies included only operable cancer (or, in a few

TABLE 1 Characteristics of 61 Studies Presenting and/or Validating Prognostic Models for Breast Cancer Patients

Study characteristics	n	%
Dates of start and end of recruitment and end of follow-up all given	13	21
Study design		
Prospective (including four randomized trials)	10	16
Retrospective	48	79
Unclear	3	5
Justification of sample size	0	0
Inclusion criteria stated explicitly	23	38
Menopausal status		
Pre- and postmenopausal	39	64
Postmenopausal only	1	2
Not stated	21	34
Adjuvant therapy (at least some patients)		
Chemotherapy	30	49
Hormone therapy	23	38
Radiotherapy	26	43
Immunotherapy	1	2
Patient endpoints analyzed		
Explicitly any death	13	21
Not explicitly any death (includes three reporting "overall survival")	22	35
Specifically cancer death	16	26
Relapse (including recurrence, progression or disease free survival) (includes 15 studies where it was unclear if death was taken as an event or censored)	29	48
Any event (death or relapse)	2	3
Time origin specified	17	29
Summary of length of follow-up		
Median (or mean) and range	15	25
Median (or mean) only	19	31
Other	11	18
Not stated	16	26
Median (or mean) follow-up		
<5 yr	9	15
5–9.9 yr	22	36
10 + yr	7	11
Not stated	23	38
Clear statement on number of patients lost to follow-up[a]	14	23
Clear statement on how loss to follow-up treated was in analysis[a]	11	18
Discussion in text of missing data? (includes six studies with no missing data)	19	32
Number of excluded patients due to missing data was reported (includes six studies with no missing data)	29	48

[a]Including two studies that stated that no patients were lost.

cases, did not specify). In 33 studies, all patients were reported as having surgery but this information was missing for 23 studies. Some studies gave no information at all about patient characteristics (30,31).

Endpoints for Outcome Analysis

The majority of papers (56/61) analyzed two outcomes in multivariate analyses, usually death and recurrence, each defined in various ways. Most papers (51/61)

TABLE 2 Characteristics of Studies Developing Prognostic Models for Breast Cancer Patients ($n = 54$ Unless Otherwise Stated)

Study characteristics	n	%
Number of candidate prognostic variables used in developing the model		
2–5	6	11
6–10	30	56
11–20	10	19
21–30	3	6
>30	3	6
Not stated	2	4
Multivariate method used (six studies used two different methods)		
Cox PH (including one using a time-dependent model)	45	83
Accelerated failure time	3	6
Classification tree/recursive partitioning	1	2
Logistic regression	2	4
Discriminant analysis	1	2
Artificial neural network	6	11
None	1	2
Choice of variables to include		
All available variables/all used in univariate analyses	34/53	64
All variables with $P < 0.05$ in univariate	10/53	19
Other	5/53	9
Unclear	4/53	8
Strategy for building the multivariate model		
Stepwise selection (unspecified)	25/53	47
All significant in univariate (no further selection)	5/53	9
Other	6/53	11
Unclear	12/53	23
Not relevant	5/53	9
Forced inclusion in full model of variables known a priori to affect survival	2/53	4
Model assumptions discussed	9/53	17
Model assumptions assessed	9/53	17
Goodness-of-fit assessed	8/53	15
How continuous prognostic variables were treated in multivariate analysis		
No continuous variables	3/53	6
All kept continuous	13/53	24
Some or all categorized (of which five used a data-dependent method)	34/53	64
Unclear	4/53	7
Regression coefficients presented	30/49	61
Hazard ratios (relative risks) presented	19/49	39
SE or CI of regression coefficients or risk/hazard ratios presented	24/49	49
P-values from final model (eight partially)	39/49	80
Calculation of PI	28/49	57
Risk groups created	32	59
Two groups	6	11
Three groups	11	21
Four groups	11	21
Five + groups	3	6
Method used to create risk groups		
Count of factors present	5/32	16
Data-dependent	6/32	19
Equal size (e.g., at quartiles)	3/32	9
Other non-data-dependent method	8/32	25
Unclear	10/32	31

(*Continued*)

TABLE 2   Characteristics of Studies Developing Prognostic Models for Breast Cancer Patients ($n = 54$ Unless Otherwise Stated) (*Continued*)

Study characteristics	n	%
Graph presented showing expected survival for risk groups	29	54
Full model was specified (so it could be applied to new patients)		
Yes	13	24
No	32	59
Unclear	9	17

Abbreviations: ANN, artificial neural network; PI, prognostic index; PH, prognostic hazard.

included models for survival, but for only about a quarter (13/51) was it unambiguous that the authors were including deaths from any cause. In 16 studies (26%), the outcome was explicitly death from cancer. Similar ambiguity afflicted the reporting of analyses of time to recurrence.

Data Quality
Data completeness was generally poorly described. In several studies, absence of missing data was an inclusion criterion, but the number excluded for that reason was usually not stated. In other papers, the initial number of patients was reported but the number included in the final model was not stated. It was thus usually impossible to tell how representative the analyzed sample was of the original cohort.

Handling of Continuous Variables
The handling of continuous variables was generally reported poorly. All continuous variables were kept continuous in only 13 studies (24%). The large majority of studies categorized some or all of the continuous variables, in 13 cases by dichotomizing all of them. The method for choosing cutpoints was usually not specified, but in at least five studies the cutpoints were chosen in a data-dependent way. In contrast, a few studies carefully examined alternative models for modeling continuous data.

Multivariate Analysis
Fifty three of 54 papers presented the results of a multivariate analysis. Most studies (83%) reported the results of Cox regression analysis. Of these, five also investigated one or more additional models. One-third of studies used all the available variables as candidates in the multivariate analysis, but 10 (19%) included only those significant with $P < 0.05$ in univariate analyses. Five studies simply took as their prognostic model all the variables that were statistically significant in univariate analysis, a highly questionable approach. About half the studies (25/53) used stepwise selection to derive a final prognostic model. The final model had between two and eight variables apart from three models with more than 10 variables; two-thirds of models included three to five variables.

Presentation of Multivariate Model
Many authors (32/54) used their prognostic model to create risk groups, typically three or four groups (22/32). These groups were created in a variety of ways with six studies choosing cutpoints in some data-dependent manner. One-third

of studies (10/32) did not indicate how the risk groups were created. Many papers did not note explicitly how many patients fell into each of their risk groups. Most papers (29/32) included plots of survival in the different risk groups.

To be of any potential value to other investigators or clinicians, a model needs to be presented adequately, with regression coefficients (or hazard ratios) for all variables in the model—this was the case for only 13/54 studies (24%). We note, though, that the regression coefficients allow only statements about relative survival of different patients. To enable an estimate of survival of individual patients ("absolute" rather than relative survival), the baseline hazard function is needed. No study gave this information (and indeed it is very rare in the medical literature at large). The baseline hazard function used in a Cox model cannot be specified simply; there is a clear advantage here (in principle) for parametric models.

Findings

Despite considerable heterogeneity of clinical characteristics, the variables studied, and the statistical approach to deriving a model, some clear features could be seen. A relatively small number of variables featured in more than one or two of the models. The most common variables were nodal status, tumor size, and grade. Other variables often included were age, estrogen receptor (ER) status, and progestrogen receptor (PgR) status. Quite a few variables featured in just one published model. In many cases those studies were the only papers to investigate those particular factors, and presumably their inclusion reflected a particular research interest of that group. Although age featured quite often for the endpoints of death and recurrence, it was rarely important in models for predicting cancer death. It is not simple to summarize the discriminatory ability of the many published prognostic models, partly because of a lack of a standard metric used in all papers, and partly because such measures could be influenced by major variations in case-mix.

The Nottingham Prognostic Index (NPI) (32) merits comment. It is one of the oldest indices proposed for breast cancer patients and is one of the relatively few such indices that is actually used in clinical practice (especially in the United Kingdom). Likely explanations for its wide uptake include its simplicity, clinical credibility, and especially the demonstration that it performs well in different populations (validation) (3). After simplification, the NPI was expressed as $I = 0.2 \times$ tumor size (cm) + lymph node stage + tumor grade, where lymph node stage and tumor grade were coded 1 to 3. The authors' suggested cutpoints of 3.4 and 5.4 have become standard when using the NPI.

Subsequent publications from the same group (33,34) revisited the NPI using an extended database. These analyses supported the original model, but the authors made the important suggestion that lymph node stage could be replaced in the NPI by the number of involved nodes (33). They suggested using groups of 0, 1–3, and 4+ involved nodes. Aspects of the design and analysis of the study in which the NPI was developed can be criticized. However, "clinical validity" is more important than "statistical validity" (4), and the NPI clearly has very good discrimination both in the original sample and in subsequent evaluations elsewhere (see below).

Validation of Prognostic Models

Given the need to demonstrate that a model does indeed have prognostic value, those models that have been evaluated in separate data sets are of particular importance. Only 19 validation studies were identified, of which only three models had been evaluated on new data from different locations.

In addition to two studies mentioned already (33,34), several other groups have evaluated the NPI and confirmed its prognostic value (35–40). Hansen et al. (38) found that vascular grade added significant prognostic information to the NPI. Collett et al. (40) concluded that adding estrogen and progestrogen receptors to the NPI gave additional prognostic information, but did not present a model including those variables.

Just three papers reported validation studies of two models other than the NPI, and only one was not by the group who developed the model. The study by Collan et al. (41), of just 120 women, was the only independent evaluation identified of any prognostic model other than the NPI. These authors (41) found that the model of Baak et al. (42) did not perform particularly well with about two-thirds of patients correctly predicted as dead or alive at 5.5 years.

DISCUSSION

Over 60 published studies were reviewed in which authors have presented one or more prognostic models for women with newly diagnosed operable breast cancer. There was no attempt to assess the quality of these studies, although there are clear pointers to both the heterogeneity of the methodology and overall poor quality of reporting. Such findings are consistent with reviews in other cancers (43–46) and in other disease areas (47).

For example, Vollmer (43) summarized the findings of 54 multivariate analyses of survival from melanoma. He observed:

> In spite of 54 studies using multivariate techniques, there remain uncertainties about which prognostic factors to use in melanoma and how well we can predict the course of this disease. To some degree we must blame the methods of these studies. ... They seldom published the coefficients of their models so that others could validate the results, and they almost never validated their models with their own test data.

Interpretation of the literature is further hindered by variability in the clinical aspects of the studies. Some studies focused on only node negative or node positive cancers, or considered these groups separately, whereas most studies included both, with nodal status included in the modeling. The variables examined seem to have been largely determined by the data that had already been collected.

The most common endpoints were death from all causes and recurrence (also known as disease-free survival), each with variations. Some studies examined both of these endpoints, some just one, and others examined different endpoints either instead of or as well as these—most common of these was cancer death. There was no consensus on definitions of clinical endpoints. In some papers it was not completely clear which endpoint was used; when the endpoint was death, it was often unclear if all deaths or only cancer deaths were considered, and when the endpoint was recurrence of disease it was often unclear whether deaths without recurrence were treated as events or censored.

The failure to be specific perhaps indicates an implicit view that the choice of endpoint is not important, because the factors that are predictive of recurrence are the same as those predictive of death. Indeed, some authors have validated previously published models using a different clinical endpoint from the one used to develop the model. The assumption that the same factors apply to all endpoints may be reasonable, but it is generally made without comment and there does not seem to be clear evidence to support or refute the idea.

Few of the studies reviewed can be considered to be of high methodological quality. A lot of the problems stem from the general need to carry out retrospective studies using data that have been collected for clinical purposes. Such databases are often deficient with regard to data completeness, may have problems of standardization of measurements, and the quality of the follow-up information may not be good. The potential impact of missing data has rarely been appreciated. The standard approach is to omit women without complete data; but, as well as reducing the sample size, this approach will give biased results in some circumstances. The possibility of imputing missing data (48) and the advantages and disadvantages of doing so need wider appreciation, and these methods need more empirical investigation in this context.

Nonetheless, many studies compound the difficulties of less-than-ideal data with less-than-ideal statistical methods. Many researchers have developed models on data sets that are too small. Further, when some form of variable selection is used, as was the case in most of these studies, there is a considerable risk of over-optimism—that is, the results are biased to show too much prognostic discrimination. Such problems can be alleviated by having a very large sample, by starting with a small number of important predictors, by not reducing the number of variables, and by not making data-dependent choices regarding the modeling of continuous variables. Bootstrap investigation can help to investigate the stability of a prognostic model (49). In addition, models should be evaluated in independent data, preferably in a different location, as discussed later.

One particular statistical issue is the handling of continuous covariates. Tumor size, age, and most tumor markers are continuous variables, yet the majority of studies categorize these variables, and many dichotomize all continuous variables. Much of the same remarks apply to the number of affected lymph nodes. Categorization of variables greatly reduces the power of a study (which is probably not large enough in the first place), and will diminish the apparent prognostic importance of those variables (21). Cutpoints derived by selecting the value that minimizes the P-value are seriously biased and will lead to highly misleading models.

Given the long survival of many women with operable breast cancer, prospective studies are difficult. The main way to avoid the problems associated with database studies is to embed the collection of prognostic information and/or the collection of tissue and blood samples within large randomized trials as a resource for future research.

Methodological deficiencies in published studies are often compounded by deficiencies in reporting. Regardless of the specific details of a study, studies should be reported completely and accurately. It is clear that the reporting quality of the studies in this sample share many of the deficiencies seen in previous reviews (50,51). All papers should provide basic information about important aspects of the study, including the sample selection, patient characteristics, markers examined, clinical endpoints, statistical methods of analysis, and the results of model fitting. Journals should ensure that reports of prognostic studies adhere to basic requirements for sound scientific reporting (52).

Evidence on which variables are prognostic in newly diagnosed breast cancer patients is to some extent constrained by the variables that have been investigated.

Some variables featured in the majority of prognostic models—in particular nodal status (number of positive nodes), tumor size, and grade followed by age, ER, and PgR. Few other variables were explored in more than a handful of studies, and some factors have been studied in only one publication. Some of the studies did not investigate all of the most common prognostic variables, with a few focusing on a specific subset of possible prognostic information—for example, Parham et al. (53) investigated only histological information.

A (long-term) goal is to be able to make precise forecasts of the prognosis of individual patients. Whether this could ever be achieved remains open to serious doubt. Nonetheless, prognostic models are undoubtedly useful for classifying groups of patients, for example to help choose appropriate adjuvant therapy. The extent to which a prognostic model is clinically useful has thus far not been considered objectively, reflecting the lack of an agreed metric for judging the value of a prognostic model. As noted by Graf et al. (54), a measure of inaccuracy that aims to assess the value of a given prognostic model should compare the estimated event-free probabilities with the observed individual outcome. They observed that various ad hoc measures commonly used are only of limited value, in particular, methods associated with ROC curves that have been borrowed from the evaluation of diagnostic tests. A recently developed index of separation, which can be used for grouped or continuous prognostic scores, may offer a valuable step forward in this regard (29).

Regardless of how well a model is able to identify groups with differing prognosis, it has to be said that no model is of any use if it is not published in enough detail. For regression models, this means that the regression equation should be published—either the hazard ratios or log hazard ratios should be quoted for all variables in the model. In addition, it is essential that the exact definition and numerical coding of each variable is specified (3). The familiar Cox model is not easily transported in full. The part of the model that is generally provided, the "prognostic model," indicates the relative risk of different patients according to prognostic factors. Assessment of a patient's actual risk also requires the baseline hazard function, which is never published.

Parametric models allow a parsimonious description of the full model to allow both absolute and relative survival to be predicted. Such models are thus eminently more transportable to other settings. The wide preference for Cox models thus militates against useful transfer of models between clinical settings. Remarkably few published prognostic models have been re-examined by independent groups in independent settings. The few validation studies have been carried out on ill-defined samples, sometimes of smaller size and short follow-up, and authors, in general, are unclear about how to summarize the performance. Overall, the only clear message from the published validation studies is support for the prognostic value of the NPI.

Despite much research effort over two decades, no new prognostic factors have been shown to add substantially to those identified in the 1980s. As Haybittle (55) noted, "Any improvement [on the NPI] in prediction must now depend on finding factors which are as important as, but independent of, lymphnode stage and pathological grade." The NPI remains a useful clinical tool, although additional factors may enhance its use. Such factors have proved surprisingly elusive (56) as is evidenced by the continued widespread use of the NPI in clinical practice.

Nor has any other prognostic model yet emerged that is clearly superior to the NPI. That said, it seems clear that there is a small set of prognostic variables, perhaps especially ER (even though it is more often viewed as having predictive value), that may usefully add to the variables included in the NPI: grade, tumor size, and positive lymph nodes.

ACKNOWLEDGMENT

Douglas G. Altman is funded by Cancer Research UK. The project that includes this review was funded by the UK NHS Health Technology Assessment program.

REFERENCES

1. Clark GM. Do we really need prognostic factors for breast cancer? Breast Cancer Res Treat 1994; 30(2):117–126.
2. Williams C, Brunskill S, Altman D, et al. Cost effectiveness of using prognostic information to select women with breast cancer for adjuvant systemic therapy of breast cancer. Health Technol Assess 2006; 10(34):1–222.
3. Wyatt JC, Altman DG. Commentary: prognostic models: clinically useful or quickly forgotten? Brit Med J 1995; 311:1539–1541.
4. Altman DG, Royston P. What do we mean by validating a prognostic model? Stat Med 2000; 19:453–473.
5. Vergouwe Y, Steyerberg EW, Eijkemans MJ, Habbema JD. Validity of prognostic models: when is a model clinically useful? Semin Urol Oncol 2002; 20(2):96–107.
6. Redelmeier DA, Lustig AJ. Prognostic indices in clinical practice. J Am Med Assoc 2001; 285(23):3024–3025.
7. Concato J, Feinstein AR, Holford TR. The risk of determining risk with multivariate models. Ann Intern Med 1993; 118(201):210.
8. Simon R, Altman DG. Statistical aspects of prognostic factor studies in oncology. Br J Cancer 1994; 69(6):979–985.
9. Altman DG, Lyman GH. Methodological challenges in the evaluation of prognostic factors in breast cancer. Breast Cancer Res Treat 1998; 52:289–303.
10. Schumacher M, Holländer N, Schwarzer G, Sauerbrei W. Prognostic factor studies. In: Crowley J, ed. Handbook of Statistics in Clinical Oncology. New York: Marcel Dekker, 2001:321–378.
11. Schmoor C, Sauerbrei W, Schumacher M. Sample size considerations for the evaluation of prognostic factors in survival analysis. Stat Med 2000; 19:441–452.
12. McShane LM, Simon R. Statistical methods for the analysis of prognostic factor studies. In: Gospodarowicz MK, Henson DE, Hutter RVP, et al., eds. Prognostic Factors in Cancer. New York: Wiley-Liss, 2001:37–48.
13. Harrell FE Jr, Lee KL, Matchar DB, Reichert TA. Regression models for prognostic prediction: advantages, problems, and suggested solutions. Cancer Treat Rep 1985; 69(10):1071–1077.
14. Peduzzi P, Concato J, Feinstein AR, Holford TR. Importance of events per independent variable in proportional hazards regression analysis. II. Accuracy and precision of regression estimates. J Clin Epidemiol 1995; 48(12):1503–1510.
15. Feinstein AR. Multivariable Analysis: An Introduction. New Haven: Yale University Press, 1996.
16. McGuire WL. Breast cancer prognostic factors: evaluation guidelines. J Natl Cancer Inst 1991; 83(3):154–155.
17. Hoppin JA, Tolbert PE, Taylor JA, Schroeder JC, Holly EA. Potential for selection bias with tumor tissue retrieval in molecular epidemiology studies. Ann Epidemiol 2002; 12(1):1–6.
18. Burton A, Altman D. Missing covariate data within cancer prognostic studies: a review of current reporting and proposed guidelines. Brit J Cancer 2004; 91:4–8.
19. Altman DG. Suboptimal analysis using "optimal" cutpoints. Brit J Cancer 1998; 78(4):556–557.

20. Bossard N, Descotes F, Bremond AG, et al. Keeping data continuous when analyzing the prognostic impact of a tumor marker: an example with cathepsin D in breast cancer. Breast Cancer Res Treat 2003; 82:47–59.

21. Royston P, Altman DG, Sauerbrei W. Dichotomizing continuous predictors in multiple regression: a bad idea. Stat Med 2006; 25(1):127–141.

22. Morgan TM, Elashoff FA. Effect of categorizing a continuous covariate on the comparison of survival time. J Am Stat Assoc 1986; 81:917–921.

23. Hilsenbeck SG, Clark GM, McGuire WL. Why do so many prognostic factors fail to pan out? Breast Cancer Res Treat 1992; 22(3):197–206.

24. Altman DG, Lausen B, Sauerbrei W, Schumacher M. Dangers of using "optimal" cutpoints in the evaluation of prognostic factors. J Natl Cancer Inst 1994; 86(11):829–835.

25. Bradburn MJ, Clark TG, Love SB, Altman DG. Survival analysis part II: Multivariate data analysis–an introduction to concepts and methods. Brit J Cancer 2003; 89:431–436.

26. Royston P, Parmar MK. Flexible parametric proportional-hazards and proportional-odds models for censored survival data, with application to prognostic modelling and estimation of treatment effects. Stat Med 2002; 21(15):2175–2197.

27. Nardi A, Schemper M. Comparing Cox and parametric models in clinical studies. Stat Med 2003; 22(23):3597–3610.

28. Elston EW, Ellis IO. Method for grading breast cancer. J Clin Pathol 1993; 46(2):189–190.

29. Royston P, Sauerbrei W. A new measure of prognostic separation in survival data. Stat Med 2004; 23(5):723–748.

30. Burke HB, Goodman PH, Rosen DB, et al. Artificial neural networks improve the accuracy of cancer survival prediction. Cancer 1997; 79(4):857–862.

31. Lockwood CA, Ricciardelli C, Raymond WA, Seshadri R, McCaul K, Horsfall DJ. A simple index using video image analysis to predict disease outcome in primary breast cancer. Int J Cancer 1999; 84(3):203–208.

32. Haybittle JL, Blamey RW, Elston CW, Johnson J, Doyle PJ, Campbell FC. A prognostic index in primary breast cancer. Brit J Cancer 1982; 45:361–366.

33. Galea MH, Blamey RW, Elston CW, Ellis IO. The Nottingham Prognostic Index in primary breast cancer. Breast Cancer Res Treat 1992; 22(3):207–219.

34. Todd JH, Dowle C, Williams MR, et al. Confirmation of a prognostic index in primary breast cancer. A. Brit J Cancer 1987; 56(4):489–492.

35. Guerra I, Algorta J, Diaz dO, Pelayo A, Farina J. Immunohistochemical prognostic index for breast cancer in young women. Mol Pathol 2003; 56(6):323–327.

36. Kollias J, Murphy CA, Elston CW, Ellis IO, Robertson JFR, Blamey RW. The prognosis of small primary breast cancers. Eur J Cancer 1999; 35(6):908–912.

37. Balslev I, Axelsson CK, Zedeler K, Rasmussen BB, Carstensen B, Mouridsen HT. The Nottingham Prognostic Index applied to 9149 patients from the studies of the Danish Breast Cancer Cooperative Group (DBCG). Breast Cancer Res Treat 1994; 32(3):281–290.

38. Hansen S, Grabau DA, Sorensen FB, Bak M, Vach W, Rose C. Vascular grading of angiogenesis: prognostic significance in breast cancer. Br J Cancer 2000; 82(2):339–347.

39. Sundquist M, Thorstenson S, Brudin L, Nordenskjold B. Applying the Nottingham Prognostic Index to a Swedish breast cancer population. South East Swedish Breast Cancer Study Group. Breast Cancer Res Treat 1999; 53(1):1–8.

40. Collett K, Skjaerven R, Maehle BO. The prognostic contribution of estrogen and progesterone receptor status to a modified version of the Nottingham Prognostic Index. Breast Cancer Res Treat 1998; 48(1):1–9.

41. Collan Y, Kumpusalo L, Pesonen E, Eskelinen M, Pajarinen P, Kettunen K. Prediction of survival in breast cancer: evaluation of different multivariate models. Anticancer Res 1998; 18(1B):647–650.

42. Baak JPA, Van Dop H, Kurver PHJ, Hermans J. The value of morphometry to classic prognosticators in breast cancer. Cancer 1985; 56(2):374–382.

43. Vollmer RT. Malignant melanoma. A multivariate analysis of prognostic factors. Pathol Ann 1989; 24(Pt 1):383–407.

44. Ross PL, Scardino PT, Kattan MW. A catalog of prostate cancer nomograms. J Urol 2001; 165(5):1562–1568.

45. Vollmer RT, Keetch DW, Humphrey PA. Predicting the pathology results of radical prostatectomy from preoperative information: a validation study. Cancer 1998; 83(8):1567–1580.
46. Gobbi PG, Zinzani PL, Broglia C, et al. Comparison of prognostic models in patients with advanced Hodgkin disease. Promising results from integration of the best three systems. Cancer 2001; 91(8):1467–1478.
47. Counsell C, Dennis M. Systematic reviews of prognostic models in patients with acute stroke. Cerebrovasc Dis 2001; 12:159–170.
48. Clark TG, Altman DG. Developing a prognostic model in the presence of missing data: an ovarian cancer case study. J Clin Epidemiol 2003; 56(1):28–37.
49. Sauerbrei W, Schumacher M. A bootstrap resampling procedure for model building: application to the Cox regression model. Stat Med 1992; 11(16):2093–2109.
50. Altman DG, De Stavola BL, Love SB, Stepniewska KA. Review of survival analyses published in cancer journals. Brit J Cancer 1995; 72(2):511–518.
51. Riley RD, Burchill SA, Abrams KR, et al. A systematic review of molecular and biological markers in tumours of the Ewing's sarcoma family. Eur J Cancer 2003; 39:19–30.
52. McShane LM, Altman DG, Sauerbrei W, Taube SE, Gion M, Clark GM. Reporting recommendations for tumor marker prognostic studies (REMARK). J Natl Cancer Inst 2005; 97(16):1180–1184.
53. Parham DM, Hagen N, Brown RA. Simplified method of grading primary carcinomas of the breast. J Clin Pathol 1992; 45(6):517–520.
54. Graf E, Schmoor C, Sauerbrei W, Schumacher M. Assessment and comparison of prognostic classification schemes for survival data. Stat Med 1999; 18(17/18):2529–2545.
55. Haybittle JL. Prognostic indices in breast cancer. Colloques et Seminaires 1986; 137: 779–787.
56. Blamey RW. The design and clinical use of the Nottingham prognostic index in breast cancer. Breast 1996; 5:156–157.

Challenges of Microarray Data and the Evaluation of Gene Expression Profile Signatures

Richard Simon

Biometric Research Branch, Division of Cancer Treatment and Diagnosis, National Cancer Institute, Bethesda, Maryland, U.S.A.

INTRODUCTION

The DNA microarray is a powerful technology for measuring gene expression profiles that has found broad use in basic and translational cancer research. The effective use of this technology, however, requires specialized biostatistical expertise that is not readily available for many laboratories. It is also difficult for those reading the research literature to distinguish substance from hype and to determine when findings are ready for broad clinical application. In this chapter, we will attempt to provide a summary of the key principles involved in the effective use of microarray expression profiling in translational research in terms that should be meaningful to laboratory scientists and clinicians. We will emphasize that the DNA microarray is just an assay, and its effectiveness is determined by study design and analysis principles. Because microarrays produce so much data from each specimen, they offer greater opportunities and greater dangers than traditional assays. We shall attempt to highlight both the power and the potential pitfalls involved in the microarray transcript profiling.

MICROARRAY TECHNOLOGY

DNA microarrays are assays for quantifying the types and amounts of mRNA transcripts present in a collection of cells. The mRNA is extracted from the specimen. In most cases, the mRNA is then reverse transcribed to complementary DNA (cDNA) during which a fluorescent label is incorporated into the DNA. The labeled cDNA is then placed on a solid surface on which strands of polynucleotide probes have been attached in specified positions. The labeled cDNA molecules hybridize to the probes to which they share sufficient sequence complementarity. After allowing sufficient time for the hybridization reaction, the excess sample is washed off the solid surface.

The quantity of cDNA bound to each polynucleotide probe is quantified by illuminating the solid surface with laser light of a frequency tuned to the fluorescent label employed, and then measuring the intensity of fluorescence over each probe on the array. This intensity of fluorescence should be proportional to the number of molecules of cDNA bound to the probe.

Microarrays differ in many important details. cDNA microarrays usually consist of probes of cDNA robotically printed on a coated microscope slide. Because the cDNAs are generally several hundred bases long, cross-reactivity is limited. However, robotic printing often results in substantial variability in the size and shape of corresponding probes on different arrays. With cDNA arrays, there is also substantial variability in sample distribution across the face of different arrays. Hence, direct comparison of intensities of corresponding probes on different arrays is problematic. Much of this variability can be controlled by co-hybridizing two samples on the same array. The two cDNA samples are labeled with different fluorescent dyes. By using two laser beams, one can measure the intensity of fluorescence in each of the two frequency channels over each probe. This approach is also used for printed oligonucleotides. The second sample may represent either a specimen whose expression profile relative to the first specimen is of biological interest or a reference sample, used on all arrays in order to control experimental variability.

Affymetrix GeneChip^{TM} arrays have oligonucleotide probes lithographically synthesized directly on the silicon surface of the array. Probe geometry is more reproducible on GeneChips relative to cDNA arrays. Interarray variability due to sample distribution effects is also minimized in GeneChips because the samples are circulated inside the GeneChip during hybridization. Because of these reductions in interarray variability, a single sample is usually hybridized to GeneChips.

OBJECTIVES OF MICROARRAY STUDIES

Effective microarray experiments require careful planning. Careful planning begins with a clear objective. The objective drives the selection of specimens and the specification of an appropriate analysis strategy (1). The large numbers of genes whose expressions can be measured in a single hybridization creates an even greater than usual need for careful planning of the methods of analysis so that biologically meaningful conclusions, rather than spurious associations are reported.

The objectives of many studies utilizing DNA microarrays can be categorized as "class comparison," "class prediction," or "class discovery." Class comparison focuses on determining which genes are differentially expressed among samples representative of predefined classes. The classes may represent different tissue types, diseased tissue or normal tissue of the same cell type or the same tissue under different experimental conditions. In cancer studies, the classes often represent different categories of tumors, differing with regard to stage, primary site, genetic mutations present, or response to therapy. The specimens may represent tissue taken before or after treatment or experimental intervention. The defining characteristic of class comparison is that the classes are predefined independently of the expression profiles. For example, Korn et al. (2) evaluated expression profiles from breast tumors pre- and postchemotherapy to identify those genes whose expression was modified by treatment. Yang et al. (3) studied gene expression changes in metastatic breast tumors pre- and post-Erlotinib treatment. Sotiriou et al. (4) evaluated genes whose expression was correlated with clinico-pathological characteristics of breast tumors. Desai et al. (5) evaluated genes differentially expressed among different transgenic mouse models of breast cancer.

Class prediction is similar to class comparison except that the emphasis is on developing a mathematical function that can predict which class a new specimen belongs to based on its expression profile. This usually requires identifying which genes are effective for distinguishing the predefined classes, estimating the parameters of the mathematical function used and the accuracy of the predictor (6,7). Class prediction is important for medical problems of diagnostic classification, prognostic prediction, and treatment selection. For example, van't Veer et al. (8) and Vijver et al. (9) developed and evaluated predictors of which patients with primary breast cancer are at high risk for recurrence after local treatment alone. Ma et al. (10) developed such a predictor for patients with estrogen receptor (ER)-positive primary breast cancer who received tamoxifen monotherapy after local therapy. Ayers et al. (11) developed a predictor of complete pathological response to neo-adjuvant chemotherapy in patients with breast cancer. Jansen et al. (12) developed a predictor of response to tamoxifen for patients with metastatic breast cancer.

Class discovery involves the grouping together of specimens based on their expression profiles across the set of genes represented on the array or the grouping together of genes with regard to their expression profiles across the samples assayed. "Cluster analysis" is generally used for generating the groups. Cluster analysis algorithms are called "unsupervised" because the grouping is not driven by any phenotype external to the expression profiles, such as tissue type, stage, grade or response to treatment. The objective of clustering expression profiles of tumors is to determine new disease classifications or identification of novel sub-types of specimens within a population. For example, Perou et al. (13) characterized expression profiles of primary breast tumors into four patterns which they called basal-like, luminal-like, Erb-B2+, and normal-like. Cluster analysis is an explora-tory analysis method, however, and even random expression profiles can be clus-tered. It is generally difficult to evaluate the meaningfulness of a set of clusters except by comparing them with regard to existing phenotypes. Cluster analysis is greatly overutilized. This is true in large part because investigators have access to cluster analysis software and the results can be displayed in colorful ways. Most cancer studies involving microarray expression profiling really have class comparison or class prediction objectives. For such studies, "supervised methods" are much more appropriate (14).

CLASS COMPARISON

In the earliest microarray studies, investigators performed class comparison by examining fold change differences for each gene between a microarray of a single specimen from one class and a specimen of the other class. This is not really mean-ingful, however, because the comparison may reflect sample differences, rather than class differences. Using replicate arrays for measuring expression for one sample from each of two classes does not help much. Such "technical replicates" do not satisfy the crucial need for studying multiple tumors of each type, that is, for "biological replicates." Usually, the biological variation between individuals will be much larger than the assay variation and it will be inefficient to perform replicate arrays using specimens from a small number of individuals rather than performing single arrays from a larger number of individuals. Individual micro-arrays of independent biological replicates from each phenotype class of interest is generally needed, not assay replicates of the same RNA specimen or microarrays of pooled biological replicates (1).

Standard statistical methods are commonly used to compare expression levels among independent biological replicate samples of the classes. This com-parison is generally done one gene at a time for each gene represented on the array. Although standard statistical methods like t-tests are often used, the strik-ingly non-standard aspect of this analysis that must be taken into account is that there are generally tens of thousands of genes analyzed. Hence, more stringent standards of statistical significance for claiming differential expression must be used. If, for example, there are 10,000 genes represented on the array, then in comparing expression for samples from two classes, one would expect 500 false-positive claims of statistical significance at the traditional 5% significance level ($0.05 \times 10,000$). This is not acceptable, and hence more stringent standards for claiming differential expression are needed.

In comparing gene expression profiles among classes, biostatisticians today prefer reporting the "false discovery rate" (FDR) for the comparison as a whole rather than the statistical significance level for individual comparisons (15). The FDR is the proportion of false positives among the genes claimed to be differentially expressed among the classes. For example, suppose that one claims a gene to be differentially expressed if the univariate significance level is less than 0.001. Then for 10,000 genes analyzed, the expected number of false positives is about 10 (since most of the 10,000 of genes are not expected to be differentially expressed). If there are 40 genes for which the univariate significance level is less than 0.001, then the FDR is about $10/40$ or 25%, that is, one in four of the reported genes are likely to be false positives. There are powerful multivariate methods for comparing expression profiles between classes and identifying differentially expressed genes in a manner that controls the FDR and takes into account the correlation among the genes (2,16).

Cluster analysis is often used in a potentially misleading way in identification of differentially expressed genes. Investigators may generate a gene list using an inadequately stringent univariate significance level of 0.05 or 0.01. The samples are then clustered with regard to the expression profiles for the selected genes. The fact that the samples from the classes are separated in this cluster analysis is taken as validation that the genes are really differentially expressed. This supervised form of cluster analysis is invalid. If one generates expression profiles for two classes using random numbers with no real difference between the two classes, there will be about 500 false positives per 10,000 genes. If one clusters the randomly generated samples with regard to those selected genes that were found significant at the 0.05 level, the samples will be separated.

One problem encountered in the analysis of gene expression data is biologically interpreting and understanding lists of genes identified as differentially expressed among compared classes. This is a serious challenge for a variety of reasons. Many investigators using microarrays are not expert tumor biologists, and the functions of many genes are incompletely understood. State-of-the-art software for the analysis of gene expression data such as BRB-ArrayTools (17) generally provides links to genomic annotations to assist investigators in interpreting gene lists. Recently, a new approach to class comparison has been introduced in which classes are compared with regard to the expression of predefined meaningful gene sets rather than the expression of individual genes. There are a variety of such methods, called gene set expression analysis methods (18,19), which provide a score for differential expression for each gene set. The commonly used gene sets are based on gene ontology classification, annotated metabolic or signaling pathways, chromosome arm, or experimentally determined signature of response to pathway activation or some other cellular intervention. Since the number of gene sets tested is generally much less than the number of genes represented on the array, the magnitude of the multiple comparison problem is reduced. Also, expression patterns of genes in a gene set can reinforce each other and do not have to be individually significant at a very stringent level as required for the post hoc annotation methods. Consequently, these kinds of methods are increasingly popular. State-of-the-art software packages such as BRB-ArrayTools incorporate this new approach (17).

CLASS PREDICTION

A class predictor, or classifier, is a function that predicts a class from an expression profile. Specification of a class predictor requires specification of (*i*) the mathematical form used to translate the vector of expression levels to the class indicator, (*ii*) the genes whose expression levels are utilized in the prediction, and (*iii*) the parameters such as weights placed on expression levels of individual genes and threshold values used in the prediction (6,20). The development of a class predictor is similar to that of a statistical regression function, except that the former predicts class identifier rather than a continuous value. Statistical regression models are generally built using data in which the number of cases (n) is large relative to the number of variables (p) that are evaluated for inclusion in the regression. In the development of class predictors using gene expression data, however, the number of candidate predictors is generally orders of magnitude greater than the number of cases. This has two important implications. One is that only simple class prediction functions should be considered (21). The other is that the data used for evaluating the class predictor must be distinct from the data used for developing it. It is almost always possible to develop a class predictor even on completely random data which will fit that same data almost perfectly but be completely useless for prediction with independent data (14).

The most straightforward method of estimating the accuracy of a class predictor is the split-sample method of partitioning the set of samples into a training set and a test set. Rosenwald et al. (22) used this approach successfully in their international study of prognostic prediction for large B cell lymphoma. They used two-thirds of their samples as a training set. Multiple kinds of predictors were studied on the training set. When the collaborators of that study agreed on a single fully specified prediction model, they accessed the test set for the first time. On the test set, there was no adjustment of the model or fitting of parameters. They merely used the samples in the test set to evaluate the predictions of the model that was completely specified using only the training data.

The split-sample method is often used with so few samples in the test set, however, that the validation is almost meaningless. One can evaluate the adequacy of the size of the test set by computing the statistical significance of the classification error rate on the test set or by computing a confidence interval for the test set error rate.

Michiels et al. (23) suggested that multiple training-test partitions be used, rather than just one. The split-sample approach is mostly useful, however, when one does not have a well-defined algorithm for developing the classifier. When there is a single training set–test set partition, one can perform numerous unplanned analyses on the training set to develop a classifier and then test that classifier on the test set. With multiple training–test partitions, however, that type of flexible approach to model development cannot be used. If one has an algorithm for classifier development, it is generally better to use one of the cross-validation or bootstrap resampling approaches to estimate error rate (discussed subsequently) because the split-sample approach does not provide an efficient use of the available data (24).

Cross-validation is an alternative to the split-sample method of estimating prediction accuracy (20). Molinaro et al. (24) describe and evaluate many variants of cross-validation and bootstrap resampling for classification problems where the number of candidate predictors vastly exceeds the number of cases. The cross-validated prediction error is an estimate of the prediction error associated with application of the algorithm for model building to the entire data set.

Simon et al. (14) showed that cross-validating the fitting of the prediction model after selection of differentially expressed genes from the full data set results in a highly biased estimate of prediction accuracy. Their results underscore the importance of cross-validating all steps of predictor construction in estimating the error rate. It can also be useful to compute the statistical significance of the cross-validated estimate of classification error. This determines the probability of obtaining a cross-validated classification error as small as actually achieved if there were no relationship between the expression data and class identifiers. A flexible method for computing this statistical significance was described by Radmacher et al. (20). This method of computing statistical significance of cross-validated error rate for a wide variety of classifier functions is implemented in the BRB-ArrayTools software (17).

VALIDATION AND CLINICAL UTILITY

In trying to determine whether the results of a published microarray-based patient classifier is ready for prime time, it is important to distinguish developmental from validation studies (7,25,26). A developmental study is one that develops a classifier, whereas a validation study uses a classifier developed previously. For a variety of reasons, just using a split-sample or cross-validation analysis does not make a developmental study into a validation study. There are many factors that may influence the predictive accuracy of a classifier, which are not represented in artificially subdividing the cases from a single study. These factors include differences in patients from different centers, the nature of their diseases and prior treatments, differences in tissue handling, and differences in assay performance over time and location. Developmental studies are often conducted based on specimens available at one or a very limited number of centers, and the results may not be applicable to patients more generally. Developmental studies also often have the assay performed at one time in one research laboratory and may not reflect important sources of variation involved in real-world sample collection, tissue handling, and assay performance.

Following the performance of a successful developmental study, it is often appropriate to address whether the original assay platform is suitable for broad application of the classifier. If not, then a recalibration of the classifier for its new platform is necessary before conducting the validation study. Dobbin et al. (27) reported that in order to ensure good interlaboratory reproducibility in using the Affymetrix GeneChip system, a pilot study and development of a common protocol were necessary. In classifying the risk of recurrence for patients with node-negative and ER-positive breast cancer receiving tamoxifen treatment, the investigators utilized DNA microarray gene expression profiling to identify the informative genes, but then transferred to an RT–PCR platform based on primers for use with paraffin-embedded formalin-fixed tissue. They performed detailed studies on sources of variation of the assay in order to assure reproducibility of results (28).

Validation studies should address clinical utility of the classifier, not just predictive accuracy. Most prognostic factor studies are conducted based on convenience samples of available specimens. Consequently, they often include a heterogeneous group of patients who have received a variety of treatments (29). For example, many prognostic factor studies in breast cancer include node-negative and node-positive ER-negative and ER-positive patients, those who received cytotoxic chemotherapy and those who received tamoxifen alone. Showing that a new classifier is prognostic for such a mixed group generally has little or no therapeutic value and such classifiers are rarely used (30). It does not matter whether one shows from a multivariate analysis that the new classifier is more statistically significant than standard prognostic variables, because therapeutic strategies have often been developed based on the established variables.

Although prognostic factors are rarely used in oncology, we do need predictive factors, that is, biological measurements and classifiers that identify which patients respond to specific treatments. Predictive factors are needed because we often overtreat the majority of patients with the hope of benefitting the minority. This is true for adjuvant studies where the majority of patients may be cured by local therapy alone and for advanced disease studies where expensive molecularly targeted drugs may benefit only a minority of patients.

Developing classifiers of which patients are most likely to respond to a new drug can dramatically improve the efficiency of clinical trials for establishing the effectiveness of that drug. This was shown theoretically by Simon and Maitournam (31,32). Targeted development of Trastuzumab is an important example of the effectiveness of this approach. Recent experience with the use of Trastuzumab in women with node-positive breast cancer has shown how the use of classifiers for selecting the right drug for the right patient can dramatically increase the proportion of treated patients who benefit from the drug.

It is very desirable for classifier development and validation to use patients who received a treatment in a single clinical trial because it helps ensure that the classifier developed is a therapeutically relevant predictive classifier, not just a prognostic factor. Both developmental and validation studies should address therapeutically meaningful sets of patients.

Establishing the "validity" of a classifier for identifying which patients have tumors responsive to a new drug is ideally accomplished by conducting a prospective randomized trial of the new drug versus control treatment in patients who are predicted to be responsive (classifier positive) and in those predicted to be non-responsive (classifier negative) (33). Demonstrating that the new drug is more effective than control in the classifier-positive patients but not in the classifier-negative patients establishes the utility of the classifier and the effectiveness of the drug. Generally, it is essential that the classifier be completely specified based on data external to the prospective clinical trial. Developing the classifier on the same data used to evaluate its utility is invalid unless highly structured prospectively defined approaches are used (34).

In some cases where the classifier is biologically linked to the known mechanism of action of the drug and there is compelling evidence based on the mechanism of action of the drug that the drug will not work in classifier-negative patients, it may not be possible to include classifier-negative patients in the prospective study. This was the case for Trastuzumab, for example.

The clinical utility of a classifier for use of an established treatment depends on a variety of factors including other treatments available for those patients and the availability of other more easily measured predictive factors (35). In general, establishing clinical utility requires demonstrating that a clinically meaningful measure of patient benefit is improved based on using the new classifier compared with not using the classifier. One approach is to randomize patients to treatment selection based on conventional practice guidelines or based on the genomic classifier. The genomic classifier has clinical utility if treatment outcome is improved overall for the group randomized to classifier-based treatment assignment. The genomic classifier also has clinical utility if outcome is the same for the two randomized groups, but the patients randomized to classifier determined treatment have reduced adverse events, inconvenience, or cost. This kind of prospective clinical trial design generally requires a very large sample size, however, because many patients in both randomization groups receive the same treatment (36,37). An alternative design is to measure the classifier on all eligible patients and determine before randomization whether the recommended treatment assignment would differ between conventional practice guidelines and the classifier-based strategy. Then, the only patients randomized are those for whom the two strategies result in different treatment assignments. This approach entails the cost of measuring the classifier on all patients, but results in a much smaller clinical trial than that described above (26,35).

In some cases, it may be possible to utilize archived tumor samples from patients treated in a randomized clinical trial to simulate the analysis that would have been performed in a prospective trial. This is a viable strategy only when archived specimens are available for almost all patients in the randomized trial. Otherwise, there will be concern about whether the patients for whom samples are available are representative of the whole. The retrospective strategy is also not credible unless the plan for the retrospective analysis is completely specified in writing prior to performing assays on the archived specimens. The classifier must be completely determined by data external to the clinical trial used for retrospective analysis (33). Even if these considerations are satisfied, retrospective classification of archived specimens may not accurately reflect the challenges of tissue handling and assay performance encountered prospectively in a time frame that enables the real-world treatment selection. Consequently, with retrospective analysis for establishing clinical utility, it is important to separately establish technical assay reproducibility and robustness to real-world tissue handling.

REFERENCES

1. Simon RM, Korn EL, McShane LM, Radmacher MD, Wright GW, Zhao Y. Design and Analysis of DNA Microarray Investigations. New York: Springer, 2003.
2. Korn EL, McShane LM, Troendle JF, Rosenwald A, Simon R. Identifying pre-post chemotherapy differences in gene expression in breast tumors: a statistical method appropriate for this aim. Br J Cancer 2002; 86:1093–1096.
3. Yang SX, Simon RM, Tan AR, Nguyen D, Swain SM. Gene expression patterns and profile changes pre- and post-Erlotinib treatment in patients with metastatic breast cancer. Clin Cancer Res 2005; 11:6226–6232.
4. Sotiriou C, Neo SY, McShane LM, et al. Breast cancer classification and prognosis based on gene expression profiles from a population based study. Proc Natl Acad Sci USA 2003; 100(18):10393–10398.
5. Desai KV, Xiao N, Wang W, et al. Initiating oncogenic event determines gene-expression patterns of human breast cancer models. Proc Natl Acad Sci USA 2002; 99:6967–6972.

6. Simon R. Diagnostic and prognostic prediction using gene expression profiles in high dimensional microarray data. Br J Cancer 2003; 89:1599–1604.
7. Simon R. Development and validation of therapeutically relevant multi-gene biomarker classifiers. J Natl Cancer Inst 2005; 97:866–867.
8. van't Veer LJ, Dai H, Vijver MJvd, et al. Gene expression profiling predicts clinical outcome of breast cancer. Nature 2002; 415:530–536.
9. Vijver MJvD, He YD, Veer LJvt, et al. A gene-expression signature as a predictor of survival in breast cancer. New Engl J Med 2002; 347(25):1999–2009.
10. Ma XJ, Wang Z, Ryan PD, et al. A two-gene expression ratio predicts clinical outcome in breast cancer patients treated with tamoxifen. Cancer Cell 2004; 5:1–10.
11. Ayers M, Symmans WF, Stec J, et al. Gene expression profiles predict complete patholo-gic response to neoadjuvant paclitaxel and fluorouracil, doxorubicin and cyclophos-phamide chemotherapy in breast cancer. J Clin Oncol 2005; 22(12):2284–2293.
12. Jansen MPHM, Foekens JA, Staveren ILv, et al. Molecular classification of Tamoxifen-resistant breast carcinomas by gene expression profiling. J Clin Oncol 2005; 23(4): 732–740.
13. Perou CM, Sorlie T, Eisen MB, et al. Molecular portraits of human breast tumors. Nature 2000; 406:747–752.
14. Simon R, Radmacher MD, Dobbin K, McShane LM. Pitfalls in the analysis of DNA microarray data: class prediction methods. J Natl Cancer Inst 2003; 95:14–18.
15. Benjamini Y, Hochberg Y. Controlling the false discovery rate: A practical and powerful approach to multiple testing. J Roy Stat Soc, Ser B 1995; 57:289–300.
16. Tusher VG, Tibshirani R, Chu G. Significance analysis of microarrays applied to the ionizing radiation response. Proc Natl Acad Sci 2001; 98:5116–5121.
17. Simon R, Lam AP. BRB-ArrayTools Users Guide (Version 3.4). Bethesda, MD: Biometric Research Branch National Cancer Institute, 2005. Technical Report 46, http://linus.nci. nih.gov./brb.
18. Subramanian A, Tamayo P, Mootha VK. Gene set enrichment analysis: a knowledge-based approach for interpreting genome-wide expression profiles. Proc Natl Acad Sci USA 2005; 102(43):15545–15550.
19. Tian L, Greenberg SA, Kong SW, Altschuler J, Kohane IS, Park PJ. Discovering statisti-cally significant pathways in expression profiling studies. Proc Natl Acad Sci USA 2005; 102(38):13544–13549.
20. Radmacher MD, McShane LM, Simon R. A paradigm for class prediction using gene expression profiles. J Comput Biol 2002; 9:505–511.
21. Dudoit S, Fridlyand J. Classification in microarray experiments. In: Speed T, ed. Statisti-cal Analysis of Gene Expression Microarray Data. New York: Chapman & Hall/CRC, 2003:93–158.
22. Rosenwald A, Wright G, Chan WC, et al. The use of molecular profiling to predict sur-vival after chemotherapy for diffuse large-B-cell lymphoma. New Engl J Med 2002; 346:1937–1947.
23. Michiels S, Koscielny S, Hill C. Prediction of cancer outcome with microarrays: a multiple random validation strategy. Lancet 2005; 365:488–492.
24. Molinaro AM, Simon R, Pfeiffer RM. Prediction error estimation: a comparison of resampling methods. Bioinformatics 2005; 21(15):3301–3307.
25. Simon R. When is a genomic classifier ready for prime time? Nat Clin Pract Oncol 2004; 1(1):2–3.
26. Simon R. A roadmap for developing and validating therapeutically relevant genomic classifiers. J Clin Oncol 2005; 23:7332–7341.
27. Dobbin K, Beer DG, Meyerson M, et al. Inter-laboratory comparability study of cancer gene expression analysis using oligonucleotide microarrays. Clin Cancer Res 2005; 11:565–572.
28. Paik S, Shak S, Tang G, et al. A multigene assay to predict recurrence of tamoxifen-treated, node-negative breast cancer. New Engl J Med 2004; 351:2817–2826.
29. Simon R, Altman DG. Statistical aspects of prognostic factor studies in oncology. Br J Cancer 1994; 69:979–985.
30. Bast RC, Ravdin P, Hayes DF, et al. 2000 update of recommendations for the use of tumor markers in breast and colorectal cancer: clinical practice guidelines of the American Society of Clinical Oncology. J Clin Oncol 2001; 19:1865–1878.

31. Simon R, Maitournam A. Evaluating the efficiency of targeted designs for randomized clinical trials. Clin Cancer Res 2004; 10:6759–6763, supplement and correction 2006; 12:3229.
32. Maitournam A, Simon R. On the efficiency of targeted clinical trials. Stat Med 2005; 24:329–339.
33. Simon R, Wang SJ. Use of genomic signatures in therapeutics development. Pharmacogenomics J 2006; 6:166–173.
34. Freidlin B, Simon R. Adaptive signature design: an adaptive clinical trial design for generating and prospectively testing a gene expression signature for sensitive patients. Clin Cancer Res 2005; 11:7872–7878.
35. Simon R. Guidelines for the design of clinical studies for development and validation of therapeutically relevant biomarkers and biomarker based classification systems. In: Hayes DF, Gasparini G, eds. Biomarkers in Breast Cancer: Molecular Diagnostics for Predicting and Monitoring Therapeutic Effect. New York: Humana Press, 2005:3–16.
36. Sargent DJ, Conley BA, Allegra C, Collette L. Clinical trial designs for predictive marker validation in cancer treatment trials. J Clin Oncol 2005; 23(9):2020–2027.
37. Pusztai L, Hess KR. Clinical trial design for microarray predictive marker discovery and assessment. Ann Oncol 2004; 15:1731–1737.

4 Preoperative Therapy as a Model for Translational Research in Breast Cancer

Harold J. Burstein

Dana-Farber Cancer Institute, Harvard Medical School, Boston, Massachusetts, U.S.A.

INTRODUCTION

Preoperative (sometimes called neoadjuvant or primary) treatment for breast cancer is well established as a treatment for locally advanced tumors (1). Early results, principally with chemotherapy, suggested that neoadjuvant chemotherapy could effectively cytoreduce bulky tumors, rendering operable women with extensive primary tumors, including inflammatory breast cancer. On the basis of these results, and the growing literature on adjuvant chemotherapy, neoadjuvant chemotherapy became the standard of care for locally advanced breast cancer.

Neoadjuvant chemotherapy has also been studied among women with earlier stages of breast cancer. The landmark National Surgical Adjuvant Breast and Bowel Project Protocol (NSAPB) B-18 trial randomized women with operable breast cancer to either adjuvant or neoadjuvant chemotherapy (2). This study proved several important treatment principles for preoperative chemotherapy that have been validated in other randomized clinical trials. First, neoadjuvant therapy was tolerable and did not interfere with other treatment modalities, such as surgery or radiation therapy. Secondly, neoadjuvant therapy provided equivalent long-term disease outcomes as adjuvant therapy. Distant disease-free and local–regional disease recurrence rates were equal with either strategy. Third, neoadjuvant therapy had the advantage of surgical downstaging some patients. That is, patients who might otherwise have needed a mastectomy could in some instances have sufficient tumor shrinkage to facilitate breast-conserving surgery. Fourth, neoadjuvant therapy appeared to identify a new prognostic feature, the pathological complete response (pCR). While most patients had tumor response to treatment, only a small fraction—10% to 20%—had complete eradication of detectable tumor within the breast or regional lymph nodes. Those patients who did achieve pCR had a superior long-term breast cancer outcome compared to patients with residual tumor in the breast at the time of surgery. This suggested that pCR following neoadjuvant chemotherapy could be an effective surrogate marker for long-term cancer results.

Because the breast tumor is clinically detectable, measurable, and accessible for tissue sampling or radiological assessment, preoperative treatment offers unparalleled opportunities to study breast cancer biology. In addition, treatment in the preoperative setting is relatively short, and results are available quickly. The potential for pCR to serve as a surrogate for late recurrence risk invites the possibility that long follow-up, which is time-consuming and expensive, might be unnecessary for identifying better treatments. From a methodological viewpoint, preoperative treatment trials may require smaller number of patients. The sample size for clinical studies is governed by the number of "events." In adjuvant trials, events are tumor recurrences that happen in only a fraction of patients. In contrast, events, such as response or pCR in preoperative studies, happen in a larger fraction of patients, potentially lowering the number of needed patients. For all these reasons, preoperative treatment has emerged as a favored model for translational clinical trials.

A challenge for preoperative research has been to define adequately the nature of response to treatment. A variety of criteria for pCR have been developed, as well as grading scales for measuring response less than pCR. While certain consistencies exist within various treatment reports, such as the scoring of residual in situ carcinoma, only, as equivalent to pCR, reporting practices are highly variable. For instance, definitions of pCR variously include response in the breast-alone versus breast- and lymph-node, and differences in the scoring of residual microinvasive or lymphatic/vascular invasion. The reporting of pCR is also subject to the effort made to sample the surgical specimen; the harder the pathologist searches for residual tumor, the more likely it is that tumor will be found. Treatment plans in the preoperative setting are not uniform and range from several weeks to six months or more. Finally, patient eligibility for neoadjuvant trials differs enormously from one study to another. Some studies include patients with stage I–III breast cancer; others are limited to women with locally advanced disease, only. For these reasons, it has not proven meaningful to compare rates of clinical response or pCR between different clinical trials.

Recent studies utilizing preoperative therapy can be broadly divided into several categories, each with different primary endpoints. Larger, randomized trials have sought to define new standards of treatment suitable for adjuvant therapy. Smaller phase 2 trials have attempted to define the efficacy of specific regimens, including those that incorporate novel agents, in the preoperative setting. Biomarker trials have attempted to analyze serial changes in tumor biology in response to treatment, with the goals of identifying predictors of benefit/response using conventional therapies. Finally, there are "exposure" studies in which patients are offered short treatments with novel therapies in an effort to identify mechanisms of action, relevant biomarkers, or efficacy signals that would be evaluated further in larger trials. The remainder of this chapter discusses some of these recent findings with focus on the methodological lessons that have emerged.

RANDOMIZED PREOPERATIVE TRIALS: IS PATHOLOGICAL COMPLETE RESPONSE A WORTHY SURROGATE?

The great virtue of preoperative treatment is the ability to assess the response within the breast. The great limitation of preoperative treatment as a translational study model is the nature of the relationship among in-breast response, biomarker outcomes, and long-term clinical outcomes that matter to patients. The key issue yet to be proven in the preoperative literature is whether step-wise improvement in pCR would in fact translate into improvement in long-term prevention of breast cancer recurrence. This concept is of critical importance to the preoperative field. Historically, standards of care for adjuvant treatment have been defined based on long-term diseases-related results—recurrence and survival. The replacement of adjuvant trials with neoadjuvant trials as "standard-defining regimens" depends on the proof of a suitable surrogate for late cancer events. To date, pCR appears to be the best available measure of long-term recurrence risk in patients receiving neoadjuvant chemotherapy (2,3). For this reason, NSABP B-27 sought in part to determine the correlation of pCR with long-term recurrence risk (4). Patients were randomized to treatment with preoperative anthracycline and cyclophospha-mide (AC) chemotherapy alone or AC followed by docetaxel. The pivotal findings were that the addition of docetaxel improved the pCR rate from 13% to 26%. Patients who achieved pCR continue to show lower risk of recurrence than patients with residual tumor. However, to date, the 100% increase in pCR has not translated into longer-term improvement in disease-free survival. This is probably for several reasons: first, the difference in pCR rate was still modest in absolute terms. Second, breast cancer heterogeneity affects the interpretation of the results. Tumors that are strongly hormone-sensitive probably get little gain from chemotherapy, but do benefit from adjuvant endocrine treatment given after preoperative therapy. Patients with tumors that do dramatically respond to neoadjuvant chemotherapy tend to fare well in the longer term; however, residual tumor after neoadjuvant treatment identifies a group of patients with a particularly poor prognosis down the road, contributing substantial events. For all these reasons, the NSABP B-27 result still begs the question as to whether better response rates in the neoadjuvant setting are an adequate substitute for disease-free survival in the adjuvant setting. It remains a fundamental challenge for preoperative therapy to demonstrate that the short-term clinical measures of efficacy are acceptable for defining regimens for use when long-term outcomes remain the driving force for most adjuvant decision-making.

Another instance of exploration of pCR as suitable surrogate was a random-ized trial of preoperative chemotherapy alone versus chemotherapy plus trastuzu-mab as treatment for HER2 overexpressing breast cancer (5). This study, led by MD Anderson Cancer Center, was planned as a mid-sized phase 2 trial involving several hundred women. The study was stopped prematurely, having accrued only 42 patients, when preliminary data suggested tremendous improvement in pCR with use of trastuzumab; the pCR rate went from 26% to 65% with use of tras-tuzumab. This provocative result proved to be a foreshadowing of the major improvements seen with adjuvant trastuzumab. However, because the study was so small and lacked long-term follow, this result did not transform adjuvant prac-tice. Trastuzumab was widely adopted only once when the reports from the large, phase 3 adjuvant trials were available.

A final limitation to use of pCR is that not all therapeutic agents are likely to work via short-term tumor regression, or accomplish pCR. Endocrine therapy, for instance, is critical for adjuvant treatment of estrogen-receptor positive breast cancer. While there are responses to neoadjuvant endocrine therapy, endocrine therapy almost never achieves a pCR in neoadjuvant trials that have studied three to six month's duration of treatment. Thus, pCR fails as a predictor of benefit for endocrine treatment. For newer agents like angiogenesis inhibitors, the relationship between tumor response and control of tumor progression is again not straightforward. In trials of metastatic cancer, the benefits of antiangio-genesis therapy are not limited to those patients with objective tumor response. Thus, in neoadjuvant trials of antiangiogenesis drugs, response or pCR over a period of several months may not be a relevant marker of activity or may not correlate in magnitude with the potential long-term disease control benefits.

These experiences underscore the difficulties of using neoadjuvant therapy as a vehicle for defining standard treatments for early stage breast cancer. While cooperative groups continue to explore neoadjuvant treatment regimens, they are cognizant of the potential limits of this approach for altering the adjuvant land-scape. It seems likely that preoperative treatment can be used to define compelling standards of care when the novel intervention has phenomenal clinical activity compared with standard therapy, or when more modest advantage is achieved with modest alteration in side effects/tolerability of therapy.

Preoperative Phase 2 Trials

Preoperative therapy has been studied in innumerable single- or multi-center phase 2 trials using novel treatment strategies for breast cancer. These studies have often established the feasibility of new therapies in the early or preoperative setting, but have not in any instance identified regimens that define clinical practice. In this regard, these studies are similar to most phase 2 trials in advanced breast cancer, which serve mainly to document activity and safety of various regimens.

Nonetheless, preoperative treatment results have proven interesting for justification of further research in a field (Table 1). Neoadjuvant phase 2 studies have yielded the first glimpses into the role of novel biological therapies, such as trastuzumab and bevacizumab, in the adjuvant setting. They have been used to generate exciting hypotheses about the role of Epidermal Growth Factor Receptor (EGFR) and HER2 growth factors as predictors of outcome for endocrine therapy.

Preoperative treatment programs have also been enormously valuable in helping to define clinically important subsets of breast cancer. In particular, phase 2 trials using anthracycline- and taxane-based chemotherapy have demonstrated different rates of pCR among the different subsets defined by hormone-receptor and HER2 status. Retrospective analyses of neoadjuvant chemotherapy trials at the MD Anderson Center have shown that tumors that are estrogen receptor (ER) positive have far lower pCR rates (5%) than ER-negative tumors (20%), suggesting that ER-positive breast cancers derive less benefit from chemotherapy than ER-negative tumors (6), and suggesting that pCR may not be an equally suitable surrogate for all types of breast cancer. This observation extends into subsets defined by gene expression arrays, as well (Table 2) (7). Tumors classified as

TABLE 1 Recent Examples of Preoperative Phase 2 Trials of Note

Study	Patient population	Treatment/finding
Burstein et al. (8)	HER2+ breast cancer	Feasibility and clinical effects of neoadjuvant chemotherapy plus trastuzumab
Buzdar et al. (5)	HER2+ breast cancer	Adding trastuzumab to chemotherapy improves pCR
Eiermann et al. (9)	ER+ breast cancer	Comparison of neoadjuvant tamoxifen versus aromatase inhibitor (letrozole)
Cataliotti et al. (10), PROACT trial	ER + breast cancer	Comparison of neoadjuvant tamoxifen versus aromatase inhibitor (anastrozole)
Smith et al. (11), IMPACT trial	ER+ breast cancer	Comparison of neoadjuvant tamoxifen versus aromatase inhibitor (anastrozole) versus combination
Wedam et al. (12)	Locally advanced/ inflammatory breast cancer	Feasibility, clinical, and biological effects of bevacizumab
Buzdar et al. (13)	Operable breast cancer	Comparison of taxane versus anthracycline-based neoadjuvant chemotherapy

Abbreviations: IMPACT, Immediate Preoperative Anastrozole, Tamoxifen, or Combined with Tamoxifen; ER, estrogen receptor; pCR, pathological complete response; PROACT, Preoperative "Arimidex" Compared to Tamoxifen.

TABLE 2 Pathological Complete Response to Neoadjuvant Chemotherapy in Breast Cancer Subsets Defined by Gene Expression Arrays

Molecular subset	Clinical features	Number of patients	Rate of pCR (%)
Luminal A/B	ER+, HER2−	30	7
Normal breast-like	ER+, HER2−	10	0
HER2 +	HER2 +	20	45
Basaloid	ER, PR, and HER2−, generally high grade	22	45

Abbreviations: ER, estrogen receptor; PR, progesterone receptor; pCR, pathological complete response.
Source: Adapted from Ref. 7.

basal-like (lacking hormone-receptor and HER2 expression) or HER2-positive tumors are quite likely to response to neoadjuvant chemotherapy with pCR. In contrast, the so-called luminal and normal breast-like tumors, which express hormone-receptors, are in fact very unlikely to response to neoadjuvant chemotherapy with pCR. These observations have fueled the re-assessment of the benefits of adjuvant chemotherapy among clinically relevant subsets of breast cancer.

PREOPERATIVE THERAPY: THE SEARCH FOR BIOMARKERS

Breast cancers are among the most accessible tumor tissues encountered in solid tumor oncology. The accessibility lends itself to serial biopsy of tumors at the time of diagnosis, at the time of definitive breast surgery, and potentially at several opportune moments in between during the course of neoadjuvant treatment. This access to "before and after" tumor specimens has been successfully exploited by investigators in a search for novel biomarkers of treatment activity and insights into the mechanism of action for new agents. Table 3 lists several

TABLE 3 Biomarker Results from Preoperative Treatment Trials: Key Examples

Study	Intervention	Biomarker findings
Ellis et al. (14)	Randomized treatment with tamoxifen or AI	Different response rates for AI versus tamoxifen in ER+ tumor subsets defined by EGFR/HER2 status
Dowsett et al. (15), IMPACT trial	Randomized treatment with tamoxifen or AI or both	Characterization of differential effects of tamoxifen or AI therapy on markers of tumor differentiation and proliferation
Archer et al. (16)	Neoadjuvant chemotherapy	Characterization of apoptosis induction and changes in proliferation as marker of response to chemotherapy
Mohsin et al. (17)	Neoadjuvant trastuzumab	Demonstration of apoptosis induction by neoadjuvant therapy identifies mechanism of action
Gianni et al. (18)	Neoadjuvant chemotherapy	Molecular prognostic tool based on gene expression array predicts likelihood of pCR
Chang et al. (19)	Neoadjuvant taxane chemotherapy	Gene expression array signature predicts likelihood of response

Abbreviations: AI; aromatase inhibitor; EGFR, epidermal growth factor receptor; ER, estrogen receptor; IMPACT, Immediate Preoperative Anastrozole, Tamoxifen, or Combined with Tamoxifen; pCR, pathological complete response.

recent examples where investigators have exploited neoadjuvant treatment to examine key biological changes in tumors with therapy. The hope is that ongoing work in this vein will identify new target pathways, and provide early insights into whether new treatments are actually achieving the desired changes within tumors.

"WINDOW OF OPPORTUNITY" TRIALS

A final clinical trial strategy for neoadjuvant studies has been brief exposure trials to novel agents, with a goal of defining very short-term biological effects. In such trials, patients are offered limited courses of treatment—typically one to three weeks—prior to their breast surgery, without established therapeutic intent. This approach seems most suitable for nontoxic treatments that are unlikely to interfere with planned surgical treatment, as the goal of therapy is not therapeutic but exploratory. However, there are trials underway designed to investigate this strategy. If successful, it would establish a new paradigm of drug discovery, where direct drug activity is measured in these short exposures without true therapeutic intent.

SUMMARY

Preoperative treatment is a mainstay of clinical care and research for women with breast cancer. Unique among solid tumors, the use of neoadjuvant treatment has been extensively studied in breast cancer patients, with many beneficial and provocative clinical results. It is an outstanding model for translational research, because of the accessibility of tumor tissue, and the opportunity to obtain tissue at serial time points before, during, and after treatment.

The largest challenge confronting the use of neoadjuvant therapy as a definitive model for treatment of early stage disease remains the difficulty in convincingly relating the short-term surrogate (response, pCR) with the long-term endpoint of tumor control or recurrence. In the meanwhile, the use of response/pCR as endpoints should allow novel strategies to be quickly evaluated in the neoadjuvant setting, identified approaches that clearly warrant (or not) large-scale study in randomized phase 3 adjuvant trials. Preoperative treatment also holds promise for identifying biological pathways and biological effects of new cancer drugs. Insights from such translational studies may allow for accelerated recognition of biologically relevant compounds, or pairs of compounds, that can verify or refute other laboratory-based models of cancer treatment. This information—uniquely available from preoperative studies because of the availability of tumor samples—should dramatically inform evolving clinical practice in the years ahead.

REFERENCES

1. Kaufmann M, Hortobagyi GN, Goldhirsch A, et al. Recommendations from an international expert panel on the use of neoadjuvant (primary) systemic treatment of operable breast cancer: an update. J Clin Oncol 2006 Apr 20; 24(12):1940–1949.
2. Fisher B, Bryant J, Wolmark N, et al. Effect of preoperative chemotherapy on the outcome of women with operable breast cancer. J Clin Oncol 1998 Aug; 16(8):2672–2685.
3. Kuerer HM, Newman LA, Smith TL, et al. Clinical course of breast cancer patients with complete pathologic primary tumor and axillary lymph node response to doxorubicin-based neoadjuvant chemotherapy. J Clin Oncol 1999 Feb; 17(2):460–469.

4. Bear HD, Anderson S, Brown A, et al.; National Surgical Adjuvant Breast and Bowel Project Protocol B-27. The effect on tumor response of adding sequential preoperative docetaxel to preoperative doxorubicin and cyclophosphamide: preliminary results from National Surgical Adjuvant Breast and Bowel Project Protocol B-27. J Clin Oncol 2003 Nov 15; 21(22):4165–4174.

5. Buzdar AU, Ibrahim NK, Francis D, et al. Significantly higher pathologic complete remission rate after neoadjuvant therapy with trastuzumab, paclitaxel, and epirubicin chemotherapy: results of a randomized trial in human epidermal growth factor receptor 2-positive operable breast cancer. J Clin Oncol 2005 Jun 1; 23(16):3676–3685.

6. Buzdar AU, Valero V, Theriault RL, et al. Pathological complete response to chemotherapy is related to hormone receptor status. San Antonio Breast Cancer Symposium 2003, abstract 302.

7. Rouzier R, Perou CM, Symmans WF, et al. Breast cancer molecular subtypes respond differently to preoperative chemotherapy. Clin Cancer Res 2005 Aug 15; 11(16):5678–5685.

8. Burstein HJ, Harris LN, Gelman R, et al. Preoperative therapy with trastuzumab and paclitaxel followed by sequential adjuvant doxorubicin/cyclophosphamide for HER2 overexpressing stage II or III breast cancer: a pilot study. J Clin Oncol 2003 Jan 1; 21(1):46–53.

9. Eiermann W, Paepke S, Appfelstaedt J, et al.; Letrozole Neo-Adjuvant Breast Cancer Study Group. Preoperative treatment of postmenopausal breast cancer patients with letrozole: a randomized double-blind multicenter study. Ann Oncol 2001 Nov; 12(11):1527–1532.

10. Cataliotti L, Buzdar AU, Noguchi S, et al. Comparison of anastrozole versus tamoxifen as preoperative therapy in postmenopausal women with hormone receptor-positive breast cancer: the Pre-Operative "Arimidex" Compared to Tamoxifen (PROACT) trial. Cancer 2006 May 15; 106(10):2095–2103.

11. Smith IE, Dowsett M, Ebbs SR, et al.; IMPACT Trialists Group. Neoadjuvant treatment of postmenopausal breast cancer with anastrozole, tamoxifen, or both in combination: the Immediate Preoperative Anastrozole, Tamoxifen, or Combined with Tamoxifen (IMPACT) multicenter double-blind randomized trial. J Clin Oncol 2005 Aug 1; 23(22):5108–5116.

12. Wedam SB, Low JA, Yang SX, et al. Antiangiogenic and antitumor effects of bevacizumab in patients with inflammatory and locally advanced breast cancer. J Clin Oncol 2006 Feb 10; 24(5):769–777.

13. Buzdar AU, Singletary SE, Theriault RL, et al. Prospective evaluation of paclitaxel versus combination chemotherapy with fluorouracil, doxorubicin, and cyclophosphamide as neoadjuvant therapy in patients with operable breast cancer. J Clin Oncol 1999 Nov; 17(11):3412–3417.

14. Ellis MJ, Coop A, Singh B, et al. Letrozole is more effective neoadjuvant endocrine therapy than amoxifen for ErbB-1- and/or ErbB-2-positive, estrogen receptor-positive primary breast cancer: evidence from a phase III randomized trial. J Clin Oncol 2001 Sep 15; 19(18):3808–3816.

15. Dowsett M, Ebbs SR, Dixon JM, et al. Biomarker changes during neoadjuvant anastrozole, tamoxifen, or the combination: influence of hormonal status and HER-2 in breast cancer—a study from the IMPACT trialists. J Clin Oncol 2005 Apr 10; 23(11):2477–2492.

16. Archer CD, Parton M, Smith IE, et al. Early changes in apoptosis and proliferation following primary chemotherapy for breast cancer. Br J Cancer 2003 Sep 15; 89(6):1035–1041.

17. Mohsin SK, Weiss HL, Gutierrez MC, et al. Neoadjuvant trastuzumab induces apoptosis in primary breast cancers. J Clin Oncol 2005 Apr 10; 23(11):2460–2468.

18. Gianni L, Zambetti M, Clark K, et al. Gene expression profiles in paraffin-embedded core biopsy tissue predict response to chemotherapy in women with locally advanced breast cancer. J Clin Oncol 2005 Oct 10; 23(29):7265–7277.

19. Chang JC, Wooten EC, Tsimelzon A, et al. Gene expression profiling for the prediction of therapeutic response to docetaxel in patients with breast cancer. Lancet 2003; 362: 362–369.

Pharmacology and Pharmacogenetics of Chemotherapeutic Agents

Shaheenah Dawood
Department of Oncology, Dubai Hospital, Dubai, United Arab Emirates

Brian Leyland-Jones
Departments of Oncology and Medicine, McGill University, Montreal, Quebec, Canada

INTRODUCTION

"If it were not for the great variability among individuals medicine might as well be a science and not an art." The words of Sir William Osler (1892) describe the practice of medicine over the last 100 years reflecting the lack of data available to aid physicians in their pursuit of individualized therapy. Only recently, with greater understanding of the mechanisms behind the heterogeneity observed across patient populations, both in terms of efficacy and toxicity of a variety of therapeutic agents, are we now able to shift our practice from art to science with the ultimate goal of creating an era of "personalized medicine."

PRINCIPLES OF PERSONALIZED MEDICINE

In recent times, the field of oncology has seen remarkable progress with respect to the development of a number of chemotherapeutic drugs. Despite such progress, the benefits achieved have been modest at best. The choice of chemotherapeutic agent is often empirical and geared to fit the average patient with the unfortunate result that ~40% of patients may be receiving the wrong drug (1). The problem faced is the varied efficacy, ranging from success to failure, and unpredictable treatment-associated toxicity, ranging from no effect to a lethal event, seen with the administration of the same dose of a given anticancer drug to a population of patients with apparently the same malignancy (2).

Varying efficacy and toxicity have implications not only for the patient but also for the health-care system. Currently available anticancer drugs show limited efficacy in as many as 70% of treated patients, and adverse drug reactions caused by the failure to predict individual drug toxicity or toxic drug–drug interactions now accounts for 100,000 patient deaths and two million hospitalizations in the United States every year (3). Serious adverse drug reactions are the sixth leading cause of death in the United States (4), which costs the health-care system billions of dollars (5). Identifying drug-specific predictive markers would help individualize therapy, ensuring cost-effective management that has maximal therapeutic efficacy with minimal toxicity.

Pharmacoepidemiology is a field that focuses on understanding why individuals respond differently to drug therapy, in terms of both beneficial and adverse events. Because of the narrow therapeutic index of chemotherapeutic agents, it has become even more important to identify the causes of the observed interindividual differences. Such observed differences are due to a complex interplay of a number of factors, including the patient's age, sex, diet, comorbid conditions, performance status, and, last but not least, the genetic profile of the patient and tumor. On the basis of these differences, four groups of patients can be identified: (*i*) responders, (*ii*) nonresponders, (*iii*) toxic responders, and (*iv*) toxic nonresponders (Fig. 1).

Pharmacogenetics, a term first coined by Friedrich Vogel (6) in 1959, focuses on identifying genetic factors that influence drug response. Genetic variants of the drug target, drug metabolizing enzymes, or disease pathway genes may all be used as predictors of drug efficacy or toxicity. Ideally, an easily accessible and relatively inexpensive genetic test that could be used to detect these variants on a readily obtainable biological sample (i.e., tissue or peripheral blood) could be used to predict efficacy or toxicity. However, before development of such a test, one would need to compare its clinical value against current predictive tests. At present, the ability to predict response in cancer is low, such that the clinical value of such a pharmacogenetic test would be high (Fig. 2).

Molecular markers, both predictive and prognostic (associated with disease outcome independent of therapy), will play an important role in the therapeutic decision-making process. Specific DNA polymorphisms used to predict therapeutic efficacy or toxicity are static markers, whereas those identified using gene expression (mRNA), protein expression, or protein function are dynamic predictive markers which will change through the progression of the disease or under the influence of chemotherapy. Predictive markers (dependent on specific treatments) will not only identify the best chemotherapeutic agent to be used for a specific malignancy but will also guide the amount that should be administered in order to stay within the therapeutic window of the drug.

CLINICAL PREDICTORS OF TOXIC EFFECTS

When we administer a drug to a patient, we assume that the patient will achieve maximal benefit from the drug with minimal toxicity. As drugs used for the treatment of cancer have the narrowest therapeutic index in all of medicine, delivering

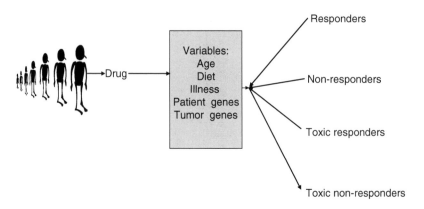

FIGURE 1 Variability of response.

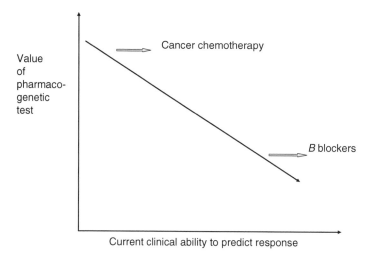

FIGURE 2 Value of pharmacogenetic test is high in cancer. *Source*: Adapted from Ref. 37.

the right dose is crucial if morbidity is to be avoided. Thus, understanding the mechanisms behind the variability in response and toxicity profile seen with these medications is even more important when dealing with a cancer patient. At the clinical level, variability of the drug can be understood by considering both its pharmacokinetic and pharmacodynamic profiles (Fig. 3). Pharmacokinetics, simply described, is "what the body does to the drug." It describes the relationship between time and plasma concentration of the drug metabolites being affected by variables such as absorption, distribution, metabolism, and excretion of the drug. Pharmacodynamics tells us "what the drug does to the body" in terms of effect (drug response and toxicity) allowing us to monitor events clinically that take place at the molecular level.

Pharmacokinetics and pharmacodynamics can be considered as a spectrum of continuous events starting with the ingestion of the drug and ending with a clinical effect seen in the patient. Thus, variability in the processes of absorption, distribution, metabolism, and excretion may be associated with either an increase or a decrease in a pharmacodynamic effect. Figure 4 illustrates the relationship between the two parameters. As the plasma concentration of the drug increases, so does its effect, illustrating how most of the toxicity that a patient experiences is not idiosyncratic but predictable on a concentration–response curve.

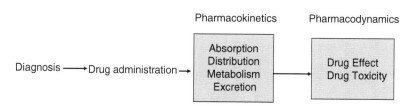

FIGURE 3 Drug processing.

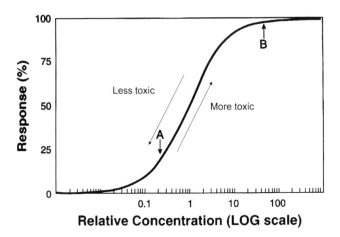

FIGURE 4   Mathematical representation of pharmacokinetic and pharmacodynamic relationship.

Concentrations of drugs will predictably be altered in a number of special population groups (Table 1). Patients with organ dysfunction will be unable to metabolize or excrete (depending on the drug administered) drugs properly resulting in either an increase or a decrease in effect (response and toxicity). One such example is the use of carboplatin in patients with renal dysfunction. Carboplatin is excreted primarily by the kidney. Early pharmacological studies of carboplatin demonstrated a close relationship between its thrombocytopenic effect and the area under the curve (AUC) in the individual, a parameter that is closely related to the renal function. On the basis of these observations, a number of formulas (6,7) have been derived using creatinine clearance either to predict the percentage change in platelet count or to determine the target AUC, thereby avoiding unacceptable thrombocytopenia while maximizing dose intensity in the individual being treated.

Taxanes are primarily metabolized and excreted in the liver with their main hematological toxicity being neutropenia. Patients with hepatic dysfunction are particularly sensitive to the taxanes, experiencing severe neutropenia if given regular doses (Fig. 5). Liver function tests, however, are not very reliable for individualized dosing, but this could be improved upon by testing the function of specific enzymes, which would be more accurate. However, such tests are not readily available. There are two tests that can be used to evaluate the activity of the hepatic isoenzyme CYP3A that is involved in the metabolism of docetaxel. They include the midazolam clearance test and the C14 erythromycin breath test; however, both are not routinely used in clinical practice. Currently in the clinic, we rely upon

TABLE 1   Populations with Altered PK/PD

Groups	Examples
Renal dysfunction	Carboplatin, cisplatin
Hepatic dysfunction	Paclitaxel, docetaxel
Hypoalbuminemia	Coumadin, paclitaxel, docetaxel
Elderly patients	Fewer reserves
Obese patients	Increased volume of distribution, fatty liver
Female patients	Less clearance of gemcitabine, doxorubicin

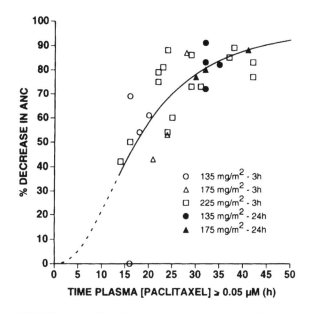

FIGURE 5 Relationship of paclitaxel and neutropenia.

basic liver function tests; although inconsistent, they have been useful in preventing excessive toxicity with taxanes. In addition, due to the significant amount of plasma protein binding of taxanes, patients with low protein levels are also more sensitive to taxanes.

Elderly patients also represent a special population group where individual dosing is important due to reduced physiological reserves, especially in terms of both hepatic and renal function. In addition, interindividual variability plays a role in this group of patients as illustrated by the paclitaxel pharmacokinetic trial conducted by CALGB (8). This prospective study looked at the pharmacokinetic parameters and toxicity profile of paclitaxel administered to patients greater than 55 years of age. The study showed that with increasing age there was a decrease in total body clearance of paclitaxel, an increase in AUC, and an increase in grades 3 and 4 neutropenia. However, the altered pharmacokinetic and pharmaco-dynamic parameters did not translate into a statistically significant increase in the rate of febrile neutropenia or hospitalization. More studies are thus needed before we can make definitive recommendations about individual dosing strategies for elderly patients.

Consideration of patient weight in individual dosing of drugs can also present a problem. Dosing drugs in patients who are obese using actual body weight or ideal body weight may lead to either overdosing or underdosing, respect-ively, both of which will alter the pharmacodynamic effect of the administered drug. Patient gender is also important, although it is not routinely considered in the clinic when administering chemotherapeutic agents. It is well known that the clearance of certain agents such as gemcitabine and doxorubicin is 20% less in female patients and could certainly account for their increased sensitivity.

Thus, the first step to individualizing therapy is to consider dose modification based on simple clinical variables that influence the various parameters of the

TABLE 2   Genes Affecting Therapeutic Outcome

Gene	Malignancy
Estrogen receptor	Breast
Progesterone receptor	Breast
HER2/neu overexpression	Breast
p53	Breast
BCR/ABL	Leukemia
ALL1	Leukemia
AML1	Leukemia
PML-RARA	Leukemia
RAS	Leukemia
MDR1	Leukemia
Thymidylate synthase	Colon cancer

pharmacokinetic profile of a drug. Usually, sophisticated tests are not required for this, underlying the importance of a good clinical assessment of a patient.

GENETIC PREDICTORS OF TOXIC EFFECTS

In oncology, many genes conspire to affect therapeutic outcomes, examples of which are illustrated in Table 2. When considering genetic variants that can influence the pharmacokinetic and pharmacodynamic properties of various agents used to treat a variety of malignancies, it is important to consider genomes of both the germline and the tumor. Germline polymorphisms are determined at conception, whereas genotypic variation of the tumor is a dynamic process that evolves as the tumor grows, metastasizes, or is exposed to a variety of drugs.

Every gene contains some degree of polymorphism. Germline DNA polymorphisms are stable heritable changes that can affect the transcription and translation of genes. The simplest and most commonly studied DNA polymorphism is the single nucleotide polymorphism (SNP). SNPs occur once every 1900 bp in the three billion bases in the human genome (9). Thus far, more than 1.4 million SNPs have been identified in the human genome with more than 60,000 occurring in the coding region of genes (some being associated with variations in drug metabolism and effects) (9). Other types of polymorphisms include tandem repeats (multiple copies of repeated DNA sequences) and microsatellite repeats (sequences of as many as four nucleotides that are repeated multiple times). Polymorphisms that occur in the promoter region can effect the transcription of the gene, whereas those that occur in the exon (and intron) region and 3′-UTR of the gene will effect translation and RNA stability, respectively, ultimately resulting in either reduced or enhanced activity of the encoded protein (2). The aim is to be able to sift through the multitude of polymorphisms and identify those occurring in gene regulatory or coding regions that have clinical relevance. To some extent, SNPs have already been associated with substantial changes in the metabolism or effects of medications and some are now being used to predict clinical response.

Two approaches have been used to identify clinically relevant polymorphisms. The reverse genetic approach involves giving a particular drug to a group of individuals, observing the variability in response or toxicity, prioritizing the phenotypes of clinical importance and then identifying the biochemical and molecular nature of the variability through extensive resequencing techniques that will link the polymorphisms with the observed phenotypes. A more cost-effective method is the forward genetic approach that can be used to pinpoint genomic variability at specific loci in a group of individuals, formulate hypotheses regarding these polymorphisms causing phenotypic variability, and finally investigate the subsequent clinical consequences. In oncology, SNP technology has focused on detecting the predisposition of cancer, predicting drug toxicity and, to a lesser extent, drug efficacy. In the following sections, common examples of polymorphisms that result in increased toxicity of a number of chemotherapeutic agents used in oncology are discussed.

N-Acetyltransferase

Almost all polymorphisms studied to date differ in frequency among ethnic and racial groups, a phenomenon shown early on in individuals receiving isoniazid for the treatment of tuberculosis. Polymorphisms of N-acetyltransferase, a phase II conjugating liver enzyme required for the metabolism of isoniazid, are responsible for the interindividual and interethnic differences observed in toxicity and efficacy related to the drug. During the development of isoniazid, a bimodal distribution in its plasma concentration was observed and individuals with the highest plasma concentrations were generally slow acetylators suffering from peripheral nerve damage, whereas fast acetylators (having low plasma concentrations of isoniazid) were not affected (10). In addition, studies showed that the slow acetylator phenotype is inherited as an autosomal recessive trait with large variations among ethnic groups (40% to 70% of Caucasions and African Americans, 10% to 20% of Japanese, and more than 80% of Egyptians) (11,12).

Amonafide (13), a topoisomerase II inhibitor, is another substrate of N-acetyl transferase whose clinical development has been hampered by highly variable and unpredictable toxicity caused, at least in part, by interindividual differences in N-acetylation (fast acetylators experienced greater myelosuppression than did slow acetylators). This illustrates the potential importance of pharmacogenetic determinants on pharmacokinetics and pharmacodynamics.

The Acute Lymphoblastic Leukemia Story

Remarkable progress has been made in the treatment of acute lymphoblastic leukemia (ALL) with cure rates increasing from a mere 10% (four decades ago) to nearly 80% in children and 40% in adults (14). This progress was made through increasing the optimization of the use of antileukemic drugs allowing for better therapeutic efficacy with minimal toxicity. One such drug is mercaptopurine, a thiopurine prodrug that is converted into thioguanine nucleotides that are subsequently incorporated into DNA, inducing an antileukemic effect. Thiopurine methyltransferase (TPMT) is an enzyme that converts the thiopurine prodrugs into inactive methylated metabolites. Patients with an inherited TPMT deficiency suffer severe, potentially fatal hematopoietic toxicity when exposed to standard doses of mercaptopurine (and other thiopurine prodrugs such as azathioprine and thioguanine).

TPMT deficiency is an autosomal recessive trait and occurs in about 1 in 300 people, whereas the heterozygous form (resulting in intermediate levels of enzyme activity) occurs in about 10% of the population (15). Only three nonsynonymous SNPs account for nearly 90% of the clinically relevant TPMT mutant alleles that result in enzymes with low or absent activity (16) rendering it feasible to determine TPMT activity via a single blood test and thereby individualize dosage to avoid

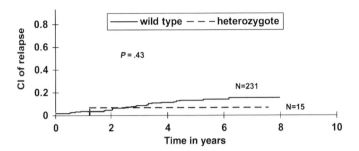

FIGURE 6 Dosage individualization according to thiopurine methyltransferase status does not affect cumulative incidence of relapse. *Source*: From Ref. 17.

excessive toxicity. One such pharmacogenetic test developed at St. Jude Hospital classifies patients according to normal, intermediate, and deficient levels of TPMT activity and has a concordance rate of 100% between genotype and phenotype. Questions have arisen as to whether such attempts to minimize toxicity would have an impact on the efficacy of thiopurine drugs. A study by Relling and coworkers (17) revealed that there were no long-term outcome changes related to dosage individualization based on the TPMT status of a patient (Fig. 6), illustrating how the clinical application of pharmacogenetics can be used to minimize toxicity without compromising efficacy.

Methyltetrahydrofolate reductase (MTHFR) is an important enzyme in the metabolism of folic acid. It catalyzes the reduction of 5,10-methylenetetrahydrofolate to 5-methyltetrahydrofolate (the predominant circulatory form of folate and the carbon donor for the demethylation of homocysteine to methionine). Methotrexate (a drug used extensively in the treatment of ALL) not only increases the levels of homocysteine but its active polyglutamate metabolite also inhibits MTHFR function. As a result, patients with a low level of MTHFR function are at an increased risk of methotrexate-induced toxicities such as oral mucosities. Two polymorphisms associated with reduced MTHFR activity have been identified with the 677C > T (substitution of thymine for cytosine at nucleotide 677) being the most common with 10% of the population being homozygous (have 30% enzyme activity) and 40% being heterozygous (have 60% enzyme activity) for this genotype (18). In addition to increasing the risk of methotrexate toxicity, recent findings have suggested that MTHFR polymorphisms may in fact protect against the development of both adult and pediatric ALL (19).

Tamoxifen

Tamoxifen is one of the most widely used drugs in the treatment and prevention of breast cancer. When given in the adjuvant setting to patients with estrogen receptor positive breast cancer for a period of five years, it reduces the annual recurrence rate of breast cancer by half and the breast cancer mortality rate by one-third (20). Tamoxifen undergoes extensive metabolism with the production of endoxifen and to a lesser extent 4-hydroxytamoxifen (21). These metabolites play an important role in the anticancer effect of tamoxifen through their high affinity binding to estrogen receptors and suppression of estradiol-stimulated cell proliferation (22).

The clinical effects of tamoxifen pertaining to its efficacy and toxicity are highly variable with roughly 35% of individuals with advanced breast cancer not responding to tamoxifen (23). This variability has been attributed to the variability seen in the plasma levels of the more potent metabolites of tamoxifen. The metabolism of tamoxifen to endoxifen is primarily mediated by CYP2D6-mediated oxidation of *N*-desmethyl tamoxifen, whereas its conversion to 4-hydroxy tamoxifen is catalyzed by multiple enzymes (24). Thus, the endoxifen plasma concentration is sensitive to the CYP2D6 genotype (most common allele associated with CYP2D6 poor metabolizer phenotype is CYP2D6*4) with one prospective trial revealing that women, receiving tamoxifen, who carry genetic variants associated with low or absent CYP2D6 activity had lower levels of endoxifen (25). In addition, this trial also showed that the concomitant administration of medications known to inhibit the activity of CYP2D6 also resulted in lower plasma levels of endoxifen. Whether the reduced levels of endoxifen had a clinically relevant pharmacodynamic impact was answered in a study that used tissue samples obtained from tamoxifen-treated women enrolled onto the North Central Cancer Treatment Group adjuvant breast cancer trial (26). The study showed that women with a homozygous CYP2D6 phenotype tended to have a higher risk of disease relapse and a lower incidence of hot flashes.

Polymorphisms associated with the activity of the metabolites of tamoxifen teach us two important lessons. First, the interindividual variability in the response to tamoxifen is explained both by genetic variation in CYP2D6 and by the coadministration of drugs that inhibit the activity of CYP2D6. Second, the toxicity associated with the drug can help identify responders.

Irinotecan

Irinotecan, a topoisomerase I inhibitor used extensively in the treatment of colorectal cancer, is a prodrug that is activated by systemic carboxylesterases to its active metabolite SN-38. SN-38 is then subsequently inactivated by glucuronide conjugation, catalyzed by UGT1A1 (uridine diphosphate glucuronosyltransferase), to form the inactive SN-38-glucuronide that is then excreted via the renal pathway. Polymorphisms of UGT1A1 (27) resulting in its decreased activity will result in increased levels of the SN-38 which is then excreted via the bile causing damage to the intestinal lining resulting in prolonged bouts of diarrhea that can be fatal. A phenotyping procedure for UGT1A1 has not been identified and genotyping of the UGT1A1 promoter in patients receiving irinotecan may identify patients at increased risk of toxicity. Clinical trials are currently ongoing to demonstrate the predictive significance of UGT1A1 genotyping for irinotecan effect.

5-Fluorouracil

5-Fluorouracil (5-FU) is a uracil analog that is widely used to treat solid malignancies and remains one of the most commonly prescribed chemotherapeutic agents in oncology (28). Approximately 5% of administered 5-FU is converted into its active form, 5-fluoro-2-deoxyuridine monophosphate (5-FdUMP), which is responsible for its antitumor activity through inhibition of thymidalate synthetase. The bulk of the drug (85%) is inactivated in the liver by dihydropyrimidine dehydrogenase (DPD), an enzyme that exhibits up to 20-fold variation in activity among individuals (29), with the remainder of the drug being excreted into the urine unchanged. Up to 20 mutations (30) that cause inactivation of DPD have been identified, with 3% to 5% of individuals in the general population being heterozygous carriers and 0.1% being homozygous carriers (31). The DPYD*2A allele has been associated with severe toxicity due to its inability to inactivate 5-FU leading to excessive amounts of 5-FdUMP, thereby causing gastrointestinal, hematopoietic, and neurological toxicities that are potentially fatal (32).

Despite identification of polymorphisms associated with DPD inactivation, a number of patients still exhibit severe 5-FU toxicity with no detectable mutations in the coding region of the DPD gene, indicative of the complex nature of genetic control of the molecular mechanisms regulating DPD activity. This also complicates the implementation of DPD pharmacogenetics in the prospective identification of high-risk patients for severe 5-FU toxicity.

5-FU exerts antitumor activity through the inhibition of thymidylate synthase (TS) by FdUMP. TS is a critical enzyme required for the synthesis of thymidylate, a precursor required for DNA synthesis and repair (33). Genetic polymorphism in the gene encoding TS has also been shown to influence the response to 5-FU therapy and is one of the few examples of a germline polymorphism that is associated with the genetic makeup of the tumor. Levels of both TS mRNA and protein are inversely related to clinical antitumor response with clinical resistance linked to over expression of TS (34). In vivo, the expression of TS appears to be controlled by a polymorphism that is characterized by tandem repeats in the TS promoter enhancer region (TSER) of the gene. Higher levels of TS expression and enzyme activity are observed with increasing copies of tandem repeats resulting in a lower response rate to 5-FU (35). One study revealed that the increased number of tandem repeats in patients with metastatic colorectal tumors receiving 5-FU-based chemotherapy not only correlated to response (two tandem repeats were nearly twice as common in responders than in nonresponders), but also to median survival (16 months for patients with two tandem repeats and 12 months for patients with three tandem repeats) (36).

Polymorphisms of TS that result in 5-FU variability of its pharmacodynamic and pharmacokinetic properties illustrate the important fact that cancer, being a polygenic disease, will need a polygenic solution to guide therapy. In order to accurately select patients who are most likely to tolerate and respond to 5-FU therapy, one needs to use combined genotyping of DPYD and TSER functional variants as well as take into account the nongenetic factors.

CONCLUSION

Adverse drug reactions impose a huge burden not only on the patient but also on the health-care system. With the narrow therapeutic index of most agents used to treat cancer and the marked heterogeneity observed across cancer patient populations, adverse drug reactions are a reality that must be dealt with. A better understanding of the clinical and genetic factors that influence the pharmacokinetic profile of a chemotherapeutic agent is needed to optimize drug-dosing regimens to obtain maximal efficacy with minimal toxicity. Moreover, promising advancements in the field of pharmacogenetics will enable the development of effective agents that will make their way to the clinic in a timely manner. With the remarkable rate of progress seen in the field of cancer therapeutics, the application of "personalized cancer chemotherapy" to routine clinical practice will be a reality in the not too distant future.

REFERENCES

1. Bordet R, Gautier S, Le Louet H, et al. Analysis of the direct cost of adverse drug reactions in hospitalized patients. Eur J Clin Pharmacol 2001; 56:935–941.
2. Evans WE, Relling MV. Pharmacogenomics: translating functional genomics into rational therapeutics. Science 1999; 286:487–491.
3. Jeffrey S, Ross MD, David P, et al. Pharmacogenomics. Adv Anat Pathol 2004; 11: 211–220.
4. Lazarou J, Pomeranz BH, Corey PN. Incidence of adverse drug reactions in hospitalized patients—a meta-analysis of prospective studies. JAMA 1998; 279:1200–1205.
5. Johnson JA, Bootman JL. Drug-related morbidity and mortality. A cost-of-illness model. Arch Intern Med 1995; 155:1949–1956.
6. Egorin M, Echo DV, Olman E, et al. Prospective validation of a pharmacologically based dosing scheme for the cisdiamminedichloroplatinum (II) analogue diamminecylobutane dicarboxylato platinum. Cancer Res 1985; 45:6502.
7. Calvert A, Newell D, Gumbrell L, et al. Carboplatin dosage: prospective evaluation of a simple formula based on renal function. J Clin Oncol 1989; 7:1748.
8. Lichtman SM, Hollis D, Miller AA, et al. Prospective evaluation of the relationship of patient age and paclitaxel clinical pharmacology: Cancer and Leukemia Group B (CALGB 9762). J Clin Oncol 2006; 24:1846–1851.
9. Sachidanadam R, Weissman D, Schmidt SC, et al. A map of human genome sequence variation containing 1.42 million single nucleotide polymorphisms. Nature 2001; 409:928–933.
10. Evans DA, Manley KA, McKusch VA, et al. Genetic control of isoniazid metabolism in man. Br Med J 1960; 2:485–491.
11. Knight RA, Selin MJ, Harris HW, et al. Genetic factors influencing isoniazid blood levels in humans. Trans Conf Chemother Tuberc 1959; 8:52–56.
12. Evans DA. Survey of human acetylator polymorphism in spontaneous disorders. J Med Genet 1984; 21:243–253.
13. Ratain MJ, Mick R, Berezin F, et al. Paradoxical relationship between acetylator phenotype and amonafide toxicity. Clin Pharmacol Ther 1991; 50:573–579.
14. Pui C-H, Evans WE. Acute lymphoblastic leukemia. New Engl J Med 1998; 339: 605–615.
15. Krynetski EY, Tai HL, Yates CR, et al. Genetic polymorphisms of thiopurine S-methyltransferase: clinical importance and molecular mechanisms. Pharmacogenetics 1996; 6:279–290.
16. McLeod HL, Coulthard S, Thomas AE, et al. Analysis of thiopurine methyltransferase variant alleles in childhood acute lymphoblastic leukemia. Br J Hematol 1999; 105:696–700.
17. Pui C-H, Relling MV, Cheng Cheng, et al. Thiopurine methyltransferase in acute lymphoblastic leukemia. Blood 2006; 107:843–844.
18. Molloy AM, Daly S, Mills JL, et al. Thermolabile variant of 5,10-methylenetetrahydrofolate reductase associated with low red-cell folates: implications for folate intake recommendations. Lancet 1997; 349:1591–1593.
19. Franco RF, Simoes BP, Tone LG, et al. The methylenetetrahydrofolate reductase C677T gene polymorphism decreases the risk of childhood acute lymphocytic leukemia. Br J Haematol 2001; 115:616–618.
20. Effects of chemotherapy and hormonal therapy for early breast cancer on recurrence and 15-year survival: an overview of the randomized trials. Lancet 2005; 365: 1687–1717.
21. Lonning PE, Lien EA, Lundgren S, et al. Clinical pharmacokinetics of endocrine agents used in advanced breast cancer. Clin Pharmacokinet 1992; 22:327–358.
22. Stearns V, Johnson MD, Rae JM, et al. Active tamoxifen metabolite plasma concentrations after co administration of tamoxifen and the selective serotonin reuptake inhibitor paroxetine. J Natl Cancer Inst 2003; 95:1758–1764.
23. Osborne CK. Tamoxifen in the treatment of breast cancer. N Engl J Med 1998; 339: 1609–1618.

24. Desta Z, Ward BA, Soukhova NV, et al. Comprehensive evaluation of tamoxifen sequential biotransformation by the human cytochrome P450 system in vitro: prominent roles for CYP3A and CYP2D J Pharmacol Exp Ther 2004; 310:1062–1075.

25. Jin Y, Desta Z, Stearns V, et al. CYP2D6 genotype, antidepressant use, and tamoxifen metabolism during adjuvant breast cancer treatment. J Natl Cancer Inst 2005; 97:30–39.

26. Goetz MP, Rae JM, Suman VJ, et al. Pharmacogenetics of tamoxifen biotransformation is associated with clinical outcomes of efficacy and hot flashes. J Clin Oncol 2005; 23:9312–9318.

27. Iyer L, King CD, Whitington PF, et al. Genetic predisposition to the metabolism of irinotecan (CPT-11). Role of uridine diphosphate glucuronosyltransferase isoform 1A1 in the glucuronidation of its active metabolite (SN-38) in human liver microsomes. J Clin Invest 1998; 101:847–854.

28. Heidelberger C, Chaudhuri NK, Danneberg P, et al. Fluorinated pyrimidines, a new class of tumor-inhibitory compounds. Nature 1957; 179:663–666.

29. Etienne MC, Lagrange JL, Dassonville O, et al. Population study of dihydropyrimidine dehydrogenase in cancer patients. J Clin Oncol 1994; 12:2248–2253.

30. McLeod HL, Collie-Duguid ES, Vreken P, et al. Nomenclature for human DPYD alleles. Pharmacogenetics 1998; 8:455–459.

31. Lu A, Zhang R, Diasio RB. Dihydropyrimadine dehydrogenase activity in human peripheral blood mononuclear cells and liver: population characteristics, newly identified deficient patients, and clinical implication in 5-fluorouracil chemotherapy. Cancer Res 1993; 53:5433–5438.

32. Raida M, Schwabe W, Hausler P, et al. Prevalence of a common point mutation in the dihydropyrimidine dehydrogenase (DPD) gene within the 5′-splice donor site of intron 14 in patients with severe 5-fluorouracil (5-FU)-related toxicity compared with controls. Clin Cancer Res 2001; 7:2832–2839.

33. Grem JL. 5-Fluorouracil: forty-plus and still ticking. A review of its preclinical and clinical development. Invest New Drugs 200; 18:299–313.

34. Leichman CG, Lenz HJ, Leichman L, et al. Quantitation of intratumoral thymidylate synthase expression predicts for disseminated colorectal cancer response and resistance to protracted-infusion fluorouracil and weekly leucovorin. J Clin Oncol 1997; 15: 3223–3229.

35. Horie N, Aiba H, Oguro K, et al. Functional analysis and DNA polymorphism of the tandemly repeated sequences in the 5′-terminal regulatory region of the human gene for thymidylate synthase. Cell Struct Funct 1995; 20:191–197.

36. Marsh S, Mckay JA, Cassidy J, Mcleod HL. Polymorphism in the thymidylate synthase promoter enhancer region in colorectal cancer. Int J Oncol 2001; 19:383–386.

37. Flochart DA. Pharmacogenomics in the endocrine treatment of breast cancer. San Antonio Breast Cancer Symposium, MINI Symposium 4; 2005.

6 Aging, Cancer, and Translational Research

Lodovico Balducci

Senior Adult Oncology Program, H. Lee Moffitt Cancer Center and Research Institute, Tampa, Florida, U.S.A.

INTRODUCTION

Cancer in the older aged person is becoming increasingly common. Currently, individuals aged 65 and over account for 12% of the whole U.S. population and for 50% of all neoplasms; by the year 2030, they are expected to account for 20% of the population and 70% of the cancers (Fig. 1) (1). Furthermore, cancer is the number one cause of death for Americans up to age 85 (2). Clearly, only a decline of cancer-related mortality in older individuals would represent effective cancer control.

The advent of safer forms of cancer treatment and of antidotes to chemotherapy-related toxicity, especially of myelopoietic growth factors, has reduced the treatment-related morbidity and mortality and might have improved the survival of elderly patients affected by common malignancies, such as non-Hodgkin's lymphoma (NHL), cancer of the breast, of the large bowel, and of the prostate (3–6). Despite these advancements, a number of problems remain unsolved:

1. lack of effective and safe forms of cancer chemoprevention
2. reduced tolerance of the complications of cancer treatment by many older patients
3. difficulty in estimating benefits and risks of cancer treatment in individual situations, based on life expectancy and treatment tolerance

New insights in the biology of cancer and aging allow us to address these issues with translational research. This chapter explores the role of translational research in the management of cancer of the older aged person, after an overview of biological and clinical interactions of aging and cancer.

BIOLOGY OF AGING
Toward a Biological Definition of Aging

Aging may be defined as a progressive loss of entropy and fractality (7). In clinical terms, the loss of entropy indicates a progressive decline in a person's functional reserve of different organs and systems; loss of fractality implies increasing difficulty in negotiating the living environment, due mainly to inadequate coordination of different functions. The increasing frequency of falls in the older aged person, despite the absence of focal neurological deficits and muscular weakness, may be considered an example of loss of fractality. A number of biological, physiological, medical, and functional changes underlie the loss of entropy and fractality.

Cellular and Molecular Changes of Aging
Cellular aging may be associated with changes typical of early stage carcinogenesis and include epigenetic changes, such as DNA hypermethylation, formation of

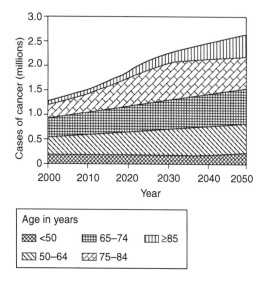

FIGURE 1   Current and projected cases of cancer in the elderly.

DNA adducts, point mutation, and chromosomal translocation (8). Other changes may prevent carcinogenesis and include progressive shortening of telomeres and reduced cell proliferation and cell survival (9). The origin of these changes is not clear and may include exposure to environmental carcinogens, micro-environmental changes, including chronic inflammation (10), and emergence of apoptosis-resistant genotypes with more prolonged cellular survival as normal genotypes, which are more common then progressively wane as an effect of apoptosis (11). In experimental animals, where they were mostly studied, these changes are, to some extent, tissue-specific and are particularly common in the skin and lymphatic system (8).

Of special interest is the proliferative senescence of fibroblasts "in vitro" (12). At the same time they lose their self-replicative ability, these cells seem to lose the ability to undergo apoptosis, and they start producing a number of tumor growth factors and lytic enzymes (metalloproteinase) that may promote the growth and spread of cancer.

Systemic Changes of Aging
These include chronic inflammation, immune senescence, endocrine senescence, and possibly increased levels of circulating growth factors and metalloproteinases from senescent stromal fibroblasts.

The role of chronic inflammation in aging is well established, and according to some investigators, aging is a chronic and progressive inflammation (10). Interleukin 6 (IL6) has been the most studied of inflammatory markers. Circulating levels of IL6 are elevated in the presence of several geriatric syndromes, including dementia, osteoporosis, failure to thrive, unexplained anemia, sarcopenia, and functional disability (13,14). Other inflammatory cytokines were found elevated in the circulation of individuals affected by different forms of cognitive disorders (15). In home-dwelling individuals aged 70 and over, increased circulating levels of IL6 and of D-dimer heralded the increased risk of death and of functional dependence (14). It has recently been shown that chronic inflammation may favor the development of precancerous genomic abnormalities; so, it is not far-fetched to assume that chronic inflammation may underlie some of the genomic changes of aging (16). The cancer preventative effects of COX 1 and 2 inhibitors may be explained, in part, by the antiflogistic effect of these substances.

Reduced production of sexual hormones by the gonads is the most obvious manifestation of endocrine senescence and may affect development and growth of hormone-dependent tumors, such as prostatic, mammary, and endometrial cancer. It is important to remember that the activity of sexual hormones is also influenced by body size and shape. With aging, abdominal deposition of fat becomes more common and is associated with increased aromatization of androgens and circulating levels of estrogens (17). In addition, abdominal obesity is associated with decreased concentrations of sexual hormone–binding proteins in the circulation (17). For this reason, obesity may favor the development of breast cancer in postmenopausal women and favor its recurrence after surgery. Obesity may also be associated with increased insulin resistance, increased circulating levels of insulin and, consequently, of growth hormone and of insulin-like growth factor 1 (IGF-1), that is, a powerful growth stimulator of several tumors (18). The circulating levels of corticosteroids appear increased in the older person, probably as a result of chronic inflammation (19).

Immune senescence involves an accumulation of so-called "memory" cells and a decline of T-cell mediated immunity and possibly of antigen presenting cells activity (20). The effects of immune senescence on tumor growth appear variable. In the experimental system, immune senescence appears to be associated with accelerated growth of highly immunogenic tumors, such as radiation-induced sarcoma, but with decreased growth of poorly immunogenic tumors, such as Lewis lung carcinoma (LLC) or B16 melanoma (21).

Physiological Changes of Aging
The physiological changes of aging include a reduced functional reserve of multiple organs and systems and, consequently, increased susceptibility to different forms of stress. These may comprise cancer treatment with surgery, radiation therapy, or cytotoxic chemotherapy. Of special interest is the decline in function of organs that are involved in drug metabolism and excretion or that are targets of drug toxicity. For example, the glomerular filtration rate is almost universally reduced with age, which indicates adjustments of the doses of medications excreted through the kidneys (22). Likewise, hepatic uptake and metabolism of drugs become altered with age, but the pharmacokinetics implications in cancer treatment are not well appreciated.

The organs and systems that are more vulnerable to the toxicity of chemotherapy with aging include the hemopoietic system, the mucosas, the heart, and the peripheral and central nervous systems (22).

The Concept of Frailty
The term frailty is commonly associated with the idea of aging. It is important to note that no agreement exists on the definition of frailty and that this term has been used to indicate two very different situations. One situation involves a critical reduction of functional reserve that does not impair the independence of the person, but makes the person more susceptible to the consequence of stress (23). This is the term that is gaining more general acceptance and may be utilized in

the future in oncology to designate individuals for whom special care is indicated to minimize the complications of treatment. The other situation is one where the functional reserve is so critically reduced that it is barely sufficient to keep the person alive (24). In this case, symptom management is the only reasonable form of treatment, as the patient would not be able to tolerate even minimal stress. This disagreement on the meaning of frailty reflects some general agreement on how aging should be construed and approached clinically: aging represents a progressive loss of functional reserve; loss of functional reserve may lead to loss of independence, that is, an older person may become unable to live without social support.

Some important landmarks may be recognized on the trajectory of aging that may influence medical as well as social intervention. These include a situation

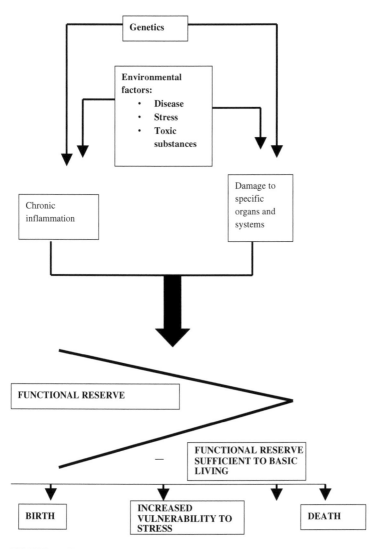

FIGURE 2 Trajectory of aging.

of increased vulnerability to environmental stress, including aggressive medical treatment, and a condition in which the functional reserve is almost exhausted and in which preservation of comfort is the only realistic goal. The recognition of these landmarks and the definition of situations in between are one of the most important challenges in the management of older individuals. Current methods of evaluation include medical, functional, and performance evaluation and, more recently, some laboratory tests including the determination of circulating levels of inflammatory cytokines (25). Figure 2 summarizes the concepts described in this section.

BIOLOGICAL INTERACTIONS OF AGING AND CANCER

To define the potential roles of translational research in geriatric oncology, it is useful to identify the biological interactions of cancer and aging, which occur at the level of carcinogenesis, cancer growth, and cancer treatment.

Aging and Carcinogenesis

The increased incidence of cancer with age may be explained by the three, non-mutually exclusive mechanisms (1):

1. Duration of carcinogenesis: As carcinogenesis is lengthy and may extend over decades, it is reasonable to expect that cancer becomes more common with aging.
2. Increased susceptibility of aging tissues to environmental carcinogens due to the similarity of molecular changes of aging and carcinogenesis.
3. Changes in bodily environment that may favor the growth of cancer, including immune senescence and proliferative senescence of fibroblasts.

Aging and Tumor Growth

Tumor growth may be altered by two nonmutually exclusive mechanisms. Thinking of cancer as a tree, the growth of the tree may be influenced by the nature of the "seed," or the tumor cell, and of the "soil," or the tumor host. In rodents, the influence of the tumor host has been clearly established: when the same tumor load of B16 melanoma and LLC was injected in older and younger animals, the younger animals died earlier and with increased number of lung metastases (21).

In humans, the biology of cancer appears to change with age in at least some tumors (Table 1), and both seed and soil mechanisms appear to be involved (25).

Aging and Cancer Control

Any decision related to cancer prevention and treatment in older individuals is predicated upon the following questions.

1. Is the patient going to die of cancer or with cancer?
2. Is the cancer going to affect the patient's welfare during the patient's lifetime?
3. Is the patient able to tolerate the treatment?

The answer to these questions implies the estimate of the patient's life expectancy and functional reserve, of the aggressiveness of the tumor, and of the availability of effective treatment.

Currently, the estimate of life expectancy and functional reserve is based mainly on clinical data, provided by some forms of geriatric assessment, evaluation

TABLE 1 Human Cancers Whose Clinical Behavior May Change with Age

Tumor	Change in prognosis	Change in tumor behavior	Mechanism
Acute myeloid leukemia	Worse	Decreased responsiveness to chemotherapy	Seed: Increased prevalence of multidrug resistance Increased prevalence of unfavorable cytogenetics changes Increased prevalence of multilineage leukemia
NHL	Worse	Increased risk of recurrence after remission	Soil: Increased concentration of Il6 in the circulation?
Breast cancer	Better	More indolent course	Seed: Increased prevalence of well differentiated, hormone-receptor rich cancers Soil: Endocrine senescence and possibly immune senescence
Celomic cancer of the ovary	Worse	Decreased responsiveness to chemotherapy Decreased disease-free survival	Unknown
Nonsmall cell cancer of the lung	Better?	More indolent course?	Seed: More common cancer in ex-smokers?

Abbreviation: NHL, non-Hodgkin's lymphoma.

of laboratory parameters, or proof of physical functions (Table 2) (26–28). These forms of assessment have been extremely helpful in several areas including:

1. Recognition of individuals who are unable to tolerate even minimal stress due to exhausted functional reserve

TABLE 2 Examples of Instruments Currently Used to Estimate an Older Person's Life Expectancy and Functional Reserve

Clinical geriatric assessment	Laboratory tests	Proofs of physical function
CGA Function Comorbidity Nutrition Polypharmacy Mental status Social support Abbreviated forms of geriatric assessment Vulnerable elderly survey (VES-13) CHS San Francisco VA assessment	Il-6 D-dimer C-reactive protein Hemoglobin	Timed "get-up and go" test Strength of upper and lower extremities

Abbreviations: CGA, comprehensive geriatric assessment; CHS, cardiovascular health study.

2. Recognition of individuals whose function and life expectancy may be improved by treatment of underlying diseases, social support, management of nutrition, and polypharmacy and physical rehabilitation
3. Estimate of short- and long-term mortalities
4. Risk of short- and long-term disabilities

The main limitations of these forms of assessment include labor intensity, in the case of the comprehensive geriatric assessment (CGA), redundancy, and, most importantly, inability to provide more precise information as to the risk of death, disability, and treatment complications of each individual.

For what concerns tumor aggressiveness, it is assumed that current prognostic factors, such as histologic differentiation, s-phase, proteomics, and genomics, have the same value in all patients irrespective of age. The role of the tumor host (the soil) in modulating tumor growth is unestablished, however.

TRANSLATIONAL RESEARCH AND CANCER MANAGEMENT IN THE OLDER PERSON

Translational research has improved enormously the management of cancer in older individuals already, as shown in the following examples:

1. Development of antidotes to the toxicity of cytotoxic chemotherapy. Filgrastim and pegfilgrastim have reduced by more than 50% the incidence of neutropenic infections in older individuals receiving cytotoxic chemotherapy and have allowed a large portion of these patients to receive treatment at full doses (22). At the same time, erythropoietic growth factors have contributed to the preservation of quality of life and functional independence of older cancer patients (22).
2. Development of so-called "targeted" therapy. By targeting a specific neoplastic process, new drugs promise to improve the outcome of treatment and reduce the risk of damage to normal tissues in all patients. As they are at increased risk of therapeutic complications, older individuals may benefit most by targeted therapy.
3. Development of prognostic indices based on genomic and proteomic tumor profile (29). These indices promise to identify individuals more likely to benefit from cytotoxic chemotherapy and limit the use and complications of these forms of treatment.

In addition to these noticeable achievements, translational research promises to benefit the management of cancer of older individuals in several areas, shown in Table 3. The importance of some of these areas, such as the recognition of early markers of carcinogenesis, development of targeted chemoprevention, and new forms of cancer treatment, is self-evident and does not need further explanation. Also, progress in these areas would be beneficial to individuals of all ages. We try to highlight here the areas that are of particular interest to the aged.

Aging and Apoptosis

Resistance to apoptosis is the hallmark of some malignancies such as the follicular lymphomas, whose incidence increases with age (30). It is also known that some cells aging in vitro such as senescent fibroblast develop resistance to apoptosis and, at the same time, that they lose the ability to replicate themselves (12). The

TABLE 3 Promising Areas for Translational Research in Older Cancer Patients

Cancer prevention	Recognition of molecular markers of early carcinogenesis, able to predict cancer risk
	Recognition of the role of the older bodily environment in carcinogenesis, targeted chemoprevention of cancer
Cancer treatment	Development of new and more specific forms of targeted therapy
	Development of new and more effective antidotes to the toxicity of cancer treatment
	Definition of the influence of the tumor host on cancer growth
Patient assessment	Development of laboratory and imaging tests capable to identify life expectancy and functional reserve of individual patients

interaction of aging and apoptosis is poorly understood and may represent a clue to the association of aging and cancer, as well as a potential target for chemoprevention. Two possibilities are particularly fascinating:

1. As it is the case with aging fibroblasts, parenchymal cells may also develop resistance to apoptosis and, at the same time, develop proliferative senescence.
2. Since birth, clones of cells are present which are resistant to apoptosis, whose population becomes more prevalent with age.

Influence of Changes in Bodily Environment on Carcinogenesis

The evidence is accumulating that age is a chronic and progressive inflammation, and the levels of some inflammatory markers, including IL-6, D-dimer, and C-reactive proteins, correlate with life expectancy, risk of disability, sarcopenia, and risk of common geriatric syndromes (10,14,28). The basic question of aging biology is whether chronic inflammation is just a marker of aging or instead is responsible for the manifestations of aging. In other words, is it possible that reversal of chronic inflammation may delay the manifestations of aging, including carcinogenesis? From the cancer standpoint, is it important to ask whether

1. chronic inflammation causes epigenetic changes characteristic both of aging and carcinogenesis;
2. chronic inflammation favors tumor growth and metastases. This effect could, in part, be mediated by immune suppression caused by chronic inflammation; or
3. chronic inflammation is a viable target for chemoprevention, as suggested by studies of COX inhibitors (31).

Other environmental changes that may favor carcinogenesis include immune and proliferative senescence.

Influence of the Aging Tumor Host on Tumor Growth

This area is poorly known and extremely important for understanding the prognosis of cancer in older individuals. It is not impossible that these effects may also become targets of prevention and treatment. Promising questions are as follows:

1. Is it demonstrable in humans, as it appears to be the case in experimental animals, that the growth of poorly immunogenic tumors is hampered and that of the highly immunogenic ones is enhanced with age? If this is the case, how can one identify highly and poorly immunogenic tumors? Can immune

competence be restored, at least to some extent, in older individuals? Is this a viable strategy of cancer prevention and cancer treatment?
2. Does the senescence of the tumor stroma favor tumor growth and metastases?
3. What is the relationship of insulin-resistance, metabolic syndromes, and tumor growth?

Prevention of Treatment-Related Toxicity in Older Individuals

The most urgent areas of translational research include the development of reliable indices of toxicity and the development of antidotes to mucositis, cardiotoxicity, and neurotoxicity of cytotoxic agents (21). Questions of larger scope include:

- Exhaustibility of organs and systems that are the major target of the toxicity of chemotherapy, especially the hemopoietic system and the mucosas. Is it possible that repeated destruction by cyclic chemotherapy of the hemopoietic system, combined with repeated growth stimulation by growth factor may lead to medullary or mucosal aplasia?
- Long-term effects of treatment. In particular, are older tissues more susceptible to the carcinogenicity of chemotherapy? Are the injuries to normal tissues less reversible in older individuals?

Assessment of the Older Person

As shown before, the most important clinical questions related to the prevention and the treatment of cancer in older individuals relate to individual life expectancy and risk of treatment-related toxicity. Current forms of assessment of the older person, listed in Table 2, are not fully satisfactory. Translational research would be extremely helpful by identifying a test or a combination of tests that are able to provide more precise estimates of life expectancy and functional reserve. These may include levels of circulating substances, such as inflammatory markers, genomic and proteomic changes in normal tissues, and imaging tests revealing these changes.

Translational Research: A Two-Way Street

The current view of translational research implies the translation of bench research into bedside practice (the so-called "bench to bedside" pathway). This incomplete view ignores the fact that, for over a century, research involved the translation of clinical findings into scientific hypotheses and bench experiments. The "bedside to the bench" pathway of translational research is still alive and well in geriatrics (32), because aging is multifactorial and can only be partially mimicked in experimental models. The interactions of different comorbidities, functional decline, polypharmacy, sensorial deprivation, and fading social support and economic resources give origin to unique clinical pictures that cannot be reproduced in a single model or even a series of models. The gist of research in geriatrics has been the recognition of common trends, such as loss of fractality and of entropy capable to quantify the individual degree of aging, or of clinical syndromes, such as frailty, reflecting landmarks in the aging trajectory. These clinical findings may feed experimental designs aimed to study the long-term consequences and reversibility of these conditions and to identify biological markers able to fine tune the diagnosis of aging in each individual.

CONCLUSIONS

Translational research has already influenced the management of cancer of older individuals, with the development of targeted therapy, of antidotes to chemotherapy-related toxicity, and of prognostic markers that allow us to individualize cancer treatment.

Promising areas of translational research involve clarifications of the mechanism associating aging and cancer and of the mechanism by which the aging tumor host may influence tumor growth, development of new antidotes to therapeutic toxicity, and more reliable estimates of individual life expectancy and functional reserve.

It is important to remember that in geriatric research, translational research is a two-way street that may go from the bedside to the bench as well as from the bench to the bedside.

REFERENCES

1. Balducci L, Ershler WB. Cancer and aging: a nexus at several levels. Nat Rev Cancer 2005; 5:655–661.
2. Jemal A, Murray T, Ward D, et al. Cancer Statistics 2005. CA: A Cancer J Physicians 2005; 50:10–30.
3. Carreca I, Balducci L, Extermann M. Cancer in the older person. Cancer Treat Rev 2005; 68:380–402.
4. Kuderer NM, Dale DC, Crawford J, et al. Mortality, morbidity, and cost associated with febrile neutropenia in adult cancer patients. Cancer 2006; 106(10):2258–2266.
5. Sargent DJ, Goldberg RM, Jacobson SD, et al. A pooled analysis of adjuvant chemotherapy for resected colon cancer in elderly patients. N Engl J Med 2001; 345(15): 1091–1097.
6. Early Breast Cancer Trialists Collaborative Group. Effects of chemotherapy and hormonal therapy for early breast cancer on recurrence and 15-year survival: an overview of the randomised trials. Lancet 2005; 365(9472):1687–1717.
7. Lipsitz LA. Physiological complexity, aging, and the path to frailty [Review]. Sci Aging Knowledge Environ 2004; 2004(16):pe16.
8. Anisimov VN. Biological interactions of aging and carcinogenesis. Cancer Treat Res 2005; 124:17–50.
9. Shin HS, Hong A, Salomon MJ, et al. The role of telomeres and telomerase in the pathology of human cancer and aging. Pathology 2006; 38(2):103–113.
10. Ferrucci L, Corsi A, Lauretani F, et al. The origins of age-related proinflammatory state. Blood 2005; 105(6):2294–2299.
11. Migliaccio E, Girgio M, Pelicci PG. Apoptosis and aging: role of p66(Shc) redox protein. Antioxid Redox Signal 2006; 8(3–4):600–608.
12. Campisi J. Senescent cells, tumor suppression, and organismal aging: good citizens, bad neighbors [Review]. Cell 2005; 120(4):513–522.
13. Kishimoto T. Interleukin-6: from basic science to medicine—40 years in immunology [Review]. Annu Rev Immunol 2005; 23:1–21.
14. Mcdermott MM, Ferrucci L, Liu K, et al. D-dimer and inflammatory markers as predictors of functional decline in men and women with and without peripheral arterial disease. J Am Geriatr Soc 2005; 53(10):1688–1696.
15. Wilson CJ, Cohen HJ, Pieper CF. Cross-linked fibrin degradation products (D-dimer), plasma cytokines, and cognitive decline in community-dwelling elderly persons. J Am Geriatr Soc 2003; 51(10):1374–1381.
16. Demierre MF, Higgins PD, Gruber SD. Statins and cancer prevention [Review]. Nat Rev Cancer 2005; 5(12):930–942.
17. Muller M, Grobbee DE, den Tonkelaar I, et al. Endogenous sex hormones and metabolic syndrome in aging men. J Clin Endocrinol Metab 2005; 90:2618–2623.

18. Hutley L, Prins JB. Fat as an endocrine organ: relationship to the metabolic syndrome. Am J Med Sci 2005; 330(6):280–289.
19. Heibronn LK, deJonge L, Frisard MI, et al. Effect of 6-month calorie restriction on biomarkers of longevity, metabolic adaptation, and oxidative stress in overweight individuals: a randomized controlled trial. JAMA 2006; 295(13):1539–1548.
20. Abedin S, Michel JJ, Lemster B, et al. Diversity of NKR expression in aging T cells and in T cells of the aged: the new frontier into the exploration of protective immunity in the elderly. Exp Gerontol 2005; 40(7):537–548.
21. Ershler WB. Influence of tumor host on the tumor growth in older patients. In: Balducci L, Lyman GH, Ershler WB, eds. Comprehensive Geriatric Oncology, 2nd ed. Taylor and Francis, 2004:238–242.
22. Balducci L, Cohen HJ, Engstrom PF, et al. Senior adult oncology clinical practice guidelines in oncology. J Natl Compr Canc Netw 2005; 3(4):572–590.
23. Bandeen Roche K, Xue QL, Ferrucci L, et al. Phenotype of frailty: characterization in the women's health and aging studies. J Gerontol A Biol Sci Med Sci 2006; 61(3):262–266.
24. Balducci L, Stanta G. Cancer in the frail patient. A coming epidemic. Hematol Oncol Clin North Am 2000; 14(1):235–250.
25. Balducci L. Management of cancer in the elderly. Oncology (Williston Park). 2006; 20(2):135–143; discussion 144, 146, 151–152.
26. Lee SJ, Lindquist K, Segal MR, et al. Development and validation of a prognostic index for 4-year mortality in older adults. JAMA 2006; 295(7):801–808.
27. Fried LP, Kronmal RA, Newman AB, et al. Risk factors for 5-year mortality in older adults: the Cardiovascular Health Study. JAMA 1998; 279(8):585–592.
28. Cohen HJ, Harris T, Pieper CF. Coagulation and activation of inflammatory pathways in the development of functional decline and mortality in the elderly. Am J Med 2003; 114:180–187.
29. Gruraraj AE, Rayala SK, Vadlamudi RK, et al. Novel mechanisms of resistance to endocrine therapy: genomic and nongenomic considerations. Clin Cancer Res 2006; 12(3 Pt 2):1001s–1007s.
30. Thomadaki H, Scorilas A, Hindmarsh JT. BCL2 family of apoptosis-related genes: functions and clinical implications in cancer. Crit Rev Clin Lab Sci 2006; 43(1):1–67.
31. Beghe C, Balducci L. Biological basis of cancer in the older person. Cancer Treat Res 2005; 124:189–221.
32. Fried LB, Headley EC, Walston JD, et al. From bedside to bench: research agenda for frailty. Sci Aging Knowledge Environ 2005; 2005(31):pe24.

The Prognostic Implications of Circulating Tumor Cells in Patients with Breast Cancer

Jeffrey B. Smerage and Daniel F. Hayes
*Department of Internal Medicine, University of Michigan,
Ann Arbor, Michigan, U.S.A.*

INTRODUCTION

Circulating tumor cells (CTCs) have been of interest to the medical and research communities for over a century (1). These cells represent an important link to the process of metastasis, and investigators have been interested in using these cells to establish the diagnosis and prognosis of cancer. In addition, these cells are a potential source of biological information that can be used to predict responsiveness to various treatment agents, monitor response to therapy, and provide tissue for further research into the mechanisms of malignant transformation and resistance. CTCs have been documented in multiple epithelial tumor types (2), but the largest body of data comes from studies of women with breast cancer.

Historically, CTC research has been limited by issues of sensitivity, specificity, and reproducibility. These limitations are primarily due to the rarity of CTCs, which occur at a frequency of one tumor cell per $1 \times 10^{5-7}$ peripheral blood mononuclear cells (3). In the 1950s and 1960s, there was great excitement surrounding the investigation of CTCs (4). However, the methodologies of the time relied almost exclusively on the microscopic properties of morphology and size as well as the physical property of density. It soon became apparent that these physical criteria alone were not sufficient for the identification of CTCs. Many of the cells identified during this era were believed to have been false positive cells that result from artifacts of sample preparation and from misclassification of immature leukocytes (5). Thus, morphological characteristics alone did not provide adequate specificity, and no further meaningful progress was made in the field of CTC research until the advent of antibody and nucleic acid technologies, which allowed the identification of biological characteristics of these cells.

METHODS OF CIRCULATING TUMOR CELL DETECTION

Research in the last 10 to 15 years has focused on the creation of methodologies with improved sensitivity and specificity. Physical techniques such as size filtration, density gradient centrifugation, and microscopic morphology continue to be used, but biological techniques such as immunomagnetic isolation, flow cytometry, immunofluorescent microscopy, reverse transcriptase–polymerase chain reaction (RT–PCR), polymerase chain reaction (PCR), and fluorescence in site hybridization (FISH) have been added to provide the required specificity. In many cases, the biological techniques have completely replaced the physical techniques in order to increase sensitivity. For example, the preparation of mononuclear cells utilizing Ficoll gradient centrifugation results in a substantial loss of CTCs. When cultured tumor cells are spiked into whole blood and then processed by density gradient centrifugation, the recovery of spiked tumor cells is only 10% to 65% (6,7). This is compared with immunomagnetic separation, which has a recovery rate of 85% (2,8).

Antibody-based techniques such as immunohistochemistry, immunofluorescent microscopy, and flow cytometry have resulted in significant progress in CTC research. They also have limitations, and these limitations must be recognized when evaluating CTC technologies. Antibodies used to identify breast cancer CTCs include epithelial and breast cancer markers such as EpCAM (6), cytokeratin (9), MUC-1 (10), and TAG-12 (11). These antibodies are also known to stain hematopoeitic cells. Some of these false-positives are due to concentration-dependent non-specific binding, and can be minimized by reducing antibody concentrations (11). Non-specific immunohistochemical staining of plasma cells can also occur due to alkaline phosphatase reaction against the normal kappa and lambda light chains expressed on the surface of the plasma cells (12). Reported false positive rates with antibody-based techniques range from 22% to 61%, and vary based upon the antibody and staining methodologies used. Many of these issues have been minimized by optimization of antibody concentration, selection of more specific monoclonal antibodies, and the use of directly labeled fluorescent monoclonal antibodies. In addition, most assays now utilize a leukocyte marker such as anti-CD45 to exclude non-specifically stained leukocytes from analysis.

The presence of CTCs can also be indirectly inferred using nucleic acid techniques such as RT–PCR and PCR. As with the antibody techniques, RT–PCR has been utilized to detect expression from multiple epithelial and breast cancer-associated genes, including cytokeratins, EGFR, mammoglobin, MUC-1, beta-HCG, c-Met, GalNac-T, Mage-3, and others (13). RT–PCR is generally reported to have higher sensitivity than antibody techniques, but this increased sensitivity comes at the cost of higher false positive rates, as documented in samples taken from normal volunteers and from patients with hematological malignancies (13). These false positives have been attributed to issues of laboratory technique, primer selection, and illegitimate expression of the genes in white blood cells. In addition, induction of the expression of breast cancer marker genes such as cytokeratin-19 and CEA can be seen in leukocytes stimulated by cytokines and growth factors (14,15). PCR can be used to detect free DNA within the plasma. However, DNA has a much longer plasma half-life than mRNA, and as a result it is not possible to determine whether the DNA is coming from CTCs or if it is simply being shed as free DNA from primary tumors, metastatic tumors, or normal tissue (13). To help distinguish DNA from tumor versus normal tissue, investigators are beginning to use methylation-specific PCR primers (16). However, this still does not allow categorization of the DNA as being from CTCs or tissue. RT–PCR and PCR still have many challenges to overcome, but they both hold promise in the analysis of CTCs.

Multiple methods have been published for the isolation and characterization of CTCs (8,9,17–28). However, these reports focus primarily on the comparison between the number of CTCs and stage of disease. These reports vary widely in methodology, definition of assay positivity, and patient populations studied. There is also significant variation in the amount and type of data presented. Thus, the ability to make direct comparisons between these studies is limited. The major finding of these studies is that the number of cells per sample and the percentage of patients with positive samples increase with increasing stage of disease.

The sensitivity in early stage breast cancer remains low (29), which currently limits the clinical use of CTCs to the metastatic setting.

Only one assay, CellSearch™ (Immunicon Corp., Huntington Valley, Pennsylvania, U.S.A.) has been cleared by the FDA for use in the clinic, and it is this assay that provides the majority of the clinical outcomes data related to the prognostic value of CTC. This assay utilizes a combination of morphological and multiple biological characteristics to identify CTCs with good sensitivity and high specificity. In addition, the system is highly automated, resulting in decreased inter-sample variability, and increased reproducibility (2). The cells are first isolated by immunomagnetic separation utilizing an iron-bound antibody against EpCAM. The sample is then fluorescently stained with the nucleic acid stain DAPI and with monoclonal antibodies directed against pan-cytokeratin and against CD-45. The sample is then visualized using a semi-automated fluorescent microscope. CTCs in this system are defined as EpCAM positive, cytokeratin positive, DAPI positive, CD-45 negative, and they must have cellular morphology including a nucleus, and a cytoplasmic diameter of at least 4 μm. This system has been shown to be highly reproducible (2). Blood samples spiked with cultured human breast cancer cells demonstrated >85% recovery, with linear recovery over a range of 55 to 1142 cells per sample ($R^2 = 0.99$). In addition, agreement between independent operators was high ($R^2 = 0.994$) as well as between duplicate samples ($R^2 = 0.975$).

PROGNOSTIC VALUE OF CIRCULATING TUMOR CELLS IN METASTATIC BREAST CANCER

Only three studies have correlated the presence of immunopurified CTCs with clinical outcome. The first by Gaforio et al. (30) evaluated a heterogeneous population of patients spanning the clinical contexts of neoadjuvant therapy, adjuvant therapy, and metastatic disease. Utilizing Kaplan–Meier analysis for progression-free survival (PFS) and overall survival (OS), they found that patients with elevated CTCs prior to therapy had worse PFS ($P = 0.058$) and OS ($P = 0.003$). However, they did not stratify for disease stage, and at the time of publication neither of the medians for PFS or OS had been reached, making interpretation of the data difficult. The second study by Bauernhofer et al. (27) evaluated CTCs in 32 patients with metastatic breast cancer. They found that patients with detectable CTCs had a significantly shorter median OS of four months, compared with 13 months for patients without CTCs ($P < 0.001$). These authors did not specify the timing of the blood draws, and they did not compare CTCs to other prognostic factors such as line of therapy, hormone receptor status, sites of disease, or performance status. Thus, it is also difficult to fully interpret the results from this second trial.

A third trial reported by Cristofanilli et al. (25,31) utilized the CellSearch methodology and demonstrated that CTCs are highly prognostic in the setting of metastatic breast cancer. In a prospective, double-blind, multi-centre trial, 177 patients with metastatic breast cancer who were beginning a new therapy were evaluated. Patients could be initiating any line of hormonal therapy or chemotherapy, and CTCs were drawn at baseline, first follow-up, and at each subsequent visit until clinical progression. Using a training set of 102 patient samples, a level of ≥5 CTC per 7.5 mL of whole blood was identified as the threshold that best distinguished PFS between the two groups. This threshold and its prognostic value were then confirmed in an independent, prospectively collected set of 75 patient samples. Elevated CTCs at baseline predicted extremely

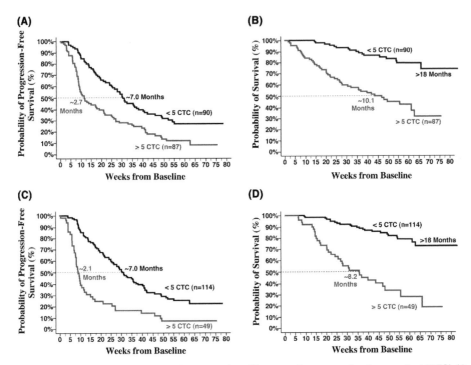

FIGURE 1 Kaplan–Meier curves demonstrating differences in progression-free survival (PFS) (**A** and **C**) and overall survival (OS) (**B** and **D**) based upon high- and low-risk circulating tumor cell (CTC) classifications. Patients with elevated CTCs at baseline (**A** and **B**) and at first follow-up after one cycle of therapy (**C** and **D**) have significantly worse median PFS and OS compared with the corresponding patients with low CTCs. *Source*: Adapted from Ref. 25.

short median PFS and OS of 3 and 10 months, respectively. This is in comparison with patients with low/negative CTCs in whom PFS and OS were 7 and 22 months, respectively (Fig. 1). Thus, elevated CTCs at baseline identify a group of high-risk patients. Even more interesting, CTC values obtained after one cycle of therapy predicted which patients were likely on ineffective therapy. Patients with elevated CTCs after one cycle of therapy had median PFS and OS of approximately 2.1 and 8.2 months, respectively, when measured from baseline (Fig. 1). In contrast, patients with low CTCs had median PFS and OS of 7.0 and 22 months, respectively. These differences in PFS and OS were all highly statistically significant ($P < 0.001$) for patients receiving chemotherapy. For patients initiating hormonal therapy, baseline CTCs were not prognostic, but CTCs evaluated at first follow-up after initiating hormonal therapy did result in substantial differences in median PFS (2.3 vs. 8.3 months, $P = 0.15$) and median OS (10.9 vs. >18 months, $P = 0.002$). Although the PFS comparison was not statistically significant, it suggests that CTCs may be able to distinguish patients who are on ineffective hormonal therapy. The subset of patients starting hormonal therapy was smaller ($n = 53$) than the group starting chemotherapy ($n = 109$). So, the analysis in hormonal therapy patients was likely underpowered and requires further investigation. Because of the lack of strong statistical significance in the hormonal therapy group, the FDA cleared indication for the CTC assay is currently limited to women undergoing chemotherapy for metastatic breast cancer.

Further analysis of this data suggests that the prognostic value is independent of the line of chemotherapy. The original publication (25) presented combined data for all patients receiving any line of therapy. Approximately half of these patients were receiving first-line therapy, and a subsequent publication demonstrated that the prognostic information was the same in patients receiving first-line therapy (Table 1) (31,32). In this report, 59 patients were initiating first-line chemotherapy. Using the cut-off of ≥ 5 CTCs, patients with elevated CTCs at baseline had significantly worse PFS (2.3 vs. 7.2 months, $P = 0.046$) and worse median OS (14.2 vs. >18 months, $P = 0.024$). Of these, 44 patients had CTC data from the first follow-up visit (three to four weeks) after initiating chemotherapy. The first follow-up CTC results were highly prognostic of PFS (2.0 vs. 8.2 months, $P = 0.008$) and OS (9.2 vs. >18 months, $P = 0.0006$), suggesting that patients who have elevated CTCs after one cycle of first line chemotherapy are on ineffective therapy.

It is particularly difficult to determine progression in women with non-measurable forms of metastatic breast cancer, such as bone-only disease. Preliminary data suggest that CTCs may also provide prognostic information in this population (33) (Table 1). To evaluate this population, 46 patients with non-measurable metastatic breast cancer underwent CTC evaluation at baseline and at first follow-up after initiating a new therapy. Patients with elevated CTCs ≥ 5 CTC) at baseline had trends toward worse median PFS at 4.4 versus 9.5 months, although this did not reach statistical significance ($P = 0.44$). Analysis of CTCs at first follow-up demonstrated an even wider difference in median PFS (3.5 vs. 14.4 months, $P = 0.032$), which was statistically significant. Median OS had not been reached for either group at the time of presentation. Again, this suggests that patients with non-measurable disease who have elevated CTCs at first follow-up are likely on ineffective therapy.

TABLE 1 Patients with Elevated Circulating Tumor Cells Have Significantly Worse Outcomes as Measured by Progression-Free Survival and Overall Survival

		Median PFS			Median OS		
		CTC count			CTC count		
	n	≥ 5	<5	*P*	≥ 5	<5	*P*
CTCs at baseline							
All patients (25,31)	177	2.7	7.0	<0.001	10.9	21.9	<0.001
Chemotherapy	54	2.3	6.8	<0.001	8.3	>18	<0.001
Hormonal therapy	118	8.1	8.3	0.44	>18	>18	0.09
First line therapy (32)	83	11.3	>18	<0.001	>18	>18	<0.001
Chemotherapy	23	2.3	7.2	0.0464	14.3	>18	0.235
Hormonal therapy	59	11.3	>18	0.148	>18	>18	0.576
Non-measurable disease (33)	46	4.4	9.5	0.44	19	>20	0.25
CTCs at first follow-up							
All patients (25)	163	2.1	7	<0.001	8.2	22	<0.0001
Chemotherapy	53	2.3	6.8	0.002	8.3	>18	<0.001
Hormonal therapy	109	2.3	8.3	0.15	10.9	>18	0.002
First line therapy (32)	60	2.1	9.5	0.006	11.1	>18	0.001
Chemotherapy	15	2.0	8.2	0.008	9.2	>18	0.001
Hormonal therapy	44	11.3	>18	0.289	>18	>18	0.670
Non-measurable disease (33)	40	3.5	14.4	0.032	NR	NR	NR

Abbreviations: CTC, circulating tumor cell; NR, not reported; PFS, progression-free survival; OS, overall survival.

FUTURE DIRECTIONS

As a result of the strong prognostic implications of elevated CTCs at first follow-up, a clinical trial has been developed in the Southwest Oncology Group (SWOG S0500) to test whether women with metastatic breast cancer and who have elevated CTCs after one cycle of first line chemotherapy have improved outcomes as a result of switching early to an alternate therapy. Current standard of care would be to continue until evidence of clinical progression. By switching prior to clinical progression, it is hypothesized that these patients will have improved outcomes by minimizing the time and toxicity spent on ineffective therapies and by spending more time on effective therapy.

In addition to enumeration, many investigators are developing methods to detect and monitor biologically important markers in CTCs. Genetic changes can be detected in CTCs, including abnormal telomerase activity (34), allelic loss, and/or amplification of multiple oncogenes not seen in normal control populations (35), and aneuploid changes in cellular chromosome content based upon FISH analysis similar to those seen in the primary tumor (36). In addition, cancer-associated protein expression by CTCs can be detected, such as HER2 (Fig. 2) (37).

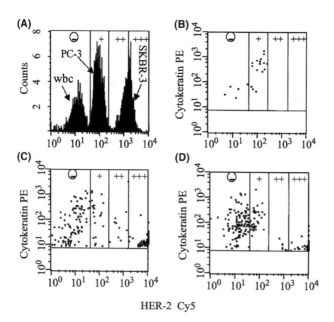

HER-2 Cy5

FIGURE 2 Quantification of HER2 density on cell lines and on CTCs of three breast cancer patients by flow cytometry. (**A**) HER2 expression of leukocytes, PC3 cells, and SKBR-3 cells immunomagnetically selected from 5 mL of blood and gated on size, CD45 expression, and cytokeratin expression. The expression levels of HER2 were subdivided into four categories (−, +, ++, +++), based on the quantitative assessment of HER2 expression on PC3 and SKBR-3 cells. (−) Designates no expression or less than 5000 receptors (WBC); (+) designates expression between 5000 and 50,000 receptors (PC-3); (++) designates expression between 50,000 and 500,000 receptors; and (+++) designates expression of more than 500,000 receptors (SKBR-3). (**B**), (**C**), and (**D**) show the expression of cytokeratin and HER2 on CTCs from three patients with breast cancer. Only the CTCs are shown in the panels. *Source:* Adapted from Ref. 37.

Interestingly, this report also suggests an inverse relationship between the level of HER2 expression and the expression of cytokeratin. Treatment-related markers such as Bcl-2 and apoptosis can also be detected in CTCs (38), and these phenotypic markers are now being investigated as possible biological indicators of target modulation and of response to treatment for the monitoring of target-directed therapy. Investigators have also demonstrated early successes in gene expression profiling (39) and multiplex RT–PCR (40) from CTCs. As each of these methodologies becomes more sophisticated, our ability to isolate, detect, and phenotype these cells will continue to improve.

SUMMARY

Modern biological techniques now allow the isolation and characterization of CTCs with improved sensitivity and with high specificity and reproducibility, and as a result it has been possible to demonstrate that elevated CTCs ($\geq$5 CTC per 7.5 mL of peripheral blood) are a clinically significant and statistically significant poor prognostic factor in women with metastatic breast cancer. Of particular interest is the poor prognosis for patients who have completed one cycle of a new therapy. This suggests that these patients are on ineffective therapy and that their treatment should be changed even if there is no clinical evidence of progression. This theory will be tested in a prospective, randomized, blinded trial that is nearing activation in the SWOG. In addition, CTCs represent a valuable source of tumor tissue that has potential in the monitoring of response. They are being approached as a minimally invasive biopsy that can be performed serially to monitor therapy through the assessment of drug targets and other biologically important cancer markers. With the evolving ability to detect protein expression with immunofluorescent microscopy, mRNA expression with RT–PCR, and gene amplification using FISH, it is expected that CTCs will provide valuable insight into biology of breast and other cancers, resulting in new treatment strategies and improved methods to monitor response to therapy.

REFERENCES

1. Ashworth TR. A case of cancer in which cells similar to those in the tumours were seen in the blood after death. Aust Med J 1869; 14:146–149.
2. Allard WJ, Matera J, Miller MC, et al. Tumor cells circulate in the peripheral blood of all major carcinomas but not in healthy subjects or patients with nonmalignant diseases. Clin Cancer Res 2004; 10(20):6897–6904.
3. Ross AA, Cooper BW, Lazarus HM, et al. Detection and viability of tumor cells in peripheral blood stem cell collections from breast cancer patients using immunocyto-chemical and clonogenic assay techniques. Blood 1993; 82(9):2605–2610.
4. Engell HC. Cancer cells in the blood; a five to nine year follow up study. Ann Surg 1959; 149(4):457–461.
5. Christopherson WM. Cancer cells in the peripheral blood: a second look. Acta Cytol 1965; 9(2):169–174.
6. Choesmel V, Pierga JY, Nos C, et al. Enrichment methods to detect bone marrow micro-metastases in breast carcinoma patients: clinical relevance. Breast Cancer Res 2004; 6(5):R556–R570.
7. Rolle A, Gunzel R, Pachmann U, et al. Increase in number of circulating disseminated epithelial cells after surgery for non-small cell lung cancer monitored by MAINTRAC(R) is a predictor for relapse: a preliminary report. World J Surg Oncol 2005; 3(1):18.

8. Witzig TE, Bossy B, Kimlinger T, et al. Detection of circulating cytokeratin-positive cells in the blood of breast cancer patients using immunomagnetic enrichment and digital microscopy. Clin Cancer Res 2002; 8(5):1085–1091.

9. Racila E, Euhus D, Weiss AJ, et al. Detection and characterization of carcinoma cells in the blood. Proc Natl Acad Sci USA 1998; 95(8):4589–4594.

10. Brugger W, Buhring HJ, Grunebach F, et al. Expression of MUC-1 epitopes on normal bone marrow: implications for the detection of micrometastatic tumor cells. J Clin Oncol 1999; 17(5):1535–1544.

11. Ahr A, Scharl A, Muller M, et al. Cross-reactive staining of normal bone-marrow cells by monoclonal antibody 2E11. Int J Cancer 1999; 84(5):502–505.

12. Borgen E, Beiske K, Trachsel S, et al. Immunocytochemical detection of isolated epithelial cells in bone marrow: non-specific staining and contribution by plasma cells directly reactive to alkaline phosphatase. J Pathol 1998; 185(4):427–434.

13. Ring A, Smith IE, Dowsett M. Circulating tumour cells in breast cancer. Lancet Oncol 2004; 5(2):79–88.

14. Jung R, Kruger W, Hosch S, et al. Specificity of reverse transcriptase polymerase chain reaction assays designed for the detection of circulating cancer cells is influenced by cytokines in vivo and in vitro. Br J Cancer 1998; 78(9):1194–1198.

15. Goeminne JC, Guillaume T, Salmon M, et al. Unreliability of carcinoembryonic antigen (CEA) reverse transcriptase-polymerase chain reaction (RT-PCR) in detecting contaminating breast cancer cells in peripheral blood stem cells due to induction of CEA by growth factors. Bone Marrow Transplant 1999; 24(7):769–775.

16. Fiegl H, Millinger S, Mueller-Holzner E, et al. Circulating tumor-specific DNA: a marker for monitoring efficacy of adjuvant therapy in cancer patients. Cancer Res 2005; 65(4):1141–1145.

17. Brandt B, Roetger A, Heidl S, et al. Isolation of blood-borne epithelium-derived c-erbB-2 oncoprotein-positive clustered cells from the peripheral blood of breast cancer patients. Int J Cancer 1998; 76(6):824–828.

18. Martin VM, Siewert C, Scharl A, et al. Immunomagnetic enrichment of disseminated epithelial tumor cells from peripheral blood by MACS. Exp Hematol 1998; 26(3): 252–264.

19. de Cremoux P, Extra JM, Denis MG, et al. Detection of MUC1-expressing mammary carcinoma cells in the peripheral blood of breast cancer patients by real-time polymerase chain reaction. Clin Cancer Res 2000; 6(8):3117–3122.

20. Kruger W, Datta C, Badbaran A, et al. Immunomagnetic tumor cell selection—implications for the detection of disseminated cancer cells. Transfusion 2000; 40(12):1489–1493.

21. Beitsch PD, Clifford E. Detection of carcinoma cells in the blood of breast cancer patients. Am J Surg 2000; 180(6):446–448; discussion 448–449.

22. Hu XC, Wang Y, Shi DR, et al. Immunomagnetic tumor cell enrichment is promising in detecting circulating breast cancer cells. Oncology 2003; 64(2):160–165.

23. Taubert H, Blumke K, Bilkenroth U, et al. Detection of disseminated tumor cells in peripheral blood of patients with breast cancer: correlation to nodal status and occurrence of metastases. Gynecol Oncol 2004; 92(1): 256–261.

24. Kahn HJ, Presta A, Yang LY, et al. Enumeration of circulating tumor cells in the blood of breast cancer patients after filtration enrichment: correlation with disease stage. Breast Cancer Res Treat 2004; 86(3):237–247.

25. Cristofanilli M, Budd GT, Ellis MJ, et al. Circulating tumor cells, disease progression, and survival in metastatic breast cancer. N Engl J Med 2004; 351(8):781–791.

26. Ring, AE, Zabaglo, L, Ormerod, MG, et al. Detection of circulating epithelial cells in the blood of patients with breast cancer: comparison of three techniques. Br J Cancer 2005; 92(5):906–912.

27. Bauernhofer T, Zenahlik S, Hofmann G, et al. Association of disease progression and poor overall survival with detection of circulating tumor cells in peripheral blood of patients with metastatic breast cancer. Oncol Rep 2005; 13(2):179–184.

28. Pachmann K, Clement JH, Schneider CP, et al. Standardized quantification of circulating peripheral tumor cells from lung and breast cancer. Clin Chem Lab Med 2005; 43(6): 617–627.

29. Almokadem S, Leitzel K, Harvey HA, et al. Circulating tumor cells in adjuvant breast cancer patients. J Clin Oncol 2005; 23(suppl 16):667.
30. Gaforio JJ, Serrano MJ, Sanchez-Rovira P, et al. Detection of breast cancer cells in the peripheral blood is positively correlated with estrogen-receptor status and predicts for poor prognosis. Int J Cancer 2003; 107(6):984–990.
31. Cristofanilli M, Budd GT, Ellis MJ, et al. Presence of circulating tumor cells (CTC) in metastatic breast cancer (MBC) predicts rapid progression and poor prognosis. J Clin Oncol 2005; 23(suppl 16):524.
32. Cristofanilli M, Hayes DF, Budd GT, et al. Circulating tumor cells: a novel prognostic factor for newly diagnosed metastatic breast cancer. J Clin Oncol 2005; 23(7):1420–1430.
33. Budd GT, Cristofanilli M, Ellis M, et al. Monitoring circulating tumor cells (CTC) in nonmeasurable metastatic breast cancer (MBC). J Clin Oncol 2005; 23(suppl 16):503.
34. Soria JC, Gauthier LR, Raymond E, et al. Molecular detection of telomerase-positive circulating epithelial cells in metastatic breast cancer patients. Clin Cancer Res 1999; 5(5):971–975.
35. Austrup F, Uciechowski P, Eder C, et al. Prognostic value of genomic alterations in minimal residual cancer cells purified from the blood of breast cancer patients. Br J Cancer 2000; 83(12):1664–1673.
36. Fehm T, Sagalowsky A, Clifford E, et al. Cytogenetic evidence that circulating epithelial cells in patients with carcinoma are malignant. Clin Cancer Res 2002; 8(7):2073–2084.
37. Hayes DF, Walker TM, Singh B, et al. Monitoring expression of HER-2 on circulating epithelial cells in patients with advanced breast cancer. Int J Oncol 2002; 21(5):1111–1117.
38. Smerage JB, Doyle GV, Budd GT, et al. The detection of apoptosis and Bcl-2 expression in circulating tumor cells (CTCs) from women being treated for metastatic breast cancer. Proc Am Assoc Cancer Res 2006; 47:187a.
39. Smirnov DA, Zweitzig DR, Foulk BW, et al. Global gene expression profiling of circulating tumor cells. Cancer Res 2005; 65(12):4993–4997.
40. O'Hara SM, Moreno JG, Zweitzig DR, et al. Multigene reverse transcription-PCR profiling of circulating tumor cells in hormone-refractory prostate cancer. Clin Chem 2004; 50(5):826–835.

8 The Prognostic Impact of Bone Marrow Micrometastases in Women with Breast Cancer

Stephan Braun, Doris Auer, and Christian Marth
Department of Obstetrics and Gynecology, Innsbruck Medical University, Innsbruck, Austria

INTRODUCTION

The genesis of overt metastases in breast cancer is based on the idea that tumor cells that dissociate from the primary cancer get access to circulation either directly into blood vessels or after transit in lymphatic channels. Thus, detection of such cells in patients with newly diagnosed solid tumors has been an appealing strategy to provide evidence for future metastases.

In the past, several models have been constructed to explain the presence of individual tumor cells in secondary organs and their influence on the subsequent course of the disease. Currently, according to the most recent transcriptome and genome analyses, circulating tumor cells (CTC) in the bloodstream and those already disseminated to secondary organs [disseminated tumor cells (DTC)] are viewed as rare and much earlier indicators of tumor cell spread, than generally assumed from the typical year-long course of cancerous diseases, such as breast cancer. Despite the observation that the numerous genetic alterations found so far in such cells are rarely identical or even similar, first, the long interval between dissemination and clinical manifest metastases; secondly, the frequently observed relative resistance of some cells to chemotherapy and; thirdly, their significant effect on disease progression despite their low abundance in secondary organs, nourish the idea that some of these cells might be progenitor cells with self-renewing properties that give rise to most of the tumor mass that is dealt with clinically.

Beyond the discussion of such models and opinions, the actual presence of tumor cells outside the primary tumor and in organs relevant for subsequent metastasis formation, such as bone and bone marrow, would serve three purposes that could be clinically useful:

1. as an unambiguous evidence for an early occult spread of tumor cells,
2. as a relevant risk factor for subsequent metastasis and, thus, a poor prognosis,
3. as a marker for monitoring treatment susceptibility.

Finally, and perhaps, as importantly in the long run, genotyping and phenotyping of these cells should provide detailed insight into the metastatic process and permit direct exploration of targeted treatment strategies.

BIOLOGY OF HEMATOGENOUS TUMOR CELL DISSEMINATION

Tumor cells evaded or shed to the blood circulation may be detectable in peripheral venous blood and, in principle, all body organs, as shown in few elegant experiments during the 1960s and 1970s (1,2). When specific monoclonal antibodies became broadly available in the 1980s, the interest in the identification of spread tumor cells was renewed. The first study groups (3–8), however, did not investigate peripheral blood, presumably because from pathophysiological considerations, the presence of tumor cells in circulation was thought to be merely temporary. For similar theoretical reasons, the initial studies did not investigate epithelial parenchymous organs, such as lung, liver, or brain, known to be frequently colonized by epithelial cancer cells, for specific antibodies available at that time largely discriminated between the histogenetic origin of cells although they were raised against tumor-associated antigens. The ability to detect non-autochthonous epithelial breast cancer cells in a mesenchymal organ environment, the physiological absence of epithelial cells, its relevance for breast cancer metastases, and the clinical convenience to explore (i.e., diagnose) the organ site of interest led to numerous studies investigating the presence and significance of hematogenously disseminated tumor cells in bone marrow samples (9–18).

In order to investigate the underlying biology of DTC in bone marrow, antibodies against tumor-associated antigens—in parallel to the (usually anticytokeratin) detection antibody—are used to profile these cells, among various reasons predominantly in order to determine what percentage of these cells are actually of neoplastic origin. Using such immunocytochemical procedures, it has been possible to identify frequent expression of urokinase-type plasminogen activator receptor (uPAR) in gastric cancer (19) and ERBB2 (also known as HER2/NEU) in breast cancer (20). In both cases, the (over-)expression was associated with poor clinical outcome, and uPAR and ERBB2, as a consequence, might be important for the survival and growth of DTC.

Detailed examination of the genome was made possible by recent technical developments, such as the combination of immunocytochemistry and fluorescence in situ hybridization, which led to the demonstration that the bone marrow contains disseminated epithelial cells of malignant origin (21). By developing a new procedure for whole-genome amplification and subsequent comparative genomic hybridization (CGH) of single immunostained cells, Klein et al. (22) demonstrated that cytokeratin-positive cells in the bone marrow of patients with epithelial breast cancer without clinical signs of overt metastases (stage M0) are genetically heterogeneous. This heterogeneity was strikingly reduced with the emergence of clinically evident metastasis (stage M1).

The stage at which individual cells leave the primary tumor is unclear. In patients with early-stage invasive breast cancer, the cytokeratin-positive cells isolated from the bone marrow had few features in common with those found in their respective primary tumors (23). A provocative interpretation of this surprising finding is that the DTC separated from their primary tumor at a very early stage. This hypothesis is also supported by the finding that only few DTC in these patients had TP53 mutations, which are associated with the later stages of tumorigenesis (22,24). DTC might therefore evolve independently into overt metastases, driven by the specific selective pressures of the bone-marrow environment (25).

Genetic analyses that compared paired primary and metastatic breast tumor samples confirm the hypothesis that DTC evolve independently from the primary tumor. The patterns of genetic alterations that are observed in overt metastases are often discordant with those of the primary tumor, and differ almost completely in approximately one-third of the cases (26). During genetic progression of the primary breast tumor, cancer cells might disseminate continuously, acquiring additional genetic alterations after migration into secondary organs such as the bone marrow.

TUMOR CELL DETECTION AND THE CLINICAL CONTEXT

When Steven Paget (27) published his theory of "seed and soil" in 1889, the idea of hematogenous tumor cell dissemination was born. More than a century later, with molecular tools being available, new clinical findings explained hitherto unexplainable phenomena, such as donor-derived cancer in recipient organ allografts (28) or detection of viable single tumor cells in secondary organs, both being descendants of a known primary tumor (29) and potential precursors of subsequent metastasis (30). The fulfillment of the request for factors enabling individual risk assessment seems to be on the horizon. Yet, in breast cancer, recent guidelines for adjuvant systemic therapy still foresee treatment recommendations for more than 90% of patients even in case of a negative lymph-node status (31,32). The risk of tumor relapse in these patients is considered high enough to recommend adjuvant therapy, even though up to 70% of early-stage breast cancer patients are cured by locoregional surgery alone.

Terminology

For their broad utilization, markers need to be implemented into current risk classification systems, such as the tumor-node-metastasis (TNM) classification. Although the decision upon implementation appears to be pending since 1990s, when DTC were mentioned for the first time in the TNM Supplement (33,34), a useful proposal for an appropriate TNM terminology has recently been made by the International Union Against Cancer (UICC) (35). The most recent TNM classification for breast cancer (36) does not qualify the presence of single cancer cells in peripheral blood or bone marrow as metastasis (stage M0), but it optionally reports the presence of such cells together with their detection method [e.g., M0(i+) or (mol+)].

Prognostic Value of Tumor Cell Detection

In order to determine the actual significance of DTC in bone marrow for the outcome and survival of breast cancer patients, the literature basis is ample. To date, most experience with bone marrow screening for DTC exists for immunocytochemical analyses. Numerous studies reported a strong prognostic impact of the presence of DTC (8,11–18,37–39), whereas other investigations failed to do so (5,6,10,40–42). One reason for the discrepant results of clinical follow-up studies is a substantial methodological variation (e.g., sensitivity and specificity of detection antibody, lower detection rate of bone marrow biopsy as compared with bone marrow aspiration, considerable variation in the number of cells analyzed) resulting in a wide range of detection rates between study populations.

However, even if only large, well-designed, and controlled studies are now considered for a summarizing statement on the prognostic significance of DTC, at least three confounding technical factors varied considerably: (*i*) consistent and blinded analysis of non-carcinoma control patients; (*ii*) diversity of antibodies used for identification of epithelial cells in bone marrow; and (*iii*) number of cells analyzed per patient sample.

In the past, two studies therefore attempted to solve this dilemma, performing meta-analyses of the published studies (43,44). However, several authors suggested that the ideal way to perform a meta-analysis of survival data would be to use individual patient data (45,46). Using individual patient data, instead, would have the advantage to include information on patient characteristics, account for differences in immunoassays, and consider variability in treatment over time. Therefore, a large pooled analysis of individual patient data of 4703 breast cancer patients from eight large studies (11,13–18,37) now provides conclusive data on the poor prognostic influence of presence of DTC on the clinical outcome and survival of stage I, II, and III breast cancer patients (30). DTC are present in one-third of patients with stage I, II, and III breast cancer. As compared with women without DTC, patients with DTC had larger tumors, tumors with a higher histological grade, lymph-node metastases, and hormone receptor-negative tumors (for all variables, $P < 0.001$). The presence of DTC was a significant prognostic factor for poor overall and breast cancer-specific survival, and disease-free and distant metastasis-free survival during the 10-year observation period (univariate mortality ratios, 2.15, 2.44, 2.13, and 2.33, respectively; for all, $P < 0.001$) (Fig. 1). In multivariable analysis, presence of DTC was an independent predictor of poor patient outcome (Table 1).

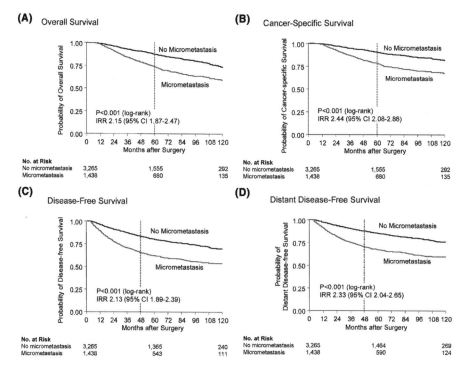

FIGURE 1 Kaplan–Meier estimates of long-term patient outcome by presence or absence of bone marrow micrometastasis. Panels show estimates of overall (**A**), cancer-specific (**B**), disease-free (**C**), and distant disease-free survival (**D**) for the complete patient group. The vertical dotted lines in (**A**) to (**D**) divide the time intervals used for piecewise Cox regression modeling. *Abbreviations*: IRR, incidence rate ratio; CI, confidence interval.

TABLE 1 Multivariable Hazards Ratios for Overall and Cancer-Specific Survival at Different Time Intervals (Adjusted for Center)

	Follow-up interval yr 0–5 (N = 3974)		Follow-up interval yr 6–10 (N = 1674)[c]	
	HR (95% CI)	P-value	HR (95% CI)	P-value
Overall survival[a]				
Bone marrow micrometastasis	1.81 (1.51–2.16)	<0.001	1.58 (1.12–2.22)	0.009
Tumor size	1.70 (1.50–1.94)[b]	<0.001	—	—
Lymph node metastasis	1.63 (1.50–1.77)[b]	<0.001	1.88 (1.61–2.21)[b]	<0.001
Tumor grade	1.72 (1.44–2.06)	<0.001	—	—
Hormone receptor	0.56 (0.47–0.68)	<0.001	—	—
Cancer-specific survival[a]				
Bone marrow micrometastasis	1.93 (1.58–2.36)	<0.001	1.63 (1.07–2.47)	0.022
Tumor size	1.67 (1.44–1.94)[b]	<0.001	—	—
Lymph node metastasis	1.71 (1.55–1.89)[b]	<0.001	1.98 (1.64–2.40)[b]	<0.001
Tumor grade	1.75 (1.43–2.15)	<0.001	—	—
Hormone receptor	0.50 (0.41–0.61)	<0.001	—	—

[a]Comparison of variable categories: bone marrow micrometastasis, negative versus positive; tumor size, T1 versus T2 versus T3/T4; lymph node metastasis, N0 versus N1 versus N2 versus N3; tumor grade: G1/G2 versus G3; hormone receptor, negative versus any receptor positive.
[b]Hazards ratio for linear trend test across categories.
[c]A separate model was fit for the second interval; blanks indicate that no-risk estimates are available for variables that dropped from the final model according to the selection process.
Abbreviations: HR, hazards ratio; CI, confidence interval.

Predictive Value of Tumor Cell Detection

Beyond merely adding another prognostic factor to the plethora of such markers in breast cancer, it needs to be emphasized that assessment of occult hematogenous tumor cell spread inherits the potential for a tool for prediction and monitoring of efficacy of systemic therapy (47–51). In contrast to lymph nodes, which are generally accepted as "indirect" marker of hematogenous tumor cell spread and, hence, risk of systemic spread but which are also generally removed at primary surgery and unavailable for follow-up evaluations, bone marrow, and blood can be obtained repeatedly in the postoperative course of the patient. Of all clinically utilized and/or established factors, the only prognostic factors available for follow-up risk assessment, in principle, are DTC or CTC. For DTC, the clinical value of such examinations has been strongly suggested by clinical studies on a total of almost 500 patients, which identified the prognostic relevance of DTC present in bone marrow several months after diagnosis or treatment when no relapse has occurred until that date (48,52,53). The potential of a surrogate marker assay that permits immediate assessment of therapy-induced cytotoxic effects on occult metastatic cells is therefore evident, as indicated previously (48). Since repeated bone marrow sampling might not be easily implemented into clinical study protocols for breast cancer, serial examinations of blood for CTC or tumor cell-associated nucleic acids might be more acceptable for most patients and clinical investigators than repeated bone marrow aspirations. The detection and characterization of CTC in peripheral blood of cancer patients has therefore received much attention in recent years and could lead to strategies for evaluation of therapeutic efficacy. This approach has been successfully realized in one study on 177 patients with metastatic breast cancer (54), but no data are available for those patients in which adjuvant therapy is applied in a curative intent.

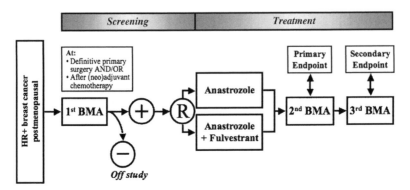

FIGURE 2 Trial design of the Austrian-German Norwegian Cooperative Trial-@fame (Adjuvant Faslodex and Arimidex against Micrometastasis). *Abbreviations*: BMA, bone marrow aspiration; HR, hormone receptor; R, randomization.

For the time being and with validated assays being available for the evaluation of bone marrow only, prospective clinical studies are now required to evaluate whether eradication of DTC in bone marrow and CTC in blood after systemic therapy translates into a longer disease-free period and overall survival. As example and an optimistic outlook one might view the start of the "Adjuvant Faslodex™ and Arimidex™ against Micrometastasis (@fame)-Trial" that investigates the effect of randomized adjuvant treatment (Fulvestrant and Anastrozole vs. Anastrozole alone) in DTC-positive, patients with hormone-receptor-positive breast cancer (55) (Fig. 2). Primary endpoint after 12 months of treatment is the number of events, defined as continued presence of DTC, any recurrence of disease, or death from any cause. As secondary endpoints, safety of the novel combination of fulvestrant and anastrozole and the number of events after 24 months are investigated. In a translational research approach, the study further addresses the question whether number of DTC before, during, and after randomized treatment for 24 months is indicative of patient outcome, or whether assessments of disseminated or circulating tumor-associated ribonucleotides as well as disseminated or circulating methylated DNA, which are analyzed in parallel DTCs, could provide similar information that might be available from more convenient and perhaps even more reliable analytical approaches.

REFERENCES

1. Zeidman I. The fate of circulating tumors cells. I. Passage of cells through capillaries. Cancer Res 1961; 21:38–39.
2. Fidler IJ. Quantitative analysis of distribution and fate of tumor emboli labeled with ^{125}I-5-iodo-2′-desoxyuridine. J Natl Cancer Inst 1970; 145:773–782.
3. Mansi JL, Berger U, Easton D, et al. Micrometastases in bone marrow in patients with primary breast cancer: evaluation as an early predictor of bone metastases. Br Med J 1987; 295:1093–1096.
4. Untch M, Harbeck N, Eiermann W. Micrometastases in bone marrow in patients with breast cancer. Br J Med 1988; 296:290.
5. Porro G, Menard S, Tagliabue E, et al. Monoclonal antibody detection of carcinoma cells in bone marrow biopsy specimens from breast cancer patients. Cancer 1988; 61:2407–2411.

6. Salvadori B, Squicciarini P, Rovini D, et al. Use of monoclonal antibody MBr1 to detect micrometastases in bone marrow specimens of breast cancer patients. Eur J Cancer 1990; 26:865–867.

7. Kirk SJ, Cooper GG, Hoper M, Watt PC, Roy AD, Olding-Smee W. The prognostic significance of marrow micrometastases in women with early breast cancer. Eur J Surg Oncol 1990; 16:481–485.

8. Cote RJ, Rosen PP, Lesser ML, Old LJ, Osborne MP. Prediction of early relapse in patients with operable breast cancer by detection of occult bone marrow micrometastases. J Clin Oncol 1991; 9:1749–1756.

9. Mansi JL, Berger U, Wilson P, Shearer R, Coombes RC. Detection of tumor cells in bone marrow of patients with prostatic carcinoma by immunocytochemical techniques. J Urol 1988; 139:545–548.

10. Funke I, Fries S, Rolle M, et al. Comparative analyses of bone marrow micrometastases in breast and gastric cancer. Int J Cancer 1996; 65:755–761.

11. Diel IJ, Kaufmann M, Costa SD, et al. Micrometastatic breast cancer cells in bone marrow at primary surgery: prognostic value in comparison with nodal status. J Natl Cancer Inst 1996; 88:1652–1664.

12. Landys K, Persson S, Kovarik J, Hultborn R, Holmberg E. Prognostic value of bone marrow biopsy in operable breast cancer patients at the time of initial diagnosis: results of a 20-year median follow-up. Breast Cancer Res Treat 1998; 49:27–33.

13. Mansi JL, Gogas H, Bliss JM, Gazet JC, Berger U, Coombes RC. Outcome of primary-breast-cancer patients with micrometastases: a long-term follow-up. Lancet 1999; 354(9174):197–202.

14. Braun S, Pantel K, Müller P, et al. Cytokeratin-positive cells in the bone marrow and survival of patients with stage I, II or III breast cancer. N Engl J Med 2000; 342(8):525–533.

15. Gebauer G, Fehm T, Merkle E, Beck EP, Lang N, Jager W. Epithelial cells in bone marrow of breast cancer patients at time of primary surgery: clinical outcome during long-term follow-up. J Clin Oncol 2001; 19(16):3669–74.

16. Gerber B, Krause A, Muller H, et al. Simultaneous immunohistochemical detection of tumor cells in lymph nodes and bone marrow aspirates in breast cancer and its correlation with other prognostic factors. J Clin Oncol 2001; 19:960–971.

17. Wiedswang G, Borgen E, Karesen R, et al. Detection of isolated tumor cells in bone marrow is an independent prognostic factor in breast cancer. J Clin Oncol 2003; 21(18):3469–3478.

18. Pierga J-Y, Bonneton C, Vincent-Salomon A, et al. Clinical significance of immunocytochemical detection of tumor cells using digital microscopy in peripheral blood and bone marrow of breast cancer patients. Clin Cancer Res 2004; 10(4):1392–1400.

19. Heiss MM, Allgayer H, Gruetzner KU, et al. Individual development and uPA-receptor expression of disseminated tumour cells in bone marrow: a reference to early systemic disease in solid cancer. Nat Med 1995; 1(10):1035–1039.

20. Braun S, Heumos I, Schlimok G, et al. ErbB2 over-expression on occult metastatic cells in bone marrow predicts poor clinical outcome of stage I-III breast cancer patients. Cancer Res 2001; 61:1890–1895.

21. Solakoglu O, Maierhofer C, Lahr G, et al. Heterogeneous proliferative potential of occult metastatic cells in bone marrow of patients with solid epithelial tumors. Proc Natl Acad Sci 2002; 99(4):2246–2251.

22. Klein CA, Blankenstein TJF, Schmidt-Kittler O, et al. Genetic heterogeneity of single disseminated tumour cells in minimal residual cancer. The Lancet 2002; 360(9334):683–689.

23. Schmidt-Kittler O, Ragg T, Daskalakis A, et al. From latent disseminated cells to overt metastasis: Genetic analysis of systemic breast cancer progression. Proc Natl Acad Sci 2003; 100:7737–7742.

24. Offner S, Schmaus W, Witter K, et al. p53 mutations are not required for early dissemination of cancer cells. Proc Natl Acad Sci USA 1999; 96:6942–6946.

25. Gray JW. Evidence emerges for early metastasis and parallel evolution of primary and metastatic tumors. Cancer Cell 2003; 4(1):4–6.

26. Kuukasjarvi T, Karhu R, Tanner M, et al. Genetic heterogeneity and clonal evolution underlying development of asynchronous metastasis in human breast cancer. Cancer Res 1997; 57(8):1597–1604.
27. Paget S. Distribution of secondary growths in cancer of the breast. Lancet 1889; 1:571.
28. Loh E, Couch FJ, Hendricksen C, et al. Development of donor-derived prostate cancer in a recipient following orthotopic heart transplantation. J Am Med Assoc 1997; 277:133–137.
29. Klein CA, Schmidt-Kittler O, Schardt JA, Pantel K, Speicher MR, Riethmüller G. Comparative genomic hybridization, loss of heterozygosity, and DNA sequence analysis of single cells. Proc Natl Acad Sci USA 1999; 96:4494–4499.
30. Braun S, Vogl* FD, Naume B, et al. A pooled analysis of bone marrow micrometastasis in breast cancer. NEJM 2005; 353(8):793–802.
31. Goldhirsch A, Glick JH, Gelber RD, Coates AS, Senn HJ. Meeting highlights: international consensus panel on the treatment of primary breast cancer. J Clin Oncol 2001; 19:3817–3827.
32. Goldhirsch A, Wood WC, Gelber RD, Coates AS, Thurlimann B, Senn H-J. Meeting highlights: updated international expert consensus on the primary therapy of early breast cancer. J Clin Oncol 2003; 21(17):3357–3365.
33. Hermanek P. What's new in TNM? Pathol Res Pract 1994; 190:97–102.
34. Hermanek P, Henson DE, Hutter RV, Sobin LH. TNM Supplement 1993. Berlin: Springer, 1993.
35. Hermanek P, Hutter RV, Sobin LH, Wittekind C. Classification of isolated tumor cells and micrometastases. Cancer 1999; 86:2668–2673.
36. Singletary SE, Allred C, Ashley P, et al. Revision of the American Joint Committee on cancer staging system for breast cancer. J Clin Oncol 2002; 20(17):3628–3636.
37. Wong GYC, Yu QQ, Osborne MP. Bone marrow micrometastasis is a significant predictor of long-term relapse-free survival for breast cancer by a non-proportional hazards model [abstr]. Breast Cancer Res Treat 2003; 82(suppl 1):S99.
38. Braun S, Cevatli BS, Assemi C, et al. Comparative analysis of micrometastasis to the bone marrow and lymph nodes of node-negative breast cancer patients receiving no adjuvant therapy. J Clin Oncol 2001; 19:1468–1475.
39. Harbeck N, Untch M, Pache L, Eiermann W. Tumour cell detection in the bone marrow of breast cancer patients at primary therapy: results of a 3-year median follow-up. Br J Cancer 1994; 69:566–571.
40. Courtemanche DJ, Worth AJ, Coupland RW, Rowell JL, MacFarlane JK. Monoclonal antibody LICR-LON-M8 does not predict the outcome of operable breast cancer. Can J Surg 1991; 34:21–26.
41. Singletary SE, Larry L, Trucker SL, Spitzer G. Detection of micrometastatic tumor cells in bone marrow of breast carcinoma patients. J Surg Oncol 1991; 47:32–36.
42. Mathieu MC, Friedman S, Bosq J, et al. Immunohistochemical staining of bone marrow biopsies for detection of occult metastasis in breast cancer. Breast Cancer Res Treat 1990; 15(1):21–26.
43. Weinschenker P, Soares HP, Otavio Clark O, Del Giglio A. Immunocytochemical detection of epithelial cells in the bone marrow of primary breast cancer patients: a meta-analysis. Breast Cancer Res Treat 2004; 87:215–224.
44. Funke I, Schraut W. Meta-analysis of studies on bone marrow micrometastases: an independent prognostic impact remains to be substantiated. J Clin Oncol 1998; 16:557–566.
45. Hunink MG, Wong JB. Meta-analysis of failure-time data with adjustment for covariates. Med Decis Mak 1994; 14:59–70.
46. Clarke MJ, Stewart LA. Obtaining data from randomised controlled trials: how much do we need for reliable and informative meta-analyses? Brit Med J 1994; 309(6960):1007–1010.
47. Thurm H, Ebel S, Kentenich C, et al. Rare expression of epithelial cell adhesion molecule on residual micrometastatic breast cancer cells after adjuvant chemotherapy. Clin Cancer Res 2003; 9(7):2598–2604.

48. Braun S, Kentenich CRM, Janni W, et al. Lack of effect of adjuvant chemotherapy on the elimination of single dormant tumor cells in bone marrow of high-risk breast cancer patients. J Clin Oncol 2000; 18:80–86.
49. Braun S, Hepp F, Kentenich CRM, et al. Monoclonal antibody therapy with edrecolomab in breast cancer patients: monitoring of elimination of disseminated cytokeratin-positive tumor cells in bone marrow. Clin Cancer Res 1999; 5:3999–4004.
50. Pantel K, Enzmann T, Köllermann J, Caprano J, Riethmüller G, Köllermann MW. Immunocytochemical monitoring of micrometastatic disease: reduction of prostate cancer cells in bone marrow by androgen deprivation. Int J Cancer 1997; 71:521–525.
51. Schlimok G, Pantel K, Loibner H, Fackler-Schwalbe I, Riethmüller G. Reduction of metastatic carcinoma cells in bone marrow by intravenously administered monoclonal antibody: towards a novel surrogate test to monitor adjuvant therapies of solid tumours. Eur J Cancer 1995; 31A:1799–1803.
52. Janni W, Rack B, Schindlbeck C, et al. The persistence of isolated tumor cells in bone marrow from patients with breast carcinoma predicts an increased risk for recurrence. Cancer 2005; 103:884–891.
53. Wiedswang G, Borgen E, Kåresen R, et al. Isolated tumor cells in bone marrow 3 years after diagnosis in disease free breast cancer patients predict unfavorable clinical outcome. Clin Cancer Res 2004; 10(16):5342–5348.
54. Cristofanilli M, Budd GT, Ellis MJ, et al. Circulating tumor cells, disease progression and survival in metastatic breast cancer. N Engl J Med 2004; 351(8):781–791.
55. (http://www.abcsg.at/abcsg/html_studien/mamma_offen.html)

9 The Prognostic Importance of Isolated Tumor Cell Clusters and Micrometastases in Sentinel Lymph Nodes

Donald L. Weaver

Department of Pathology, University of Vermont College of Medicine, Burlington, Vermont, U.S.A.

INTRODUCTION

This chapter explores the prognostic impact of nodal metastases and in particular considers the importance of sentinel lymph node biopsy in the context of enhanced detection of micrometastases and isolated tumor cell clusters (ITC). Lymph node metastases, specifically axillary nodal metastases, are considered to be one of the most important factors stratifying between good and bad prognosis breast cancers. Historically, the emphasis has been placed on the presence or absence of nodal disease. This dichotomous stratification was challenged as accumulated clinical data indicated the total number of involved lymph nodes had prognostic significance (1). Further, pathological data indicated the size of the metastatic focus had prognostic significance (2). Acknowledging these observations, the sixth edition AJCC and UICC staging manuals formally incorporated semiquantitative nodal tumor burden into the stage and substage groupings; both the number of involved lymph nodes and the size of the metastatic foci influence overall stage (3–5). This principle is consistent with quantifying primary tumor burden, the other mainstay of tumor prognosis and staging.

Tumor burden has stood the test of time as a valuable prognostic factor; however, it is a relatively crude measure when one considers that modern investigations of tumor biology can identify defects in isolated biochemical regulatory pathways. Why then in a book on translational therapeutic strategies for breast cancer are we interested in a factor as crude as nodal tumor burden? The answer to this question rests on the foundational observation that a focus of tumor in a lymph node, a metastasis in the traditional sense, represents the demonstrated capacity of a tumor to proliferate, invade, travel to a new location, proliferate in that location, and potentially spawn further metastatic foci. The critical question is when does a discovered nodal tumor deposit have clinical significance? This is not a simple question when considering micrometastases. The discussion in this chapter focuses on minimal tumor burden and how it is detected in sentinel nodes. The underlying thesis is that micrometastases and ITC clusters in lymph nodes must have less prognostic significance than macrometastases.

CHALLENGING THE DOGMA OF NODE-POSITIVE
AND NODE-NEGATIVE BREAST CANCER

Consider two patients. The first has four negative sentinel lymph nodes and the second has a 5.5 mm metastasis in one of several lymph nodes. Five years after diagnosis, the first patient develops a cerebral metastasis and the second patient has a mammographic density adjacent to the old partial mastectomy site that is fibrocystic change on biopsy. A curious pathologist performs deeper sections and cytokeratin immunohistochemistry (CK IHC) on the "negative" sentinel nodes prior to tumor board because these were not performed at the time of diagnosis. One of the sentinel nodes contains a 0.1 mm metastasis and another node contains five clusters of tumor cells ranging from one to six cells in the subcapsular sinus. Now imagine the discussion at tumor board. Someone is sure to suggest "if we had only done the deeper sections and immunos five years ago . . . ." This, of course, is the sort of magical thinking that propagates oncological myths. What are we missing in these two scenarios? Would the question still be asked if we had the whole story? The first patient was 47-years-old at the time of diagnosis and had a 2.2 cm moderately differentiated tumor she discovered on self-breast examination seven months after a negative screening mammogram. The tumor was estrogen and progesterone receptor negative and had no evidence for HER2/*neu* over-expression or amplification. She was treated with dose dense chemotherapy. The second patient was 68-years-old at the time of diagnosis. The tumor measured 1.3 cm in greatest dimension and was detected on screening mammogram. Comparison films from two previous examinations had revealed architectural distortion in the same area that was not appreciably different in size but was less dense than on the diagnostic index examination. In retrospect, it was undoubtedly a missed cancer that had been present for at least two years, probably longer. The tumor was well differentiated with strong and diffusely positive estrogen and progesterone receptors. She had been treated with tamoxifen, but did not receive chemotherapy. An astute medical student would now suggest that the younger woman had a biologically aggressive tumor and the postmenopausal woman had a biologically indolent tumor. In these two patients, the presence or absence of lymph node metastases had little influence on either treatment or outcome at five years.

These two cases are not meant to argue against the value of lymph node evaluation. Rather, they are meant to challenge the notion that lymph node status can be evaluated in a vacuum and to illustrate a fundamental principle: the intrinsic biology of a tumor is well established by the time a clinical or pathological diagnosis is established; intervention may or may not alter the ultimate outcome for any individual.

THE UNCERTAIN BIOLOGY OF SINGLE CELLS
AND MINUTE TUMOR CELL CLUSTERS

Carcinomas are heterogeneous. Some breast carcinomas exhibit tubule formation in one region, solid growth in another. They may demonstrate viable or necrotic central zones, varying degrees of tumor-induced fibrosis, and cellular differences in hormone or HER2/*neu* receptor expression. Most tumors have more mitoses and higher proliferation rates at the advancing peripheral margin. On a cellular basis, carcinomas are a mixture of differentiated cells and progenitor or stem cells (6,7). A tumor cell that can invade a lymphatic duct may not be capable of proliferation; a proliferating cell might "escape" with a nonproliferating cell. It is reasonable to assume that tumor cells or cell clusters identified within lymph nodes are also heterogeneous with respect to their proliferative or progenitor cell capacity. In fact, it is naïve to assume that they represent a homogeneous cell population. Some cell clusters that make it to the lymph node are destined to die and only a small number may survive and proliferate. In our examination of occult metastases in sentinel nodes it is fairly common, when they are detected, to observe multiple foci of minute tumor cell clusters and single tumor cells within the subcapsular and interfollicular sinuses of lymph nodes. When larger micrometastases are identified, they are more often present in only one or two locations within the node. This would suggest that only a few of the cell clusters contain progenitor cells that survive and proliferate. In the future, we may be able to determine which of the cells in a node have progenitor capacity but even that level of certainty will not absolutely resolve questions of clinical significance in sentinel nodes.

THE HEISENBERG UNCERTAINTY PRINCIPLE APPLIED TO BREAST CANCER

Heisenberg postulated that the position and momentum of a particle could not be simultaneously known. His principle led to clearer understanding of the uncertainty inherent in scientific measurement. A similar paradox exists in assessing lymph node metastases with respect to knowing where they are but not knowing where they may have been going. Even if we could assess the biological potential of a single cell, cell cluster, or micrometastasis in a sentinel node, the node has already been removed from the patient: anything removed has no capacity to harm; only disease left behind has lethal potential. By assessing the disease removed from a patient, we infer from observational experience the risk of recurrence. Implicit in any risk prediction is the assumption and probability that some quantity of tumor with proliferative capacity remains in the patient. The failure pattern, or metastatic profile, for breast cancer has not changed over the course of our transition from radical mastectomy to conservative surgical management with adjuvant radiation and multidrug combination chemotherapy. Breast cancer progenitor cells in the bone marrow, liver, brain, or other safe harbor must escape eradication during treatment and survive to proliferate and secondarily disseminate. Any prognostic value for micrometastases or minute tumor cell clusters in sentinel nodes can only be assessed by correlating the multitude of measurable factors available for both the primary tumor and nodal tumor deposits with subsequent failure patterns then determining which factors are most predictive. Imprecision in risk estimates is guaranteed because the natural history of even an aggressive tumor may be altered if detected and treated early. However, failure to eradicate even one systemic progenitor cell carries a risk of recurrence. An aggressive systemic recurrence is, for most patients, incurable and something to be avoided if possible. This fear can drive us away from the rational consideration of risk versus benefit. The question in sentinel node biopsy is whether the enhanced detection of micrometastases is "the prognostic factor" that predicts systemic recurrence. This is too high an expectation. Early data on bone marrow micrometastases suggest that a more direct measurement of occult systemic disease has greater prognostic value than occult disease in sentinel nodes (8). Overly optimistic estimates of the prognostic value for micrometastases in sentinel nodes will subject too many patients to over-treatment.

THE UNCERTAINTY INHERENT IN THE PATHOLOGICAL EVALUATION OF LYMPH NODES

When a pathologist examines a lymph node, much of what happens can be considered from a statistical frame of reference. An average lymph node is shaped like a bean and may measure 1.0 × 0.8 cm by 0.6 cm thick but there is variation from the smallest to largest nodes present in the axilla. Other variables can also change the shape, size, or appearance of a node. For example, many older or larger women have enlarged nodes that are composed of a thin rim of lymphoid tissue surrounding a central hilar zone replaced by adipose tissue. Larger nodes and nodes replaced by adipose tissue are more difficult to examine. But let us focus on the average node. A pathologist must first determine whether to slice the node or submit it intact. With modern processing equipment, the portion of tissue submitted for microscopic examination must fit into a plastic cassette that can accommodate a piece of tissue no larger than a postage stamp that is up to 5.0 mm thick. The College of American Pathologists (CAP) recommends that the entire lymph node be submitted, regardless of whether it is an axillary node or a sentinel node (9). They further recommend, as does the American Society of Clinical Oncology (ASCO), that sentinel nodes be sliced as close to 2.0 mm as possible prior to embedding in paraffin (9,10). The result is a block of tissue approximately 2.0 mm thick from which microscopic sections 0.004 to 0.006 mm thick are removed to make glass slides. Thus, it would take 330 to 500 microscopic sections to completely examine a paraffin block of nodal tissue. Most sentinel nodes can be processed, even when sliced at 2.0 mm intervals, in a single paraffin block. Larger nodes may require two or three blocks. The average number of sentinel nodes per case ranges from two to four. No sane pathologist would volunteer to look at all the possible sections that can be generated from a sentinel node biopsy. Further, as a society, we cannot afford a complete microscopic examination (11). The practical solution is to sample the lymph node. This is exactly what pathologists have been doing for decade upon decade. The difference between the pre- and postsentinel node era is that pathologists often chose to submit only part of the node for microscopic evaluation. This was a very rational approach when bulkier nodal disease was present. There was much less concern regarding the detection of micrometastases and the gross examination of the node was often sufficient to detect nodal disease; the microscopic evaluation only needed to provide the documentation of the gross impression. Primary tumors were larger and it is a fairly safe assumption that metastatic deposits were larger given the high correlation between tumor size and the presence of nodal metastases (12).

Sampling based on gross examination and impression is no longer an accepted or reasonable approach to patient stratification. Huvos et al. (2) set the bar for clinically significant nodal metastases at 2.0 mm; then Fisher and others suggested the possibility of a lower threshold (13). The current approach endorsed by both CAP and ASCO is to make sure we do not miss any metastasis larger than 2.0 mm and to document the size of the largest metastasis detected (9,10).

How is this accomplished? When a pathologist examines a sentinel node, the first step is to bisect or slice the node into sections that are no thicker than 2.0 mm. This is not the easiest task when the node is in the fresh state as required by any expectation for an intraoperative assessment. If the intraoperative assessment can be omitted, the node can be fixed in formalin for a period of time. This stiffens the tissue making it easier to thinly slice the node improving the permanent section analysis. There are also potential advantages to slicing the node in the plane that includes the two longest axes, a task more difficult than short axis sectioning. A larger number of afferent lymphatics enter the node within this plane rather than perpendicular to this plane and this tends to increase the likelihood of detecting metastases in initial microscopic sections of bisected nodes. Each slice is placed in an embedding cassette, so as to optimize the total number of cut surfaces examined. Once these are processed and embedded in paraffin, a section from the surface of each block is examined. This is the recommended standard evaluation (Fig. 1). By following this recommended strategy, we accept two repeatedly demonstrated and connected observations. The first observation is that not all "node-negative" patients are actually node-negative, metastases as large as 2.0 mm may have been missed with this

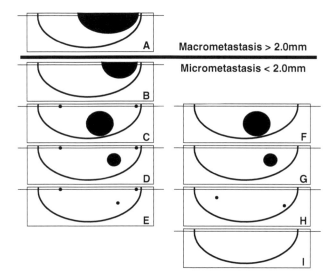

FIGURE 1 Inherent uncertainty in pathological evaluation of lymph nodes. Each panel represents a cross-section through paraffin-embedded tissue blocks containing a 2.0-mm thick section of a bisected lymph node. The horizontal line through the block represents a single microscopic section prepared from the surface of the block. This sectioning strategy was employed on NSABP B-32 and is recommended by CAP and ASCO. (**A–E**) The left panels represent positive lymph nodes. (**A**) A macrometastasis is detected. Using the described sampling strategy, virtually all metastases larger than 2.0 mm will be detected; however, metastases less than 2.0 mm may be detected or missed and the maximum size of the metastasis may be underestimated. (**B**) A micrometastasis is detected. (**C**) Isolated tumor cell (ITC) clusters are detected and an occult micrometastasis larger than 1.0 mm remains undetected. (**D**) ITC clusters are detected and an occult micrometastasis less than 1.0 mm remains undetected. (**E**) ITC clusters are detected and only occult tumor cell clusters remain undetected. (**F–I**) The right panels represent negative lymph nodes or, more accurately, lymph nodes with no metastases detected using a sampling strategy designed to exclude metastases larger than 2.0 mm. (**F**) An occult metastasis larger than 1.0 mm has been missed. (**G**) An occult metastasis smaller than 1.0 mm has been missed. (**H**) Occult ITC clusters have been missed. (**I**) A true negative lymph node. Note that the sampling strategy has excluded macrometastases from the micrometastasis and node-negative groups, but there is considerable overlap between what has been detected and what has been missed.

sampling strategy. The second observation is that any metastases smaller than 2.0 mm may have been detected by chance. Thus, for an individual patient, we cannot be sure that there is a difference between a lymph node with a detected metastasis smaller than 2.0 mm and a node with no metastases detected because of the uncertainty built into the pathology evaluation strategy (14).

PERIL IN THE MICROSCOPIC EXAMINATION

The observed increase in positive lymph nodes for patients with cancers smaller than 2.0 cm (Stage IIA) is undoubtedly attributable to sentinel node biopsy and stage shifting (14). Although it is well established that more extensive sampling detects additional micrometastases and ITC clusters, the clinical value of more extensive microscopic evaluation is still under investigation. A node and its tumor deposits are three-dimensional structures; we evaluate tissues in two dimensions. Technically, a microscopic section is three-dimensional but the 0.005 mm thickness does not evaluate much of the 2.0 mm overall thickness of each node slice. This means that the measured maximum dimension of a nodal tumor deposit on the microscopic section is not necessarily the true maximum dimension. We may be evaluating only the tip of the iceberg or we may be observing the largest dimension, uncertainty prevails again. Generally, we accept imprecision in measurement of tumor burden. This is usually accommodated by categorization such as in the AJCC and UICC stage groupings and the component tumor (T) and node (N) classifications. Even continuous or more complicated variables tend to be grouped into low, intermediate, and high risk for purposes of making treatment decisions.

Missing tumor that is or might be present is vexing or we would not have so many published studies or continue to be interested in investigating occult metastases. The fact that some studies of occult metastases have demonstrated prognostic significance, and others have not, has led us to question more carefully which tumor deposits are clinically significant. We now know that benign epithelium can be transported to axillary lymph nodes (15). It has also been demonstrated that disruption of the primary tumor can lead to progressive showering of sentinel lymph nodes with tumor cells and the frequency of nodal ITCs can be correlated with the aggressiveness of the prior biopsy procedure (16,17). Presumably, some of these detectable, showered tumor cells have no biological or clinical significance. Evidence for this can be found in the virtually nonexistent regional recurrence rates for patients with ductal carcinoma in situ and detectable occult tumor deposits in axillary lymph nodes (18). When we consider these observations, we are forced to accept that we cannot attribute prognostic significance to the mere presence of small tumor deposits in axillary or sentinel nodes; a complicated array of factors determine whether tumor cells are transported to a regional node and whether they will proliferate once present in the node. Most of these factors cannot be assessed with certainty.

DEFINING NODAL TUMOR BURDEN

Pathologically detected tumor may range from as small as a single cell to 1 or 2 cm with the average metastatic focus measuring 6.0 mm (19). Thus, the dynamic range of proven nodal tumor burden is 0.01 mm (single cells) to about 20 mm, a 2000-fold difference in maximum size. Prognostic segregation of the smallest from largest metastases was a logical improvement for classification. In 1971, Huvos et al. (2) observed that breast cancer patients with metastases no larger than 2.0 mm experienced no survival disadvantage when compared to patients with no nodal metastases detected. These smaller metastases were called micrometastases. Accordingly, metastases larger than 2.0 mm were referred to as macrometastases. Following this study, a footnote was added to the AJCC staging manuals indicating the relatively favorable prognosis when only micrometastases were detected. With the advent of sentinel node biopsy, it became easier to detect micrometastases. Compared to non-sentinel axillary nodes, metastases are four times more likely to be detected in sentinel nodes and occult micrometastases are 12 times more likely to be detected in sentinel nodes when similar detection strategies are employed for both sentinel and nonsentinel nodes (20). Hermanek et al. (21) suggested a new category of detectable tumor cell deposits that were extremely small and lacked the biological features typically associated with invasive tumors or metastases. They referred to these deposits as isolated tumor cells and cell clusters (or ITCs). The proposed biological features could not be reliably detected even in larger lymph node metastases and AJCC and UICC ultimately adopted a size criterion, 0.2 mm, to define the lower limit of micrometastases. Thus, nodal tumor deposits were divided into three logical categories: foci no larger than 0.2 mm (ITCs); foci larger than 0.2 mm but no larger than 2.0 mm (micrometastases); and foci larger than 2.0 mm (macrometastases). Note that there is approximately a 10-fold difference in maximum measurable dimension between the smallest and largest metastases in each category, whereas all three categories combined span a dynamic range from 0.02 mm (one to two cells) to 20 mm (a relatively large metastasis). The difference in tumor volume is even more profound as volume is proportional to the radius raised to the third power. For example, a single 0.2 mm tumor deposit occupies the same volume as 1000 cells each 0.02 mm in greatest dimension. Similarly, it would take 1000 deposits measuring 0.2 mm to equal the volume of a single 2.0 mm micrometastasis.

PANDORA'S OTHER BOX: OCCULT METASTASES

In 1948, the first study was published demonstrating that tumor deposits could be identified in paraffin-embedded tissue blocks of axillary lymph nodes that were initially interpreted as negative (22). These authors prepared additional histological sections from archived tissue and some sections revealed occult, or previously undetected, metastases. Following this initial study, many institutions have repeated the investigation. Most of the studies do not report the size of the occult metastases and all of the studies had no control of the initial lymph node evaluation, a critical flaw when attempting to make comparisons to current sentinel node biopsy. At the time, it was fairly common practice to sample nodes. Only a portion of the larger nodes would have been submitted for histological evaluation, whereas small nodes would probably have been submitted in their entirety. Often incorporated into these studies was a review of the initial diagnostic histological sections and as might be expected, some of these slides contained metastases that were overlooked on initial evaluation. In some instances, no distinction was made between metastases detected on original sections or those identified on newly prepared sections from deeper into the paraffin tissue blocks. Thus, two main categories of occult metastases exist: those that are missed during screening and those that are missed due to sampling. Published studies rarely stratified occult metastases according to size. However, in modern sentinel node research occult metastases can be further divided according to size. Occult ITCs, occult micrometastases, and occult macrometastases would be defined by superimposing our current staging size stratification. Each category can be further subdivided by examining whether the metastases were missed during screening or missed due to sampling.

The second wave of occult metastasis studies was driven by the introduction of immunohistochemistry (IHC) into the practice of pathology. Anti-cytokeratin antibodies or other anti-tumor-associated markers were employed to detect occult metastases. As a general rule, IHC stains detect metastases that are smaller than those identified by routine stains. It should be noted that pathologists are capable of identifying single cells on routinely stained sections; however, single cells and small clusters of cells will be more reliably, and frequently, detected when IHC is utilized. In other words, size of the tumor deposit is highly correlated but not perfectly correlated with detection by either IHC or routine stains.

What I have deliberately omitted from the discussion above is that these studies examined the clinical significance of occult metastases. The outcomes have been comprehensively reviewed elsewhere (23). As one would expect, or already knows, the results are mixed with some studies supporting a prognostic role and others failing to demonstrate clinical or statistical significance. Inconclusive results have been blamed on small study size, short follow-up, and as already mentioned, little or no documentation of occult metastasis size. Whatever the shortcomings in these studies, we can surmise that if a prognostic significance exists, it must be incrementally small compared to more easily obtainable prognostic factors of the era such as primary tumor size and larger, more easily detected nodal metastases. Further testimony to this conclusion can be found in the practical reaction of contemporary clinicians and pathologists: no change in pathological assessment of lymph nodes was adopted. The usual cited reasons are time and labor and the associated monetary expense.

The current interest in ITC clusters, micrometastases, and occult metastases is being driven by two factors: the vast majority of breast cancer patients present with negative lymph nodes and sentinel node biopsy focuses attention on the few nodes most likely to contain metastases. These two observations have created great interest in determining whether patients with occult micrometastases or ITCs may represent a group at higher risk of recurrence than patients with negative lymph nodes. In addition, IHC is widely available. The problem this creates stems from the mismatch between detection sensitivity on a microscopic slide and the ability to exclude disease based on the paraffin tissue block sampling strategy. CK IHC can detect single cells (0.01–0.02 mm) but we may be missing metastases as large as 1.0 to 2.0 mm within residual unexamined tissue in the paraffin block (Fig. 1). Pathologists are willing to sporadically find minimal disease but are unwilling to systematically exclude minimal disease because, not surprisingly, it takes too much time, labor, and expense.

I have learned several things from the retrospective literature on occult metastases. Not all lymph nodes reported as negative are actually negative. The more thoroughly a lymph node is examined, the higher the likelihood of detecting an occult tumor deposit. Some occult metastases are clinically significant; others are not. No study has demonstrated how to recognize which micrometastases are significant. In this respect, we end up back where we were 60 years ago: we know that occult metastases are present in "negative nodes"; we just do not know whether it is important to look for them. These are the main reasons why we need to control, or standardize, the lymph node evaluation, carefully document nodal tumor burden, and then collect high quality longitudinal outcome data.

TESTING THE SIGNIFICANCE OF MICROMETASTASES AND ISOLATED TUMOR CELL CLUSTERS

Ideally, this experiment would be performed on patients undergoing axillary dissection. Each lymph node identified would be entirely submitted for microscopic examination. Every tissue block would be entirely sectioned at 0.005 mm intervals. Every other section would be stained with anti-CK IHC. Patients would be stratified by primary tumor characteristics. Nodal tumor burden could then be quantified as a continuous variable. No agency would grant the money to pursue this project as the pathology and clinical data management would be far too expensive. For this reason, a sentinel node trial emerges as an attractive alternative because far fewer lymph nodes have to be evaluated. However, once we deviate from the ideal experiment, we are forced to rephrase our questions because of the inherent uncertainty in detecting minimal tumor burden when less than complete examination is performed.

Sentinel lymph node biopsy alone is being compared to axillary dissection in the National Surgical Adjuvant Breast and Bowel Project (NSABP) protocol B-32 (24). The primary endpoints are a comparison of axillary recurrence rates and overall survival between the two groups. Any patient with a positive node that had been randomized to sentinel node biopsy alone was subsequently treated with completion axillary dissection. The study cohort is 4000 node-negative patients. Half these women had an axillary dissection. An important component of the B-32 trial was prospective control over the pathological handling of sentinel nodes through a surgeon and site training program (25). Sentinel nodes were thinly sliced and totally embedded. Each tissue block was evaluated with a single routine microscopic section removed from the surface of the block. Routine use of IHC stains was prohibited but a pathologist could use IHC to evaluate suspicious findings on the routine stains. This assessment strategy creates two major groups of patients with respect to lymph node metastases. The first group has positive nodes and received, at some point in their surgical management, an axillary dissection. The second group has negative sentinel nodes or negative sentinel and axillary nodes. More accurately stated, the second group had no metastases detected utilizing the standard pathological assessment. Figure 1 is a depiction of these two groups [node-positive, left panels; node-negative (no metastases detected), right panels].

The tumor burden present in the node-positive group covers the full spectrum of expected disease from single tumor cells to large macrometastases. The precision of measurement for metastatic foci larger than 2.0 mm would be quite good considering that the nodes were sliced close to 2.0 mm intervals prior to being embedded in paraffin (Fig. 1, panel A above horizontal bar). However, measurement precision is considerably worse for tumor foci smaller than 2.0 mm for the same reasons discussed earlier. There is nearly 2.0 mm of unexamined tissue within the paraffin block implying that tumor foci as large as 2.0 mm could remain undetected. Our knowledge and precision is limited by the thickness of the unexamined tissue. We can quantify what has been identified but there is inherent imprecision in assessing minimal tumor burden.

Assessment of the tumor burden present in the "node-negative" group(s) is also imprecise and heterogeneous. The nodes may be truly negative, in which case no amount of additional evaluation will change the findings. However, because the same 2.0 mm of unexamined tissue remains in the paraffin block, a patient with no metastases detected (i.e., "node-negative") may in fact have undetected tumor foci as large as 2.0 mm (Fig. 1, panels F, G, and H). This translates to overlap in tumor burden between the "no metastases detected" group and the lower end of the node-positive spectrum where detected metastases are no larger than 2.0 mm. This uncertainty does not preclude comparing the difference in outcome between large groups of patients that fit within these tumor burden groups. The rules of statistical averages will prevail and the majority of patients in the "no metastases detected" group will in fact be node-negative. This should theoretically produce a better outcome than the statistical average of patients with minimal disease detected where no tumor deposit is larger than 2.0 mm. The real importance of this discussion is for the individual patient. For example, should a patient with no metastases detected be compared to the "node-negative" group, the isolated tumor cluster group, or the micrometastatic group? The uncertainty inherent in assessing the actual nodal tumor burden for a particular patient precludes precise comparison within the minimal nodal tumor burden groups.

At this point in time, we have no prospectively controlled outcome data to which we can compare modern patients undergoing sentinel node biopsy. When nodes are positive and the metastases are larger than 2.0 mm, we can compare with historical data. When nodes are negative or detected metastases are no larger than 2.0 mm, we can only assume that prognosis will lie between historical node-negative and node-positive patients. So, an important contribution that can be expected from a large trial such as B-32 will be an empiric assessment of absolute recurrence risk within some basic tumor (T) and node (N) classification groups in a cohort of patients undergoing sentinel node biopsy.

Assessment of outcome for sentinel node patients must be understood to be contingent upon the pathological evaluation strategy. The B-32 strategy followed a standard protocol that is virtually identical to that recommended by CAP and ASCO. That strategy was designed to detect virtually all metastases larger than 2.0 mm; some patients will have metastases detected that are smaller than 2.0 mm and some patients will have no metastases detected but we can be reasonably confident that these latter two groups do not contain patients with macrometastases larger than 2.0 mm. If a clinician or laboratory utilizes a different pathology evaluation strategy, then there would be a shift in the distribution of patients within the node (N) classification groups that would no longer be comparable. For example, routine use of IHC will shift patients out of the "no metastases detected" group and into the micrometastasis or ITC groups. These "new" groups of node-positive patients should have an outcome more favorable than the "old" stratification. Thus, the reference benchmark would need to be reassessed in yet another clinical trial setting with a large group of patients to establish new absolute outcome standards for the new evaluation strategy.

Many pathologists routinely employ additional sections and IHC stains in their assessment of sentinel lymph nodes. The extent of this practice has not been formally assessed in the United States but appears to be around 90% of laboratories in Europe (26). My own informal assessment during courses and lectures suggests 70% to 80% of labs perform an assessment "more comprehensive" than the recommendations with a slight decreasing trend more recently. It will be interesting to observe whether the ASCO recommendations further alter actual clinical practice. The B-32 protocol had anticipated the allure and potential clinical impact of a more comprehensive pathology evaluation. For sentinel node-negative patients, additional sections and anti-CK IHC stains are being evaluated. This experimental component of the study was clinically blinded; the results of the additional assessment did not influence clinical management. The standard B-32 assessment undoubtedly detected more nodal disease than historical clinical trials. Patients eligible for sentinel node trials must be clinically node-negative but also tend to have a slight selection bias towards more favorable tumors. Interestingly, the total patient accrual for B-32 had to be increased in order to obtain the target accrual of 4000 node-negative patients. The proportion of node-positive patients identified was slightly higher than anticipated suggesting conversion of patients with minimal nodal tumor burden from a historically node-negative patient group due to more comprehensive pathology assessment.

The additional experimental pathology evaluation for B-32 patients with negative sentinel nodes was designed to reassess the lymph nodes approximately 0.5 and 1.0 mm deeper into the paraffin block relative to the original surface (Fig. 2). Both routine and CK IHC stains were employed at each level. Providing

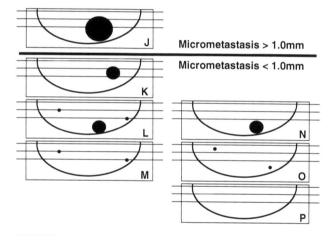

FIGURE 2 Potential node-positive and node-negative groups generated by the NSABP B-32 experimental protocol for occult metastases. Each panel represents a cross-section through paraffin-embedded tissue blocks containing a 2.0 mm-thick section of a bisected lymph node. The uppermost horizontal line represents the initial sampling performed for clinical management and is identical to the strategy in Figure 1. Note that all lymph nodes were initially reported as node-negative and virtually all metastases larger than 2.0 mm have already been detected. The second and third horizontal lines represent microscopic sections performed 0.5 mm and 1.0 mm deeper into the paraffin block. Approximately 1.0 mm of unexamined tissue may remain in the paraffin block. Tissue between the horizontal lines has been discarded without being examined. (**J–M**) The left panels represent lymph nodes with occult metastases detected. (**J**) Occult metastasis larger than 1.0 mm detected. This represents the exclusion threshold for this sampling strategy. (**K**) Occult metastasis smaller than 1.0 mm detected. (**L**) Occult ITC clusters detected and an occult metastasis smaller than 1.0 mm remains undetected. (**M**) Occult ITC clusters detected. (**N–P**) The right panels represent negative lymph nodes or, more accurately, nodes with no metastases detected using a sampling strategy that excludes occult metastases larger than 1.0 mm. (**N**) Metastasis smaller than 1.0 mm missed. (**O**) ITC clusters missed. (**P**) A true negative lymph node. Note that there is still considerable overlap between the occult node-positive and occult node-negative groups and that virtually all metastases larger than 1.0 mm have been detected.

that node slices were no thicker than 2.0 mm, this experimental protocol could leave as much as 1.0 mm of unexamined tissue within the block. The concept was to create new groups of patients within the "no metastases detected" population. The cutting protocol would identify all metastases larger than 1.0 mm, whereas the original strategy excluded patients with metastases larger than 2.0 mm. The potential occult metastasis groups include: metastases larger than 1.0 mm but no larger than 2.0 mm in greatest dimension; metastases no larger than 1.0 mm; and nodes with no metastases detected. Applying the same arguments as above, the latter group could have undetected metastases as large as 1.0 mm (Fig. 2, panel N). The addition of the 0.5 mm section from the block surface disturbs the purity of the sectioning interval but was done with purpose. Most sentinel nodes are bisected producing two hemi-ellipsoids that are then embedded in paraffin. By adding the intermediate section, a good deal more of the volume of the node has been sampled. This would tend to shift the maximum size of any missed metastases downward while enhancing the detection of metastases smaller than 0.5 mm. Despite the asymmetric sampling, the B-32 protocol should have some capacity to determine whether there is a difference in outcome for patients with micrometastases between 1.0 and 2.0 mm compared to patients with metastases no larger than 1.0 mm and to patients with no metastases detected. The other expected achievement will be to assign absolute recurrence and survival rates to these subgroups of "node-negative" patients with occult metastases detected within the context of the pathological evaluation. Any clinician or patient that desires to predict outcome based on the results of the B-32 patient subsets would have to employ the same pathological evaluation strategy for the sentinel nodes or the results would not be directly comparable.

THE FRUSTRATING REALITY OF MICROMETASTASES AND ISOLATED TUMOR CELL CLUSTERS

For me, one of the most frustrating aspects of micrometastasis research is the inability to create a continuous variable spanning the full spectrum of nodal disease from single cells to macrometastases. Hopefully, with adoption of systematic sampling strategies, we can shift the focus away from detection of the smallest tumor deposits to an emphasis on excluding disease above predetermined thresholds. With respect to providing useful information for our patients, it is far more helpful to be able to guarantee a patient we missed nothing larger than 2.0 mm than to proclaim we found a few tumor cell clusters in the subcapsular sinus. The immediate task is to determine whether we should be excluding 2.0, 1.0, 0.5 mm, or some smaller micrometastatic threshold. If readers find scientific fault with the arguments presented in this chapter, I can only hope this will stimulate further discussion and ultimately lead to an increased understanding of micrometastases as a prognostic and predictive factor.

In closing this chapter, it might be useful to restate some of its theses:

- Nodal tumor burden should be viewed as a continuum of disease that must be assessed together with primary tumor variables.
- The findings from the lymph node examination must be considered in the context of the pathological evaluation and its ability to exclude disease.
- The exclusion threshold is determined by the maximum thickness of unexamined tissue.

- Assessment of the clinical significance of pathologically detected disease that is below the exclusion threshold is confounded by the acknowledged presence of undetected disease of similar magnitude in the "node-negative" comparison group.
- It is virtually impossible to establish an absolute node-negative population for comparison.
- To identify minimal nodal tumor burden, we must remove the nodes thereby altering the natural history of the disease.
- Not all tumor deposits have progenitor capacity.
- Some detectable tumor deposits are iatrogenic.
- The biological potential of a tumor is established long before clinical detection.

All of these observations truly confound our ability to absolutely resolve the clinical significance of minimal nodal tumor burden. This is a clear call for standardizing pathological evaluation and reporting for sentinel nodes.

REFERENCES

1. Nemoto T, Vana J, Bedwani RN, et al. Management and survival of female breast cancer: results of a national survey by the American College of Surgeons. Cancer 1980; 45:2917–2924.
2. Huvos AG, Hutter RVP, Berg JW. Significance of axillary macrometastases and micrometastases in mammary cancer. Ann Surg 1971; 173:44–46.
3. Greene FL, Page DL, Fleming ID, et al. Breast AJCC Cancer Staging Manual. 6th ed. New York: Springer, 2002.
4. Sobin LH, Wittekind Ch, eds. UICC TNM Classification of Malignant Tumours. 6th ed. New York: John Wiley and Sons, 2002.
5. Singletary SE, Greene FL, Sobin LH. Classification of isolated tumor cells: clarification of the 6th edition of the American Joint Committee on Cancer Staging Manual. Cancer 2003; 98:2740–2741.
6. Al-Hajj M, Wicha MS, Benito-Hernandez A, Morrison SJ, Clarke MF. Prospective identification of tumorigenic breast cancer cells. Proc Natl Acad Sci USA 2003; 100:3547–3549.
7. Dontu G, Al-Hajj M, Abdallah WM, Clarke MF, Wicha MS. Stem cells in normal breast development and breast cancer. Cell Prolif 2003; 36(suppl 1):59–72.
8. Braun S, Cevatli BS, Assemi C, et al. Comparative analysis of micrometastasis to the bone marrow and lymph nodes of node-negative breast cancer patients receiving no adjuvant therapy. J Clin Oncol 2001; 19:1468–1475.
9. Fitzgibbons PL, Page DL, Weaver D, et al. Prognostic factors in breast cancer: College of American Pathologists Consensus Statement 1999. Arch Pathol Lab Med 2000; 124:966–978.
10. Lyman GH, Giuliano AE, Somerfield MR, et al. American Society of Clinical Oncology guideline recommendations for sentinel lymph node biopsy in early-stage breast cancer. J Clin Oncol 2005; 23(30):7703–7720.
11. Weaver DL. Sentinel lymph nodes and breast carcinoma: which micrometastases are clinically significant? Am J Surg Pathol 2003; 27:842–845.
12. Carter CL, Allen C, Henson D. Relation of tumor size, lymph node status, and survival in 24,740 breast cancer cases. Cancer 1989; 63:181–187.
13. Fisher E, Palekar A, Rockette H, Redmond C, Fisher B. Pathologic findings from the national surgical adjuvant breast project (Protocol No. 4): V. significance of axillary nodal micro- and macrometastases. Cancer 1978; 42:2032–2038.
14. Weaver DL. Pathological evaluation of sentinel lymph nodes in breast cancer: a practical academic perspective from America. Histopathology 2005; 46:702–706.
15. Carter BA, Jensen RA, Simpson JF, Page DL. Benign transport of breast epithelium into axillary lymph nodes after biopsy. Am J Clin Pathol 2000; 113:259–265.

16. Moore KH, Thaler HT, Tan LK, Borgen PI, Cody HS III. Immunohistochemically detected tumor cells in the sentinel lymph nodes of patents with breast carcinoma: biologic metastasis or procedural artifact? Cancer 2004; 100:929–934.

17. Hansen NM, Ye X, Grube BJ, Giuliano AE. Manipulation of the primary breast tumor and the incidence of sentinel node metastases from invasive breast cancer. Arch Surg 2004; 139:634–640.

18. Lara JF, Young SM, Velilla RE, Santoro EJ, Templeton SF. The relevance of occult axillary micrometastases in ductal carcinoma in situ: a clinicopathologic study with long-term follow-up. Cancer 2003; 98:2105–2113.

19. Michaelson JS, Silverstein M, Sgroi D, et al. The effect of tumor size and lymph node status on breast carcinoma lethality. Cancer 2003; 98:2133–2143.

20. Weaver DL, Krag DN, Ashikaga T, Harlow SP, O'Connell M. Pathologic analysis of sentinel and non-sentinel lymph nodes in breast carcinoma: a multicenter study. Cancer 2000; 88:1099–1107.

21. Hermanek P, Hutter RV, Sobin LH, Wittekind C. International Union against cancer. classification of isolated tumor cells and micrometastasis. Cancer 1999; 86:2668–2673.

22. Saphir O, Amromin GD. Obscure axillary lymph node metastases in carcinoma of the breast. Cancer 1948; 1:238–241.

23. Dowlatshahi K, Fan M, Snider HC, Habib FA. Lymph node micrometastases from breast carcinoma: reviewing the dilemma. Cancer 1997; 80:1188–1197.

24. Krag DN, Julian TB, Harlow SP, et al. NSABP-32: phase III randomized trial comparing axillary resection with sentinel lymph node dissection: a description of the trial. Ann Surg Oncol 2004; 11(suppl 3):208s–210s.

25. Harlow SP, Krag DN, Julian TB, et al. Prerandomization surgical training for the National Surgical Adjuvant Breast and Bowel Project (NSABP) B-32 trial: a randomized phase III clinical trial to compare sentinel node resection to conventional axillary dissection in clinically node-negative breast cancer. Ann Surg 2005; 241:48–54.

26. Cserni G, Amendoeira I, Apostolikas N, et al. Discrepancies in current practice of pathological evaluation of sentinel lymph nodes in breast cancer. Results of a questionnaire based survey of the European Working Group for Breast Screening Pathology. J Clin Pathol 2004; 57:695–701.

10 Molecular Subtypes in Breast Cancer Evaluation and Management: Divide and Conquer

Jeffrey Peppercorn, Charles M. Perou, and Lisa A. Carey
University of North Carolina, Chapel Hill, North Carolina, U.S.A.

INTRODUCTION

In the 19th century, the Scottish surgeon, Dr. Thomas Beatson, recognized that some, but not all, cases of advanced breast cancer would regress in response to "hormonal therapy," which he administered in 1896 through surgical removal of the ovaries (1). Though it was not recognized at the time, Dr. Beatson had produced the first evidence that, despite arising from the same anatomic area and having similar histological appearance, not all breast cancers were biologically the same. In the decades that followed, we have made many advances in breast cancer therapy but we have made inadequate progress in determining which patients are most likely to benefit from which therapies, and in identifying patients at highest risk for recurrence.

Standard clinical prognostic features such as patient age, tumor size, nodal status, grade, and endocrine receptor or HER2 status provide valuable information about risk of relapse, however, these clinical risk estimates are crude. For example, using a conventional mathematical model using clinical features (2), a low-risk cancer (less than 1 cm, node-negative, estrogen receptor-positive, and low grade occurring in a postmenopausal woman) will carry a 15% risk of recurrence, and a high-risk cancer (more than 5 cm, multimode-positive, estrogen receptor-negative, and high grade) will carry an 85% risk of recurrence. Thus, even in the most clinically compelling circumstances, conventional clinical prognosticators are inaccurate 15% of the time. As a result, many patients with early stage disease are treated with toxic therapies they may not need, and others are falsely reassured of a favorable prognosis based on clinical features that mask their true risk (3).

Recent evidence suggests that we can do better. Gene expression profiling, which allows simultaneous assessment of the contribution of thousands of genes in a single tumor sample, reveals a biological diversity in breast cancer that mirrors the clinical diversity in outcomes. This technique reveals that regardless of clinical features, breast cancers are several different diseases on the molecular level (4). Differences in behavior and response that seem random on the basis of known prognostic factors can be predicted by gene expression profiles that reclassify breast tumors into distinct subtypes, which should be viewed as distinct entities and managed as such. Microarray analysis of gene expression thus represents a valuable tool for assessing potential biological differences between breast cancers that may otherwise seem similar, to identify additional molecular differences between tumors with different histological characteristics, to assess the potential biological basis for commonly observed differences in outcome, and to develop better predictive models for determination of prognosis and response to therapy based on tumor biology.

This chapter explains how gene expression profiling has advanced our understanding of breast cancer biology, reviews the subtypes of breast cancer that have been identified through this new tool, and explores how these discoveries are helping us advance treatments for different classes of breast cancer. In addition, we identify some of the pitfalls of gene expression analysis and areas for future research in this field.

USE OF MICROARRAYS TO IDENTIFY BREAST CANCER SUBTYPES

Each mammalian somatic cell contains a full complement of DNA of the parent organism. Differentiation into specific tissues and cell types requires the variable expression of more than 25,000 genes contained in each cell. Using microarray technology, the relative level of expression of each gene can be determined for an individual tissue or cell type.

A gene expression microarray consists of nucleic acid sequences representing known genes fixed as either cDNA or oligonucleotide probes to a small platform or "chip" in discrete spots on a grid. A single microarray can represent thousands of distinct genes. Gene expression microarray analysis starts with purified RNA from a tumor sample and generates cDNA through reverse transcription typically using an oligo-dT primer. The sample cDNA is labeled with a fluorescent probe (red-Cy5), a reference cDNA is labeled with a different color (green-Cy3), and the two are mixed together and hybridized onto the microarray. After hybridization and washing, the microarray is scanned for the fluorescent signal and spots on the array will light up based on the amount of bound cDNA, indicating which genes from the sample were expressed and to what degree. If a particular gene or cluster of genes are over-expressed in the sample, that particular spot will appear more red; if under-expressed, the spot will appear more green.

Using microarrays as described earlier, the expression profile of a given tissue sample can be determined for genes of both known and unknown importance. Unlike traditional single-marker studies, examining genome-wide variations in expression provides a far more comprehensive, and accurate, depiction of the biology of a particular cell; moreover, it provides valuable data about the relationships between and among different genes. Given the surfeit of data that microarrays provide, the challenge becomes a meaningful analysis of massive amounts of information.

There are many methods to analyze differences in gene expression patterns between samples. In general, these involve statistical analyses to identify differentially expressed genes and to find patterns of co-expression (Fig. 1). Analysis of differential gene expression between tumor samples can be used to assess many different endpoints. For example, these can be used to evaluate differences between tumors from different patients, to identify differences between tumors that relapse or not, or to characterize patterns that predict outcomes of interest. The gene expression analyses for these different purposes have been labeled: "class discovery," "class comparison," and "class prediction" (5,6).

"Class discovery" is the most basic level of exploration in which a population of seemingly similar samples is analyzed in an unsupervised manner to determine if there are differences on the basis of genetic expression that can be used to subclassify the samples on a molecular basis. For example, a class discovery experiment

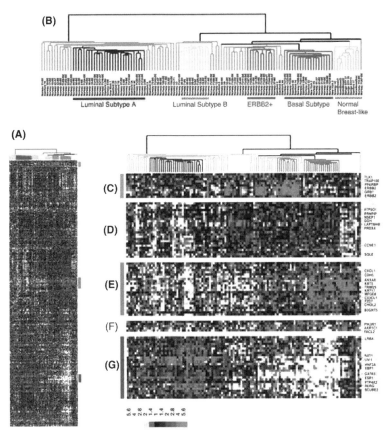

FIGURE 1   Gene expression array of breast cancer tumor samples. *Source*: From Ref. 8.

could take tumor samples from 50 consecutive breast cancer patients, determine gene expression for each sample using microarray technology as described earlier, and then use statistical tools to divide the samples into subgroups based on similarities in gene expression. Whether these groupings would have clinical significance needs to be determined by further study. In contrast, class comparison studies start with two or more groups defined by clinically meaningful endpoints, such as whether the patients did or did not develop metastatic disease, or did or did not respond to a particular therapy. The genetic expression patterns of these two groups can then be compared to determine if there is a potential biological basis for the clinical difference, and, if so, determine which genes or gene groups appear to be involved. It is important to recognize that identification of gene expression differences at this level does not mean that the genes in question caused the differential outcomes. "Class prediction" refers to the ability of a gene profile to assign an individual tumor to a particular category, for example, a particular subtype or outcome. Since the classes are already identified, class prediction often requires far fewer genes than class discovery.

BREAST CANCER MOLECULAR SUBTYPES

Unsupervised analysis and class discovery have identified several subtypes of breast cancer that differ systematically from one another and that may be considered as individual diseases under the umbrella term of "breast cancer." Given the diversity in breast cancer outcomes that is incompletely explained by known prognostic factors, and the phenotypic diversity in biological factors such as histological grade, estrogen receptor (ER) status, progesterone receptor (PgR) status, and HER2/*neu* expression (HER2), it made sense to apply newly developed gene expression techniques to breast cancer samples to study the extent to which genetic diversity explained these differences. These studies revealed that not only do differences in gene expression lead to predictable differences in phenotypic and clinical features, but also that gene expression patterns among tumors group them in a way which suggests that breast cancer is more than one discrete disease.

Initial evidence for molecular subtypes of breast cancer came from a cDNA-microarray study of gene expression among a small number of tumor samples and several benign controls. In 2000, Perou et al. (4) compared gene expression among 42 subjects consisting of 36 invasive ductal carcinomas, two invasive lobular carcinomas, one ductal carcinoma in situ, one fibroadenoma, and three normal breast biopsies. This study included 20 matched samples from the same tumor, and two matched samples from primary tumor and lymph node metastasis from the same patient. Starting with analysis of over 8000 genes, a subset of 1753 was selected based on expression levels that differed by at least four-fold across all samples. Based on these genes, computer-assisted hierarchical clustering was performed to group samples with similar patterns of expression.

Analysis of groups with similar expression patterns led to several interesting observations. First, expression patterns among matched-pair samples from the same patient revealed that differences between two different tumors were far greater than differences observed from two samples from the same tumor. In this small sample, this held true even when comparing a paired tumor and lymph node metastasis. To some extent, this validated the theory that gene expression was revealing meaningful information about the underlying biology of the tumor as opposed to random fluctuations in expression. Secondly, grouping the tumors based on 496 genes that demonstrated the greatest variation between tumors from different patients compared to samples from the same patient (termed the "intrinsic" gene set), two of the subgroups had expression patterns similar to the expression pattern of components of the normal breast epithelium, specifically basal and luminal epithelial cells. It is believed that the "basal-like" and "luminal" breast cancer subtype expression patterns reflect different cells of origin, however, further experimentation is needed to address this point. Regardless, these two groups correspond to tumors that had been clinically classified as merely ER-positive or ER-negative. The molecular profiles of these subtypes made much clearer the extent of the biological differences that separate ER-positive and ER-negative breast cancer (Table 1). Two other groups of tumors were also identified. One was characterized by strong HER2 expression and low expression of ER and its related genes. The other group displayed a genetic expression profile most similar to normal breast tissue and remains enigmatic.

Based on these findings, Perou et al. (4) proposed a novel molecular classification of breast cancer into basal-like, luminal, HER2-positive, and normal breast subgroups. In subsequent work by the same group, this classification was refined

TABLE 1   Breast Cancer Subtypes

Characteristic genes	IHC markers	Clinical features
Basal-like		
Keratin 5 and 17	ER-negative	High grade
Laminin	PgR-negative	More common among pre-menopasual African American women
Fatty acid binding protein 7	HER2-negative	Strong association with BRCA1 mutation carriers
P-Cadherin	CK5/6-positive	Higher risk of recurrence
TRIM29	Often EGFR-positive	Responsive to chemotherapy
	Ki-67 high	No known targeted treatment
HER2+/ER−		
HER2/c-erb B2	ER-negative	Usually high grade
GRB7	PgR-negative	More likely to have involved axillary lymph nodes at presentation
	HER2-positive	Higher risk of recurrence
	Ki-67 usually high	Responsive to chemotherapy
		Responsive to anti-HER2 antibody trastuzumab and EGFR/HER2 tyrosine kinase inhibitor lapatinib
Normal breast-like		
Adipose tissue enriched pattern		Potentially due to normal tissue contamination
Luminal B		
ER cluster	ER-positive and/or PgR-positive	Variable grade
Proliferation genes	Sometimes HER2-positive	Variable response to chemotherapy
	Ki-67 high compared to luminal A	Usually responsive to endocrine therapy including selective estrogen receptor modulators and aromatase inhibition
		If HER2+, responsive to anti-HER2 strategies
Luminal A		
ER alpha	ER+ and/or PgR+, HER2−	Most common form of breast cancer
GATA binding protein 3	Ki-67 low	Usually low grade
X-box binding protein 1		Lower risk of recurrence
Trefoil factor 3		Responsive to endocrine therapy
FOXA1		Often less responsive to chemotherapy
LIV-1		

Abbreviations: ER, estrogen receptor; PgR, progesterone receptor.
Source: From Ref. 7.

and expanded to distinguish between luminal A and luminal B tumor subtypes (7). Using 85 microarrays based on 78 tumors, three fibroadenomas, and four normal breast samples, they evaluated the expression of the same intrinsic genes and again grouped the samples based on hierarchical clustering analysis (Fig. 1). The five distinct subtypes of breast cancer were again identified: basal-like, HER2, normal breast-like, luminal A, and luminal B and C. Luminal B and C may be distinct subtypes but clustered differently in the test and validation data sets and had insufficiently overlapping genetic expression to warrant separate classification. The five molecular subtypes identified by Perou and Sorlie have been confirmed in independent data sets from other investigators (8) and among different ethnic groups of patients (9). The same subtypes have also been identified in inflammatory breast cancer (10). Gene expression subtype remains consistent between primary tumors and metastatic lesions from those tumors, even those that develop years later (11).

This molecular subclassification of breast cancer is based on an analysis of the gene expression patterns of a relatively small number of cancers. These distinct subtypes were also identified by high-throughput protein expression analysis using over 1000 cases of invasive breast cancer (12). In this study, 26 immunohistochemical (IHC) markers were assessed for each of 1076 tumor samples and hierarchical clustering analysis was conducted to group tumors based on IHC characteristics. Six clusters of tumors were identified, roughly corresponding to the five subtypes previously identified, and one small new group consisting of only four tumor samples. Key histological markers that differed significantly between tumor types included androgen receptor, HER2, cytokeratin 18, MUC1, Cytokeratin 5/6, p53, nuclear BRCA1, ER, and E-cadherin. This large study lends additional support to the identification of luminal A, luminal B, normal-like, HER2-positive, and basal-like cancers as discrete biological entities.

Although the gold standard for identifying breast cancer subtypes remains gene expression array analysis, this method currently requires frozen tissue, although the intrinsic gene list identifying breast cancer subtypes has recently been adapted for use across microarray platforms (13). IHC profiles for the breast cancer subtypes have been developed in fixed tissue. Exhaustive immunophenotyping on a large tissue microarray identified several luminal and basal profiles (12). Luminal breast cancers are typically positive for hormone receptors, although there currently is no accepted immunostain to separate the various luminal subtypes. The HER2+/ER- subtype over-expresses HER2 and has low to no hormone receptor expression. Nielsen et al. (14) categorized the IHC profile of basal-like breast cancers, and found that the profile of ER- and HER2-negative and either cytokeratin 5/6- or EGFR-positive was 76% sensitive and 100% specific. A slightly less accurate but reasonable proxy for basal-like breast cancers remains the "triple negative" phenotype of ER-negative, PgR-negative, and HER2-negative, of which approximately 80% to 90% are basal-like (unpublished data).

GENETIC AND ENVIRONMENTAL ASSOCIATIONS WITH BREAST CANCER SUBTYPES

Much work has gone into identifying genetic and environmental risk factors for breast cancer. Based on the recognition that breast cancer is more than one disease, it is possible that different risk factors may contribute to the development of different types of breast cancer.

One of the clearest examples of this phenomenon is the predisposition for basal-like breast cancers among carriers of BRCA1 genetic mutations. Patients with BRCA1 mutations are at high (up to 80%) lifetime risk for developing breast cancer (15). It has long been known that breast cancer arising in BRCA1 mutation carriers possess certain characteristics including ER-negativity, HER2-negativity, and certain histological characteristics (16). It has also become clear that when patients with inherited BRCA1 mutations develop breast cancer, it is virtually always basal-like (8,17–19). The reason for this segregation has not been determined, however, sporadic basal-like breast cancers also may have decreased expression of BRCA1 even though somatic BRCA1 mutations are rare (12). In addition, the basal-like subtype appears to be more common among African American women, particularly premenopausal African American women (20). Indirect evidence of an increased prevalence of the basal-like subtype of breast cancer was observed in among participants in the Women's Health Initiative, which found that African American women who develop breast cancer were more likely than white women to develop high grade ER-negative cancers. In this population-based observational study, incidence of breast cancer was evaluated among 156,570 women. Although breast cancer was less common among African American women, when cancer did develop, 32% of tumors were both high grade and ER-negative compared to 10% among white women. In multivariate analysis including age, body mass index, hormonal therapy use, socioeconomic factors and ethnicity, ethnicity remained highly predictive of these tumor characteristics (21).

Carey et al. (20) evaluated the prevalence of breast cancer subtypes among participants in the Carolina Breast Cancer Study, a population-based, case–control study of women between 20 and 74 with breast cancer designed to assess differences in breast cancer based on race and age. Breast cancer subtypes were defined based on IHC surrogates. Among 496 evaluable subjects, the basal-like phenotype was present in 39% of premenopausal African American women compared to 14% of postmenopausal African American women, and 16% of non-African American women with breast cancer. This confirmed earlier findings of an increased percentage of ER– and PgR-negative tumors among African American patients with breast cancer compared to white patients (22) and extends this observation to note that only the basal-like subtype appears to differ by race and age; the other major ER-negative subtype, the HER2+/ER– subtype, did not differ.

There may also be differences in environmental risks for development of different subtypes of breast cancer. Much of the evidence at this time is indirect and based on observed differences by hormone receptor status. For example, large epidemiological studies suggest that the risk factors for ER-negative breast cancers, which are comprised primarily of basal-like and HER2-subtypes, differ from those of ER-positive, or luminal breast cancers. Investigators from the Nurses' Health Study have found that the traditional hormonal risk factors are far more useful in predicting ER-positive breast cancer than ER-negative (23) and hormone replacement therapy is associated only with increases in ER-positive breast cancer (24). Chemoprevention with the selective estrogen receptor modulator tamoxifen reduces only ER-positive breast cancer (25). Alcohol consumption appears to correlate with increased risk of development of ER-positive, but not ER-negative tumors in some studies (26). Conversely, diet quality, particularly in vegetable intake, has been associated with ER-negative breast cancer risk (27). Long-term aspirin use has been correlated with decreased risk of ER positive tumors and increased risk of ER negative tumors (28). Folate use appears to be associated with decreased risk of ER negative tumors only (29). Whether these associations reflect causality and whether they truly correlate with molecular subtype has not yet been established. Given the biologically distinct nature of the different breast cancer subtypes, future evaluation of genetic and environmental breast cancer risks will need to address breast cancer risk factor assessment within, rather than across, subtypes.

GENE EXPRESSION PROFILES, CLINICAL CHARACTERISTICS, AND BREAST CANCER OUTCOMES

Differences in breast cancer outcomes have been attributed, in part, to differences in clinical factors such as tumor size and lymph node status that may relate to the timing of cancer detection as well as to cancer biology (30). The importance of cancer biology in the determination of outcome has been recognized by attention to histological grade, ER, PgR, and HER2. However, to a large extent, breast cancer has been viewed as a single disease, with variable features that may affect treatment and outcome. These factors do not sufficiently explain differences in outcomes, particularly among tumors that are ER-positive or intermediate grade.

In addition to the associations with race and age mentioned earlier, several tumor characteristics vary by subtype. In the population-based Carolina Breast Cancer Study, which defined the subtypes using IHC profiles that included ER, PgR, and HER2, there was no significant difference among subtypes in overall stage at presentation; however, there were marginally significant differences ($P = 0.04$) in the proportions with involved lymph nodes, with highest proportions among the HER2+/ER− (56%), followed by luminal B (47%), basal-like (41%), and luminal A (34%) (20). Infiltrating lobular carcinomas were exclusively seen among the luminal subtypes, although remained the minority comprising only 7–12%. A far more striking difference was seen in the proportions with high-grade tumors. For example, high mitotic index was seen in 87% of basal-like breast cancers, 69% of HER2+/ER−, but only 31% and 32% of luminal A and luminal B tumors, respectively. Adjusting for the other relevant variables and compared with the referent luminal A subtype, the HER2+/ER− subtype remained 2.2-fold more likely to have involved lymph nodes, 6.8-fold more likely to have marked nuclear pleomorphism, and 4.3-fold more likely to have high mitotic index. The basal-like subtype was not more likely to have involved lymph nodes, however, remained 9.7-fold more likely to have marked nuclear pleomorphism, 2.5-fold more likely to be poorly differentiated, and 11.0-fold more likely to have a high mitotic index. The luminal B subtype differed little from the luminal A in clinical characteristics, other than a higher (1.7-fold) likelihood of lymph node involvement.

Discovery of biologically distinct subtypes of breast cancer raised the question of whether these subtypes could explain the diversity of cancer behavior seen in clinical practice. To address this question, Sorlie and Perou conducted a univariate analysis of correlation between molecular subtype using gene expression array and overall survival based on the five subtypes of breast cancer identified in gene expression studies (7). They examined relapse-free and overall survival among a subset of 49 locally advanced tumors treated with doxorubicin monotherapy. With a median follow-up of 66 months, both relapse-free and overall survival differed significantly among the different breast cancer subtypes. The basal-like and HER2+/ER− subtypes had the shortest survival times and luminal A tumors the longest, with luminal B having an intermediate prognosis. This association of subtype with outcome has been confirmed in independent datasets using gene expression array and those investigators' intrinsic gene list (8). Using a panel of gene probes derived independently from those of Sorlie, Perou and colleagues, although with significant overlap, Sotiriou et al. (31) studied gene expression among 99 cases of both node-negative and node-positive invasive breast cancer and performed hierarchical clustering analysis. They again identified several subtypes demonstrating luminal or basal characteristics. The breast cancer subtype correlated significantly with survival, with superior survival for the luminal subtypes compared to basal tumors. Once again, ER status was found to correlate strongly with gene expression profile as did tumor grade. There was little correlation between expression profile and lymph node status, tumor size, or menopausal status. Studies using IHC profiling using either a large panel of antibodies (12) or a simpler intrinsic gene list-driven selection of markers (20) have found similar associations with outcome. Interestingly, some studies suggest that in addition to variability in likelihood of metastasis, the site of metastasis may vary with subtype, with basal-like more prone to visceral involvement, particularly of the lung (32,33).

Differences in outcomes that have been linked to demographic factors such as age or ethnicity, may partly be related to the differential representation of breast cancer subtypes among these populations. In other words, it may not be the race or age of a patient that conveys a bad prognosis but the fact that younger and African American patients are more likely to develop the basal-like subtype of breast cancers. As noted earlier, African American ethnicity has been associated with tumor features typical of the basal-like subtype, particularly among premenopausal women, which may in part explain poor cancer outcomes compared to those for white women (20–22). The contribution of biology to long recognized risk factors for poor outcomes is further supported by the finding that basal-like tumors were more common among younger patients, of any ethnicity, when analyzed by tissue microarray (12).

Tumor biology as reflected by gene expression appears to be an independent predictor of outcome (12). Genomics technology has also been used to develop pure prognostic panels that have been applied across subtypes. Other groups have sought to use gene expression to identify a limited set of genes correlated with a particular clinical outcome, such as recurrence, which could then be used clinically to guide decision-making. This work will be discussed in detail in a subsequent chapter but reviewed briefly here in light of associations with the breast cancer subtypes.

Researchers in the Netherlands have developed a 70-gene prognostic profile that correctly classifies 90% of tumors destined to recur within five years (19). The expression pattern of these 70 genes was shown to be a strong predictor of both distant disease-free survival and overall survival, and the "poor prognosis" signature, a stronger predictor of metastatic disease than any of the classical clinical criteria (34). Similarly, investigators from Rotterdam have developed a 76-gene prognostic profile that was recently validated in an independent group of node-negative, largely hormone receptor-positive breast cancers (35). Interestingly, the 70-gene and 76-gene prognosticators remain prognostic in multivariate analyses, but have little overlap in the genes they have identified. Paik et al. (36) identified another set of 16 genes out of a group of 250 candidate genes that correlated with prognosis in several clinical trials, including one large homogenous sample of ER-positive, node-negative tumors treated with tamoxifen in a trial from the cooperative group NSABP, trial B-20. This 16-gene model, called the Recurrence Score, was validated in tumor samples from an independent large prospective trial of patients with hormone receptor-positive, node-negative tumors treated with adjuvant tamoxifen on NSABP B-14. These studies illustrate the challenges of determining gene expression profiles of clinical importance either to predict outcomes or to identify drug targets. To some extent, the discrepancies in identified genes may reflect variations in patient population, ascertained tumors, or technical variations in array technology. An even more likely contributor is that common molecular pathways, such as apoptosis or cell cycle regulation, may involve many genes and the identification of any genes whose expression is important in this pathway may provide similar information in terms of prognosis.

Supporting data comes from comparison of several of these well-established prognostic panels with breast cancer subtypes. Using RNA from a 295-patient dataset with known clinical outcomes, investigators at the University of North Carolina compared the "Wound Response" prognostic model (37), the 70-gene prognostic profile (19,34), the 2-gene expression ratio profile (38), and a model replicating the 16 genes of the Recurrence Score (36) for their ability to predict recurrence and with the known breast cancer intrinsic subtypes (39). The Recurrence Score and 2-gene ratio predictors were designed only for ER-positive patients, and therefore, were tested on the 225 ER+ patients from the dataset and on all 295 patients. The investigators found that all models except the 2-gene ratio provided significant accuracy for estimating recurrence risk, and provided prognostic information that was independent of classical factors. Classification of tumors into high-risk and low-risk groups by the 70-gene model and the 16 genes used in the Recurrence Score were identical in 81% of all cases, even though the models overlap by only one gene (39) As before, the intrinsic subtypes also provided independent prognostic information. Comparison of the prognostic profiles by subtype was intriguing. There were 53 basal-like and 35 HER2+/ER− tumors in the dataset; in these subtypes over 90% had high Recurrence Scores, "poor prognosis" 70-gene signatures, were wound response "activated." Fifty-five luminal B tumors similarly gave fairly uniform poor prognosis signatures, 50 (91%) had high Recurrence Scores, 46 (84%) had poor 70-gene signatures, and 51 (93%) were wound response-activated. The group with the greatest disparity in prognostic profiles was the luminal A subtype. Of 123 tumors with this subtype, 36 (29%) had high Recurrence Scores and poor 70-gene signatures, and 78 (63%) had activated wound response signatures. This study is reassuring in that multiple disparate array-based molecular prognostic assays appear to be capturing similar biological information and are making similar outcome predictions. Among poor-prognosis subtypes such as the HER2+/ER−, basal-like, and luminal B, these assays do not provide additional information, suggesting that new assays that can prognosticate within these groups might be useful. For patients with the luminal A intrinsic groups, the Recurrence Score, 70-gene, and wound-response assays did appear to provide additional information that could be used to guide treatment decisions.

THERAPEUTIC IMPLICATIONS OF BREAST CANCER SUBTYPES

The discovery of molecular subclasses of breast cancer provides further evidence that the biological diversity of breast cancer denies a one-size-fits-all approach to therapy. Existing knowledge of the biology of breast cancer provides crude clues to therapy: luminal cancers are generally hormone receptor-positive and appropriate for endocrine therapy; the HER2+/ER− subtypes is HER2-driven and appropriate for HER2-targeted therapy such as trastuzumab. Beyond this, the power of gene expression analysis and subclassification of breast cancer to answer the questions of response to therapy is only beginning to be evaluated.

Work in this area can be divided into three broad areas: efforts to understand differences in response to therapy based on recognized therapeutic targets such as ER, PgR, and HER2; efforts to identify gene expression signatures that predict response or resistance to specific therapies; and efforts to identify novel targets within breast cancer subtypes. Increasingly, ER, PgR, and HER2 status are being recognized as both molecular targets and, as discussed earlier, surrogates for identification of specific subtypes of breast cancer. In this chapter, we will review efforts to correlate response to molecular subtypes defined by gene expression or these IHC (or FISH in the case of HER2) surrogate markers. Specific gene expression signatures for response will be discussed in a subsequent chapter.

Understanding of the response to chemotherapy based on breast cancer subtype begins with the recognition that ER-positive and ER-negative tumors respond differently to chemotherapy. In a meta-analysis of the efficacy of chemotherapy for early stage breast cancer among 145,000 women, the Early Breast Cancer Trialists' Group found that the benefit of chemotherapy in ER-poor disease was approximately twice that of ER-positive disease (40). Neoadjuvant studies demonstrate that ER-positive tumors are less responsive to chemotherapy (41,42), and that advances in chemotherapy effectiveness benefit the ER-negative subtypes more than ER-positive (43). These data emphasize the importance of evaluating response in chemotherapy trials mindful of endocrine receptor status, and the degree to which important differences in therapy for one type of breast cancer could be obscured by lesser degrees of response among a different tumor type. It seems likely that ER status serves as a marker for subtype of breast cancer with an underlying biology that is either more or less responsive to particular types of chemotherapy, rather than the estrogen receptor itself playing a major role in response to chemotherapy.

There have been few studies of response to therapy based directly on molecular subtype as determined by gene expression, but those reported to date suggest that the basal-like and HER2-positive tumor types (which happen to be primarily ER negative) are more responsive to chemotherapy than luminal breast cancer subtypes (44,45). Rouzier and colleagues evaluated response to neoadjuvant therapy among tumors in 82 patients by fine needle aspirate and determined molecular subtypes based on gene expression analysis. All patients were treated with 12 weeks of paclitaxel followed by four cycles of 5-flourouracil, doxorubicin, and cyclophosphamide. Surgery was performed after 24 weeks of neoadjuvant therapy and patients were evaluated for complete pathological response (pCR). Among the 22 patients with basal-like tumors and the 20 patients with HER2 tumors, the pCR rates were both 45%, whereas among 30 patients with luminal tumors only 6% attained a pCR. Among 10 patients with normal-like tumors there were no pCR (44). Importantly, the authors also evaluated prediction of response based on molecular subtype classification versus grade, ER status, and HER2 status and found that the predictive ability of molecular subtype was equivalent to, but not superior to the use of these factors currently available in clinical practice (44). The varying relationship of chemotherapy response to outcome by subtype was examined in a study that used ER, PgR, and HER2 immunophenotype as surrogates for the breast cancer subtypes (45) Among 107, largely stage III patients treated with neoadjuvant doxorubicin and cyclophosphamide, pCR was seen in 36% of HER2+/ER− patients, 26% of basal-like patients, and 8% of luminal patients. Despite the lower rates of response to therapy, disease-free survival was still better for patients with luminal tumors, most of whom went on to receive endocrine-based adjuvant therapy. Interestingly, the poorer outcome among basal-like and HER2+/ER− tumors was due to a significantly higher risk of early relapse among patients who did not achieve pCR. A larger study examining hormone receptor status only also found a higher pCR among ER-negative tumors despite poorer outcome. Within hormone receptor subsets, however, the relationship of pCR to outcome was maintained (42). These studies illustrate the need to account for varying subtype proportions when comparing pCR statistics across trials.

More work needs to be done in this area to identify which regimens are most effective in which breast cancer subtypes. Those tumor types predicting greatest risk for recurrence appear most responsive to chemotherapy, justifying a more aggressive approach to use of chemotherapy in these patients. Intriguing preclinical studies have suggested that the same chemotherapy agents may have differential mechanisms of action in different breast cancer subtypes (46). Strategies exploiting such biological variability may provide therapeutic approaches in the future.

Recognition of the existence and importance of molecular subtypes of breast cancer can also lead to improved insights into the biology of these tumor types and identification of single genes, clusters of genes, or molecular pathways responsible for clinical behavior of a given tumor. Such identification can lead to targeted therapy. Recognition of the importance of HER2 for tumor behavior preceded recognition of the so-called HER2+/ER− subtype of breast cancer. HER2-driven breast cancer provides an example of a tumor subtype with unique biology that has been successfully targeted for therapeutic intervention. The development of trastuzumab, a monoclonal antibody against HER2, and its proven effectiveness against metastatic and early stages of HER2 positive breast cancer, serves as an example of how outcomes for patients can be transformed by recognition of the underlying biological processes responsible for tumor behavior and targeting of those processes. More recent studies have successfully employed combined EGFR/HER2-targeted strategies in trastuzumab-resistant breast cancer, suggesting that combined blockade strategies using biological agents may prove to be the future of therapy in this subtype (47,48).

A major challenge, currently, is to identify such targets for the basal-like subtype of breast cancer, which is not responsive to endocrine therapy or trastuzumab. Identification of the basal-like subtype has allowed us to make some observations about this form of breast cancer, but we have not yet identified the specific genes that drive the behavior of this tumor in the way that ER does for luminal tumors or HER2 for the HER2+/ER− subtype. As noted earlier, basal-like tumors are commonly seen in BRCA1 carriers (8,17,18) and the BRCA1 pathway may also be involved in sporadic basal-like tumors (12). Some authors suggest that aberrant BRCA1 function in DNA repair and cell cycle checkpoint responses may alter sensitivity to particular cytotoxic chemotherapy agents with sensitivity to DNA damaging agents and resistance to spindle poisons (49). Regarding targeted options in this subtype, although none have yet been clinically proven some preclinical studies suggest that this subtype may be EGFR-driven (14,50,51). Several therapeutic strategies already exist for EGFR-driven cancers, including cetuximab, gefititnb, or erlotinib. It is possible, however, that the mechanisms driving proliferation in these tumors may require a combined blockade approach (52).

Another potential target in basal-like breast cancer is c-kit, which is over-expressed in up to 31% of basal-like breast cancers. However, the activating kit mutation that conveys sensitivity to imatinib, has not been seen among breast cancers over-expressing c-Kit (53). Imatinib was not effective in a single phase II study conducted among unselected patients with metastatic breast cancer (54), but whether this strategy might be more successful within the basal-like subtype has not yet been tested. The importance of selecting patients appropriately for clinical trials of targeted therapy based on the presence and/or over-expression of the specified target cannot be overemphasized. Depending on the prevalence of over-expression of the target in the broader population of breast cancer patients, an effective therapy among a subgroup of patients could be abandoned due to poor trial design. Identification of additional potential molecular targets among basal-like breast cancers will be crucial to improving outcomes for patients with this distinct form of cancer.

PROBLEMS WITH GENE EXPRESSION ANALYSIS METHODOLOGY

Despite the promise of this technology, the methods currently required for processing samples and determining molecular subclass based on gene expression analysis are relatively complicated and work intensive compared to standard pathological analysis of breast cancer samples. Due to the requirement for tissue samples, the gene expression studies discussed earlier are based on small cohorts of patients (55). Prospective collection of tissue specimens in banks for future research will be an important component of advancing research in this area. Increasingly, such samples are being collected in breast cancer clinical trials, and the information from these samples should prove valuable in assessing outcome and response based on subclass, and addressing other questions related to tumor gene expression.

In addition to the problem of small sample sizes, the reproducibility of gene expression patterns is a potential problem in this field. Different methods of tissue processing can yield different patterns of gene expression (55). An attempt at supervised analysis to predict a response to tamoxifen therapy found the expression of different genes to be different depending upon whether the sample was obtained by laser capture microdissection or whole tissue processing (38). Such variation may be more of a problem for attempts to define a specific small subset of genes that predict an outcome of interest compared with efforts to predict outcome or response to therapy based on molecular subtype as defined by expression of hundreds of genes (56). The current requirement for frozen tissue is likely to be solved soon where efforts at developing gene expression predictors are underway and promising that utilize other platforms and technologies (13,36).

Additional problems arise from the complicated statistical methods required to analyze gene expression. One of the potential problems arises from statistical methods that do not adequately account for similarities in gene expression based on chance alone that can lead to spurious classification of samples or alternatively, important connection may be missed. Simon et al. (57) has noted that for class prediction studies, a small number of genes may be relevant for the outcome of interest, but these genes may not adequately be taken into account by commonly used methods of unsupervised cluster analysis. They argue that supervised analysis which assigns different weights to individual genes based on their discriminative ability may be more useful, provided any model is then tested against an independent sample for validation (57). Methods to improve predictive models include thorough cross-validation from within a dataset and external validation against a large independent test dataset (57). It is important to note that connections between subclasses with low correlation coefficients may not be reliable, in contrast to correlations within groups (7). Predictive models that have been proposed without rigorous statistical evaluation or external validation should be seen as hypothesis generating only, and not sufficiently proven to affect clinical practice.

FUTURE RESEARCH

The recognition of molecular subtypes of breast cancer based on gene expression analysis creates opportunities and challenges for future clinical research. Clinical trials must be designed to evaluate results among patients with different subtypes of breast cancer. Increasingly, clinical trials may be designed to target specific subtypes such as trials among HER2-positive patients or basal-like patients only. Such trials can identify activity of novel agents and regimens among these subgroups that might be obscured in a trial including all patients with breast cancer. However, the challenge will be to recruit sufficient number of patients with the less frequent subtype in question. This will likely require increased collaboration between multiple centers, and cooperative group studies targeting the different subtypes of breast cancer. In reality, the current understanding of breast cancer subtypes is the first generation of such studies; ongoing efforts will doubtless refine our understanding of subtypes within the categories already identified. Hopefully, increasingly sophisticated understanding of biological pathways at play in individual tumors will allow for truly tailored therapy in the future.

In addition, the techniques of gene expression analysis discussed above are currently quite cumbersome. Improved techniques are needed, so that molecular subtypes of breast cancer can readily be identified in the clinic and this information can be used to guide discussions of prognosis and management decisions. This may involve development of gene array chips that can be processed rapidly in standard pathology labs or refined use of IHC surrogates that reliably differentiate molecular subtypes. One of the most important avenues of research to emerge from this work will be the identification of individual genes or groups of genes that drive cancer pathogenesis for the different subtypes. Evaluating single genes or groups of genes can lead to better understanding of the biology of cancer and may identify therapeutic targets or means of monitoring response to therapy.

Finally, recognition of the molecular subtypes should allow us to better understand the relationship between genetic and environmental causes of cancer leading to improvements in cancer detection and prevention. As with response to therapy, an environmental risk for one subtype of cancer could be obscured in a study evaluating the relationship between that risk factor and all breast cancers.

SUMMARY

Gene expression profiling has revealed that breast cancer is more than one disease. The molecular classification of breast cancer into luminal A, luminal B, normal-like, HER2+/ER-positive, and basal-like provides important prognostic information and can guide decision-making regarding therapy. The biology of breast cancer as determined by gene expression adds powerful information to understanding behavior, therapeutic responses, and outcome. Future studies should focus upon identifying individual genes and pathways that determine the behavior of these distinct tumor types, both to better understand tumor biology and to identify potential targets for therapeutic intervention, and to develop clinically applicable tools for gene expression array subtyping on fixed tissue. The diversity of outcomes and responses among patients of breast cancer has been recognized for over 100 years; the biological diversity of breast cancer as demonstrated by gene expression analysis likely explains much of that variation, and now the goal is to fully understand what this means for patients with different tumor types and to develop strategies tailored to individual tumor types in order to improve outcomes for all patients.

REFERENCES

1. Beatson G. On the treatment of inoperable cases of carcinoma of the mammary: suggestions for a new method of treatment, with illustrative cases. Lancet 1896; 104–107.
2. Ravdin PM, Siminoff LA, Davis GJ, et al. Computer program to assist in making decisions about adjuvant therapy for women with early breast cancer. J Clin Oncol 2001; 19:980–991.
3. Bergh J, Holmquist M. Who should not receive adjuvant chemotherapy? International databases. J Natl Cancer Inst Monogr 2001; 30:103–108.
4. Perou CM, Sorlie T, Eisen MB, et al. Molecular portraits of human breast tumours. Nature 2000; 406:747–752.
5. Golub TR, Slonim DK, Tamayo P, et al. Molecular classification of cancer: class discovery and class prediction by gene expression monitoring. Science 1999; 286:531–537.
6. Simon R, Radmacher MD, Dobbin K. Design of studies using DNA microarrays. Genet Epidemiol 2002; 23:21–36.
7. Sorlie T, Perou CM, Tibshirani R, et al. Gene expression patterns of breast carcinomas distinguish tumor subclasses with clinical implications. Proc Natl Acad Sci USA 2001; 98:10869–10874.
8. Sorlie T, Tibshirani R, Parker J, et al. Repeated observation of breast tumor subtypes in independent gene expression data sets. Proc Natl Acad Sci USA 2003; 100:8418–8423.
9. Yu K, Lee CH, Tan PH, et al. Conservation of breast cancer molecular subtypes and transcriptional patterns of tumor progression across distinct ethnic populations. Clin Cancer Res 2004; 10:5508–5517.
10. Van Laere SJ, Van den Eynden GG, Van der Auwera I, et al. Identification of cell-of-origin breast tumor subtypes in inflammatory breast cancer by gene expression profiling. Breast Cancer Res Treat 2006; 95(3):243–255.
11. Weigelt B, Hu Z, He X, et al. Molecular portraits and 70-gene prognosis signature are preserved throughout the metastatic process of breast cancer. Cancer Res 2005; 65:9155–9158.
12. Abd El-Rehim DM, Ball G, Pinder SE, et al. High-throughput protein expression analysis using tissue microarray technology of a large well-characterised series identifies biologically distinct classes of breast cancer confirming recent cDNA expression analyses. Int J Cancer 2005; 116:340–350.
13. Hu Z, Fan C, Oh DS, et al. The molecular portraits of breast tumors are conserved across microarray platforms. BMC Genom 2006; 7:96.
14. Nielsen TO, Hsu FD, Jensen K, et al. Immunohistochemical and clinical characterization of the basal-like subtype of invasive breast carcinoma. Clin Cancer Res 2004; 10:5367–5374.
15. King MC, Marks JH, Mandell JB. Breast and ovarian cancer risks due to inherited mutations in BRCA1 and BRCA2. Science 2003; 302:643–646.
16. Chappuis PO, Nethercot V, Foulkes WD. Clinico-pathological characteristics of BRCA1- and BRCA2-related breast cancer. Semin Surg Oncol 2000; 18:287–295.
17. Foulkes WD, Stefansson IM, Chappuis PO, et al. Germline BRCA1 mutations and a basal epithelial phenotype in breast cancer. J Natl Cancer Inst 2003; 95:1482–1485.
18. Olopade OI, Grushko T. Gene-expression profiles in hereditary breast cancer. N Engl J Med 2001; 344:2028–2029.
19. van 't Veer LJ, Dai H, van de Vijver MJ, et al. Gene expression profiling predicts clinical outcome of breast cancer. Nature 2002; 415:530–536.
20. Carey LA, Perou CM, Livasy CA, et al. Race, breast cancer subtypes, and survival in the Carolina Breast Cancer Study. J Am Med Assoc 2006; 295:2492–2502.

21. Chlebowski RT, Chen Z, Anderson GL, et al. Ethnicity and breast cancer: factors influencing differences in incidence and outcome. J Natl Cancer Inst 2005; 97:439–448.
22. Gapstur SM, Dupuis J, Gann P, et al. Hormone receptor status of breast tumors in black, Hispanic, and non-Hispanic white women. An analysis of 13,239 cases. Cancer 1996; 77:1465–1471.
23. Colditz GA, Rosner BA, Chen WY, et al. Risk factors for breast cancer according to estrogen and progesterone receptor status. J Natl Cancer Inst 2004; 96:218–228.
24. Chen WY, Hankinson SE, Schnitt SJ, et al. Association of hormone replacement therapy to estrogen and progesterone receptor status in invasive breast carcinoma. Cancer 2004; 101:1490–1500.
25. Fisher B, Costantino JP, Wickerham DL, et al. Tamoxifen for prevention of breast cancer: report of the National Surgical Adjuvant Breast and Bowel Project P-1 Study. J Natl Cancer Inst 1998; 90:1371–1388.
26. Suzuki R, Ye W, Rylander-Rudqvist T, et al. Alcohol and postmenopausal breast cancer risk defined by estrogen and progesterone receptor status: a prospective cohort study. J Natl Cancer Inst 2005; 97:1601–1608.
27. Fung TT, Hu FB, McCullough ML, et al. Diet quality is associated with the risk of estrogen receptor-negative breast cancer in postmenopausal women. J Nutr 2006; 136:466–472.
28. Marshall SF, Bernstein L, Anton-Culver H, et al. Nonsteroidal anti-inflammatory drug use and breast cancer risk by stage and hormone receptor status. J Natl Cancer Inst 2005; 97:805–812.
29. Zhang SM, Hankinson SE, Hunter DJ, et al. Folate intake and risk of breast cancer characterized by hormone receptor status. Cancer Epidemiol Biomarkers Prev 2005; 14:2004–2008.
30. Faneyte IF, Peterse JL, Van Tinteren H, et al. Predicting early failure after adjuvant chemotherapy in high-risk breast cancer patients with extensive lymph node involvement. Clin Cancer Res 2004; 10:4457–4463.
31. Sotiriou C, Neo SY, McShane LM, et al. Breast cancer classification and prognosis based on gene expression profiles from a population-based study. Proc Natl Acad Sci USA 2003; 100:10393–10398.
32. Rodriguez-Pinilla SM, Sarrio D, Honrado E, et al. Prognostic significance of basal-like phenotype and fascin expression in node-negative invasive breast carcinomas. Clin Cancer Res 2006; 12:1533–1539.
33. Minn AJ, Gupta GP, Siegel PM, et al. Genes that mediate breast cancer metastasis to lung. Nature 2005; 436:518–524.
34. van de Vijver MJ, He YD, van't Veer LJ, et al. A gene-expression signature as a predictor of survival in breast cancer. N Engl J Med 2002; 347:1999–2009.
35. Foekens JA, Atkins D, Zhang Y, et al. Multicenter validation of a gene expression-based prognostic signature in lymph node-negative primary breast cancer. J Clin Oncol 2006; 24:1665–1671.
36. Paik S, Shak S, Tang G, et al. A multigene assay to predict recurrence of tamoxifen-treated, node-negative breast cancer. N Engl J Med 2004; 351:2817–2826.
37. Chang HY, Nuyten DS, Sneddon JB, et al. Robustness, scalability, and integration of a wound-response gene expression signature in predicting breast cancer survival. Proc Natl Acad Sci USA 2005; 102:3738–3743.
38. Ma XJ, Wang Z, Ryan PD, et al. A two-gene expression ratio predicts clinical outcome in breast cancer patients treated with tamoxifen. Cancer Cell 2004; 5:607–616.
39. Fan C, Oh DS, Wessels L, et al. Concordance among gene-expression-based predictors for breast cancer. N Engl J Med 2006; 355(6):560–569.
40. Early Breast Cancer Trialists' Collaborative Group. Effects of chemotherapy and hormonal therapy for early breast cancer on recurrence and 15-year survival: an overview of the randomised trials. Lancet 2005; 365:1687–1717.
41. Colleoni M, Minchella I, Mazzarol G, et al. Response to primary chemotherapy in breast cancer patients with tumors not expressing estrogen and progesterone receptors. Ann Oncol 2000; 11:1057–1059.
42. Guarneri V, Broglio K, Kau SW, et al. Prognostic value of pathologic complete response after primary chemotherapy in relation to hormone receptor status and other factors. J Clin Oncol 2006; 24:1037–1044.

43. Berry DA, Cirrincione C, Henderson IC, et al. Estrogen-receptor status and outcomes of modern chemotherapy for patients with node-positive breast cancer. J Am Med Assoc 2006; 295:1658–1667.

44. Rouzier R, Perou CM, Symmans WF, et al. Breast cancer molecular subtypes respond differently to preoperative chemotherapy. Clin Cancer Res 2005; 11:5678–5685.

45. Carey LA, Dees EC, Sawyer LR, et al. The triple negative paradox: primary tumor chemosensitivity of the basal-like breast cancer (BBC) phenotype. San Antonio Breast Cancer Symposium, 2004, pp. 1023a.

46. Troester MA, Hoadley KA, Sorlie T, et al. Cell-type-specific responses to chemotherapeutics in breast cancer. Cancer Res 2004; 64:4218–4226.

47. Burris HA III, Hurwitz HI, Dees EC, et al. Phase I safety, pharmacokinetics, and clinical activity study of lapatinib (GW572016), a reversible dual inhibitor of epidermal growth factor receptor tyrosine kinases, in heavily pretreated patients with metastatic carcinomas. J Clin Oncol 2005; 23:5305–5313.

48. Konecny GE, Pegram MD, Venkatesan N, et al: Activity of the dual kinase inhibitor lapatinib (GW572016) against HER-2-overexpressing and trastuzumab-treated breast cancer cells. Cancer Res 2006; 66:1630–1639.

49. Kennedy RD, Quinn JE, Mullan PB, et al. The role of BRCA1 in the cellular response to chemotherapy. J Natl Cancer Inst 2004; 96:1659–1668.

50. Charafe-Jauffret E, Ginestier C, Monville F, et al. Gene expression profiling of breast cell lines identifies potential new basal markers. Oncogene 2006; 25:2273–2284.

51. Livasy CA, Karaca G, Nanda R, et al. Phenotypic evaluation of the basal-like subtype of invasive breast carcinoma. Mod Pathol 2006; 19:264–271.

52. Lev DC, Kim LS, Melnikova V, et al. Dual blockade of EGFR and ERK1/2 phosphorylation potentiates growth inhibition of breast cancer cells. Br J Cancer 2004; 91:795–802.

53. Simon R, Panussis S, Maurer R, et al. KIT (CD117)-positive breast cancers are infrequent and lack KIT gene mutations. Clin Cancer Res 2004; 10:178–183.

54. Modi S, Seidman AD, Dickler M, et al. A phase II trial of imatinib mesylate monotherapy in patients with metastatic breast cancer. Breast Cancer Res Treat 2005; 90:157–163.

55. Reis-Filho JS, Westbury C, Pierga JY. The impact of expression profiling on prognostic and predictive testing in breast cancer. J Clin Pathol 2006; 59:225–231.

56. Reid JF, Lusa L, De Cecco L, et al. Limits of predictive models using microarray data for breast cancer clinical treatment outcome. J Natl Cancer Inst 2005; 97:927–930.

57. Simon R, Radmacher MD, Dobbin K, et al. Pitfalls in the use of DNA microarray data for diagnostic and prognostic classification. J Natl Cancer Inst 2003; 95:14–18.

11 Development and Validation of Gene Expression Profile Signatures in Early-Stage Breast Cancer

Christine Desmedt, Christos Sotiriou, and
Martine J. Piccart-Gebhart
Department of Medical Oncology, Jules Bordet Institute, Brussels, Belgium

INTRODUCTION

With the advent of array-based technology and the sequencing of the human genome, comprehensive analysis of transcriptional variation at the genomic level has become possible. Already, the knowledge derived from gene expression profiling studies is impressive in terms of improving our understanding of the basic biology of breast cancer. Consequently, these discoveries have also challenged the currently used classification of breast cancer and the existing theories about metastatic progression. The findings of some key studies and their implications for clinical practice are discussed in this chapter.

BREAST CANCER CLASSIFICATION BASED ON GENE EXPRESSION PROFILING

By detailing the expression levels of thousands of genes simultaneously from tumor cells and their surrounding microenvironment, gene expression profiles have provided molecular "portraits" of breast cancer, distinguished by extensive differences in gene expression in breast cancer samples that were once considered homogeneous by classical diagnostic methods (1–5) (Table 1).

Using cDNA microarrays, the Stanford researchers (1,2) were the first to identify, in a series of 42 and 78 patient samples, respectively, a new molecular classification of breast cancer based on the expression levels of nearly 500 genes, called the "intrinsic" gene subset because they were found to be highly variable between different patient samples and less variable between samples taken from the same patient before and after treatment. This new classification consisted of at least five distinct subtypes of tumors: the "basal-like," the "erbB2," and the "normal-like" subgroups, which were mostly estrogen receptor (ER)-negative and characterized by the high expression of the basal/myoepithelial specific genes, and the luminal-like subgroups, composed mainly of ER-positive tumors distinguished by the expression of genes normally expressed by the breast luminal cells. The "basal-like" subgroup was characterized by high expression of keratins 5 and 17, and by laminin and fatty-acid binding protein 7; the "erbB2" subgroup by the high expression of several genes from the erbB2 amplicon. Interestingly, this study led to the recognition of several subtypes within the ER-positive "luminal-like" tumors: the "luminal-like A" was characterized by a high expression

(Text continues on page 125.)

TABLE 1 Main Microarray Studies with Prognostic Implications in Breast Cancer

Type of study	Study	Type of microarray platform	Samples (characteristics)	Informative genes	Main findings
Classification	Perou et al. (1)	cDNA (8102 features)	42 (T3, T4 tumors/20 before and after CT pairs)	Intrinsic gene subset (496 genes)	Identification of four subgroups: ER+/luminal-like, basal-like, erbB2+, normal-like
	Sorlie et al. (2)		77 (T3, T4 tumors including from Ref. 1)	Intrinsic gene subset (496 genes)	Identification of novel luminal-like subgroups A, B, and C, with luminal A having best outcome
	Sorlie et al. (3)		115 (majority T3, T4 tumors including from Ref. 2)	Intrinsic gene subset (534 genes)	Validation of Ref. 2.
	Sotiriou et al. (4)	cDNA (7650 features)	99 (53 LN+/46 LN−)	706	Identification of six subgroups: ER+/luminal-like 1, 2, and 3; ER−/basal-like 1 and 2, and HER2-*Neu*.
	Hu et al. (5)	Oligonucleotides (Agilent-17,000 genes)	105 (26 pretreatment pairs)	Intrinsic gene subset (1300 genes)	Validation of previous subgroups and identification of new "IFN" subgroup and proliferation signature. Development of a single sample predictor
"Fishing-expedition" approach	van't Veer et al. (10)	Long-oligonucleotides (Agilent Hu25K-24,479 oligonucleotides)	78 (all <55 yr old, LN− and untreated)	70-gene prognostic signature	Prediction of clinical outcome, defined as presence of distant metastases at the five-yr mark
	van de Vijver et al. (11)		295 (including 61 from previous study/both treated and untreated/151 LN− and 144 LN+)		Validation of Ref. 10.

Long-oligonucleotides (Custom-designed "Mammaprint®")	Buyse et al. (14)	307 (T1–T2 tumors from patients <61 yr old, LN–, and untreated)		Independent validation of Refs. 10,11.
Short-oligonucleotides (Affymetrix U133A-22,283 probe-sets)	Wang et al. (12)	286 (untreated LN– patients/training set: 115 and validation set: 171)	76-gene prognostic signature (60 genes for ER+ and 16 genes for ER– tumors)	Prediction of clinical outcome, defined as presence of distant metastases at the five-yr mark
Short-oligonucleotides (Custom-made Affymetrix VDX2-297 genes)	Foekens et al. (13)	180 (untreated LN–)		Validation of Ref. 12.
Short-oligonucleotides (Affymetrix U133A-22,283 probe-sets)	Desmedt et al. (15)	198 (T1–T2 tumors from patients <61 yr old, LN–, and untreated from Ref. 14)		Independent validation of Refs. 12,13.
"Hypothesis-driven" approach cDNA (43,000 features)	Chang et al. (18)	Fibroblasts from 10 anatomic sites	Fibroblast core serum response list (512 genes)	Identification of similarities between tumors and wounds
Long-oligonucleotides (Agilent Hu25K- 24,479 oligonucleotides)	Chang et al. (19)	295 (from Ref. 11)		Robustness, scalability and integration of this signature to predict survival
Short-oligonucleotides (Affymetrix U133A-22,283 probe-sets)	Sotiriou et al. (25)	189 (training set: 64 ER+ patients and validation set: 125 untreated patients)+ three publicly available data sets (from Refs. 2,4, and 11)	Gene Expression Grade Index (97 genes)	Identification of Genomic Grade associated with histological grade able to classify histological grade 2 patients into high- and low-risks of recurrence

(Continued)

TABLE 1 Main Microarray Studies with Prognostic Implications in Breast Cancer (*Continued*)

Type of study	Type of microarray platform	Study	Samples (characteristics)	Informative genes	Main findings
	Short-oligonucleotides (Affymetrix U133A-22,283 probe-sets)	Sotiriou et al. (29)	335 (ER+ both untreated and Tam-treated/86 from Ref. 25) + four publicly available data sets (from Refs. 2,4,11, and 12)	Cell proliferation signature (50 genes)	Definition of distinct subtypes of ER+ tumors with the Genomic Grade
	Long-oligonucleotides (Agilent Hu25K-24,479 oligonucleotides)	Dai et al. (27)	311 (295 samples from Refs. 11 and 16 non-redundant samples from Ref. 10)	Cell proliferation signature (50 genes)	Prognostic importance of cell-cycle genes in patients with relatively high ER expression
	Oligonucleotides (Agilent-17,000 genes)	Oh et al. (28)	MCF-7 cell line 118 (from Ref. 5+ 14 new tumors) three publicly available data sets (from Refs. 3,11, and 40)	Estrogen-induced gene set (822 genes)	Identification of two clinically relevant luminal-like groups based on this gene set

Abbreviations: CT, chemotherapy; LN, lymph node status; IFN, interferon; ER, estrogen-receptor.

of ER, GATA3, X-box binding protein trefoil factor 3, hepatocyte nuclear factor 3 alpha, and LIV-1, whereas a second subgroup that could be further divided into two smaller groups, the "luminal-like B and C," showed moderate expression of the genes expressed by the breast luminal cells.

When comparing these molecular "portraits" with the clinical behavior of these tumors, it became evident that the "basal-like" and "erbB2" subgroups were associated with the worst clinical outcome, whereas the "luminal-like A" tumors had the best relapse-free and overall survival rates. Furthermore, with regard to the "luminal-like" subgroups, "luminal-like A" revealed the best outcome when compared to the other "luminal-like" subgroups.

Also using cDNA microarrays, our group undertook to correlate gene expression patterns with known clinico-pathological characteristics and clinical outcome in 99 breast cancer tumors (4). Interestingly, our findings were similar to those of Perou and Sorlie et al. (1–3), despite differences in microarray platforms and patient populations. Indeed, ER was again the most important discriminator, and smaller subgroups were also identified within the two major groups defined by ER: the subgroups "basal-1," "basal-2," and "HER2-Neu," which were predominantly ER-negative, and the subgroups "luminal-1, 2, and 3," which were mostly ER-positive. Again, differences between these subgroups in terms of clinical outcome were evident, with a significant advantage for the luminal-subgroups compared to the others. Thus, although no differences in survival were observed between the "basal/HER2-Neu" subgroups, the luminal-subgroups appeared again to be heterogeneous with regard to clinical outcome.

When the relationship between clinical parameters and this molecular classification was examined further, we found that ER showed the strongest association with gene expression, followed by grade; in contrast, tumor size, menopausal status, and nodal status did not seem to be associated with a particular gene expression profile. These results suggested that ER and histological grade were the two clinical parameters that most affected the behavior of breast cancer.

Because microarray technology evolved since their first publications, the Stanford group created a new "intrinsic" list using Agilent oligonucleotide technology, the arrays of which included many more genes than the cDNA arrays the group had used previously (17,000 and 8000, respectively) (5). Another difference was the use of pretreatment pairs instead of before- and after-chemotherapy pairs, in order to exclude variation in profiles due to treatment.

Using a training set of 105 breast tumor samples and nine normal breast samples, the Stanford researchers derived a new intrinsic gene set that displayed a large overlap with the previous intrinsic gene list, but showed a remarkable increase in the number of genes, consistent with the greater number of genes present on the Agilent microarrays. By applying hierarchical clustering to a combined dataset of 315 samples, they identified six main subtypes: five that corresponded to the previously defined groups, "erbB2," "basal-like," "luminal-like A," "luminal-like B," and "normal-like," and one new group characterized by the high expression of interferon-regulated genes (IFN). However, the main difference with the previously reported findings was the identification of a large proliferation signature, the genes of which appeared to be highly expressed in the "erbB2," "luminal-like B," and "IFN" subgroups. Again, these subtypes appeared to be associated with significant differences in terms of both relapse-free and overall survival, the "luminal-like A" subgroup having the best outcome, whereas the "erbB2," the "basal-like," the "luminal-like B," and the "IFN" subgroups had significantly worse outcomes. Looking at the associations between the intrinsic subtypes and the clinical parameters, they also found, in addition to a strong association with ER status, a significant association with histological grade, as reported by Sotiriou et al. (4).

Although this classification based on hierarchical clustering provided interesting results, it was not suitable for clinical application, because to classify a new sample one would need to re-analyze all the samples. Therefore, the Stanford group developed an objective and stable classifier based upon the subtype mean expression profiles that could be used as a single sample predictor (SSP). This SSP was then further validated in two independent data sets to predict survival in both untreated and treated breast cancer samples, emphasizing the potential clinical applicability of this "intrinsic" subtype classification of breast tumors.

Altogether, these studies showed that tumors could be grouped according to their expression profiles and that tumor groups are often related to cellular characteristics with clear clinical relevance. These results also demonstrated that both ER and histological grade contribute significantly to breast cancer biology, suggesting that a better definition and characterization of these parameters could lead to a better understanding of the disease.

PREDICTION OF THE PROGNOSTIC POTENTIAL
OF THE PRIMARY TUMOR

In current clinical practice, the majority of patients with early breast cancer will receive some form of systemic adjuvant therapy (chemo- and/or endocrine therapy). Clinical parameters such as lymph node status, tumor size, and histological grade can provide prognostic information, and are summarized in clinical guidelines, such as the National Institutes of Health (NIH) (6) or the St. Gallen consensus criteria (7,8), in order to assist clinicians and patients in adjuvant therapy decision-making. However, risk stratification based on these guidelines is far from perfect, and much progress is needed to identify those patients who really need adjuvant systemic therapy. Several independent groups have conducted comprehensive gene expression profiling studies with the hope of improving upon traditional prognostic markers used in the clinic.

In this context, two approaches for prognostic marker discovery on a genome scale have been used: (*i*) the "fishing expedition" or "top-down" approach; and (*ii*) the hypothesis-driven or "bottom-up" approach, as illustrated by Liu (9) (Fig. 1). The first approach derives a prognostic model from the global gene expression data of a tumor set simply by seeking gene expression profiles that are associated or correlated with clinical outcome, without making any biological assumptions. The resulting gene sets may have an excellent prognostic capacity but may not carry much information about biological mechanisms. In contrast, the discovery process of the second approach starts with a specific biological hypothesis. Only once a catalog of genes has been uncovered in connection with a particular cellular process or mechanism, will the findings be linked with clinical outcome to evaluate their potential clinical applicability. Here we will present some major publications for each type of approach and discuss their implications for breast cancer patient management (Table 1).

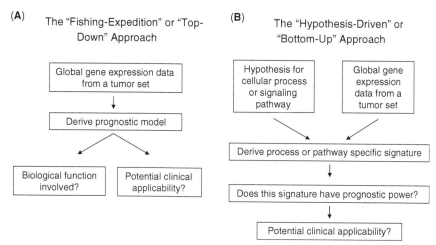

FIGURE 1   Schematic of the two different approaches of prognostic markers discovery. *Source*: Adapted from Ref. 9.

THE "FISHING EXPEDITION" OR "TOP-DOWN APPROACH"

In contrast to the previously described DNA microarray studies, which used an unsupervised analysis of gene expression data to identify a new classification of breast tumors, the studies described below used a supervised classification method to determine gene expression patterns of primary breast tumors that could predict the development of distant metastases in early breast cancer patients.

Using the Agilent platform (10), the Amsterdam group first identified a 70-gene prognostic signature in a series of 78 systemically untreated node-negative breast cancer patients younger than 55 years of age. This signature included mainly genes involved in the cell cycle, invasion, metastasis, angiogenesis, and signal transduction. This gene profile was then validated on a larger set of 295 young patients, including both node-negative and node-positive breast tumors in treated and untreated patients from the same institution (11). The signature proved to be the strongest predictor for distant metastasis-free survival, independent of adjuvant treatment (given to 44% of the patient population), tumor size, histological grade and age, both in node-negative and node-positive patients.

Using a training set of 115 breast cancer patients, Wang et al. (12) identified a 76-gene signature that could be used to predict the development of distant metastases in untreated node-negative breast cancer patients of all age groups. Importantly, and in contrast to van't Veer et al. (10), this study used Affymetrix technology to build a classification algorithm that considered ER-positive patients separately from ER-negative patients, taking into account that the mechanisms for disease progression could differ for these two ER-based subgroups of breast cancer patients. Similar to the 70-gene signature, these 76 genes were mainly associated with cell cycle and cell death, DNA replication and repair, and immune response. In the same study, Wang et al. validated the prognostic ability of their signature in an additional set of 171 node-negative untreated breast cancer patients. Recently, this same group of researchers provided additional evidence for the prognostic performance of their predictor in a multi-centric cohort of 180 node-negative untreated breast cancer patients obtained from different institutions (13).

A common feature of both signatures is that when their performance in stratifying patients according to risk classification results based is compared with one of the two traditional clinical risk classifications, namely the St. Gallen (7,8) and NIH criteria (9), both signatures were superior in correctly identifying the low-risk patients, suggesting the potential for reducing over-treatment in early breast cancer. However, the identification of high-risk patients could still be improved since half of the patients identified as high-risk did not, in fact, experience a disease recurrence.

A major challenge for gene expression profiling studies, especially those with clear clinical implications, is independent validation. Therefore, predictors should first be tested retrospectively in a large cohort of patients with a long follow-up period and then compared with established markers to assess their independent value. If confirmed, the next logical step is to evaluate their prognostic power in a large prospective study.

TRANSBIG, the translational research network created by the Breast International Group (BIG), decided to conduct an independent validation study of these two prognostic signatures in a series of 302 patients from five different centers, and across different statistical facilities (14,15). Although there was only a 3-gene overlap between the signatures, both were validated in this patient cohort, even after adjustment for clinical risk. In addition, a very interesting finding of this validation project was the heterogeneous behavior of these gene signatures over time, which could be observed given the unusually long follow-up (14 years) of the patients in the series. The signatures appeared to be strong predictors of the development of early distant metastases, while showing a decreased prognostic ability with increasing number of follow-up years. This finding, which was not observed for clinical risk, is not entirely unexpected, however, since the signatures were built to identify patients with distant metastases within five years; it suggests that different mechanisms might be associated with the development of early and late distant metastases, as already proposed by Klein and his group (16,17).

There is preliminary evidence that some tumor cells may already disseminate in a much earlier genomic state during breast cancer tumorigenesis than initially thought, and that they remain "dormant" until the microenvironment becomes favorable and advantageous aberrations are acquired in order to develop distant metastases (16,17). Therefore, by profiling primary tumor samples, we might essentially be capturing information regarding the cancer cells that disseminated from the primary tumor rather than the latent stage of the disease characterized by the presence of disseminated "young" cancer cells in a far less progressed genomic state. This may explain why these profiles may not be adequate to predict the occurrence of late metastases.

Altogether, this intensive two-year validation project has added to the growing evidence that gene expression signatures are of clinical relevance, especially in identifying patients at high-risk of early distant metastases; it also reinforced the belief that the time was right to proceed with the prospective MINDACT trial. This "Microarray for Node Negative Disease may Avoid Chemotherapy" study is a large collaborative trial conducted by the EORTC Breast Cancer Group under the TRANSBIG network that will randomize 6000 patients to investigate the benefit/risk ratio of chemotherapy when the risk

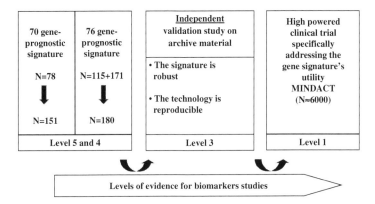

FIGURE 2 Schematic illustration of the TRANSBIG, the translational research part of the Breast International Group, validation strategy of the 70-gene signature.

assessment differs from that provided by the gene expression signature. This trial should then provide level-1 evidence about the clinical relevance of applying gene expression predictors to daily breast cancer patient management (Fig. 2).

THE "HYPOTHESIS-DRIVEN" OR "BOTTOM-UP" APPROACH
The Wound-Response Signature
The approach used by researchers at Stanford University (18) is novel compared to the studies described above in the sense that instead of selecting genes directly through their association with survival, they started with a specific physiological mechanism, namely wound healing. Indeed, wounds share many features with tumors, as in both situations cells are induced to proliferate, the extracellular matrix and connective tissues are invaded and remodeled, epithelial and stromal cells migrate, and new blood vessels are recruited. To simulate the process of wound healing, Chang and his colleagues exposed cultured fibroblasts, which are found in the connective tissue surrounding most organs and are activated when tissue is damaged, to serum, the soluble fraction of coagulated blood that is encountered only at sites of tissue injury.

The gene expression analysis of 50 fibroblast cultures derived from 10 different anatomical sites and cultured with or without serum revealed that although fibroblasts from different anatomical sites have characteristic gene expression profiles (19), in response to serum they shared a common gene expression program, made of nearly 700 genes. Most of these genes are involved in proliferation, blood coagulation, complement activation, secretory protein synthesis, angiogenesis, and proteolysis. After removing the cell-cycle genes from the list in order to improve the specificity of a wound-healing genomic signature, 512 genes remained and were defined as the fibroblast core serum response (CSR).

By examining the expression of this CSR list of genes in publicly available microarray data sets, Chang et al. found that these genes were coordinately regulated in many human tumors, including breast cancer, and those patients whose tumors had a wound-like profile had an increased risk of metastasis and death in breast, lung, and gastric carcinomas.

In a more recent article, Chang et al. (20) went several steps further to clinically operationalize this CSR list of genes. Using the series of 295 early breast cancer patients from van de Vijver et al. (11) and hierarchical clustering, they showed that patients whose tumors expressed the wound-response signature had a markedly worse clinical outcome, both in terms of distant metastasis free probability and overall survival. However, in order to allow the clinical use of this signature, the authors developed a quantitative score based on the correlation value to the gene expression centroid of the differential expression in response to serum in the cultured fibroblasts. In a multivariate analysis including a variety of clinicopathological parameters, the wound-response predictor remained the strongest predictor of metastasis and death. Similar to the findings reported previously for the 70- and 76-gene signatures (10–13), Chang et al. demonstrated that their signature improved current risk stratification based on the NIH and St. Gallen guidelines (6–9) and that it was able to identify a subset of "low-risk" patients within the clinical "high-risk" group.

As a step towards integrating diverse signatures, they compared the prognostic information provided by their CSR signature with the existing 70-gene signature (10) and with the breast cancer subtypes as defined by the intrinsic genes identified by Perou et al. (1). A little overlap was observed between these gene lists: 22 genes were common to the two signatures and 18 between the wound-response signature and the "intrinsic" gene list. In a multivariate analysis carried out on the van de Vijver dataset (11) and combining these 3-gene lists with classical clinical variables, both the wound-response and the 70-gene signatures provided independent prognostic information. Chang et al. also discovered that by combining these two signatures in a decision tree, they could further improve the prediction of metastatic disease.

Taken together, these results pointed out a strong link between wound response and cancer behavior on the genome scale, and also suggested that the wound-response signature would be a clinically useful tool for recognizing at an early stage the cancers at high risk of progression. Therefore, these studies provided an experimental model of wound-healing that could be used to study the underlying mechanisms and to develop inhibitors of this response.

BREAST CANCER GRADING
Identification of the Genomic Grade
Pathologists have traditionally used histological grade to describe distinct breast cancer phenotypes: whereas, grade I or well-differentiated tumors are composed of polarized groups of cells that form tubular or duct-like structures; grade III or undifferentiated tumors are associated with a high mitotic activity, nuclear pleomorphism, and no tubular formation; grade II tumors display intermediate characteristics. In addition, high- and low-grade tumors have been correlated with the expression of different biological markers, and several groups have also reported that mitotic/apoptotic activity is higher in high grade/poorly differentiated tumors (21). Finally, the recent results regarding the molecular classification of breast cancer have strongly pointed to an association of histological grade with particular gene expression tumor profiles (4,5).

There is growing evidence that high- and low-grade tumors should be viewed as distinct disease entities. Indeed, Roylance et al., found that the long arm of chromosome 16 is lost in 65% of grade I tumors compared to only 16% in grade III tumors, implying that the majority of well differentiated tumors do not evolve towards an undifferentiated state during tumor progression, as regain of genetic material is very unlikely (22). By investigating different markers in in situ and invasive breast cancer lesions, Warnberg et al. (23) suggested that evolution from in situ to invasive cancer likely occurs independently from tumor grade.

High- and low-grade tumors are also associated with a different clinical outcome, undifferentiated tumors being associated with the highest rate of recurrence and shorter recurrence time when compared to well-differentiated tumors (24). However, clinicians are confronted with a real problem with respect to patients carrying intermediate-grade tumors (grade II). These tumors, which represent 30% to 60% of breast cancer cases, are the major source of inter-observer discrepancy and display intermediate phenotype and survival: consequently treatment decision-making for these patients is a great challenge, with subsequent under- or over-treatment likely.

Our group decided to examine whether histological grading was associated with characteristic gene expression profiles and whether these profiles could be of use to refine histological grading in a reproducible manner (25). Using a training set of 33 histological grade I and 31 grade III ER-positive breast tumors, we identified 97 unique genes that were differentially expressed between low- and high-grade tumors. By restricting our training set to only ER-positive samples, we avoided selecting ER-related genes that would have been spuriously associated with grade. The majority of the 97 genes we identified were over-expressed in high-grade tumors and associated with cell cycle progression and proliferation. This is not surprising since histological grading is based on mitotic index, nuclear pleomorphism, and differentiation.

In order to summarize the expression of these 97 genes, we developed a score, the gene expression grade index, "GGI," in which a high index corresponds to high grade and vice-versa. In the validation sets, when comparing the gene expression profiles of intermediate-grade tumors with both high- and low-grade tumors, no distinct expression profile was observed, and the GGI of these tumors spanned the values for histological grade I and III tumors. Interestingly, when examining the prognostic value of the GGI in histological grade II tumors, we found a statistically significant difference in relapse-free survival between genomic grade I and grade III tumors, similar to the difference observed between histological grade I and III tumors. Importantly, we observed consistent results across multiple independent and heterogeneous validation sets and microarray platforms, emphasizing the reproducible behavior of the grade-associated genes.

Given the existence of other gene sets with prognostic information, we wondered how those could be compared to genomic grade. When we considered a less stringent threshold to identify genes associated with histological grade I and III tumors, we identified a larger list of 183 genes. Eleven and seven of these genes were present in the 70- and 76-gene prognostic signatures (10,12), respectively. By evaluating a predictor based on the genes common to our 97-gene genomic grade and the Amsterdam 70-gene signature (10) in their original data set, we observed a similar prognostic performance (data not shown). Also, when comparing the 70- and 76-gene signatures (10,12) with the genomic grade in the TRANSBIG validation series reported earlier (14,15), we observed consistent predictions of outcomes, both in terms of time to distant metastasis and overall survival (data not shown), indicating that proliferation-related genes appear to be an important—if not the most important—part of most prognostic gene sets.

Elucidating the Relationship Between Estrogen Receptor and Proliferation-Related Genes

When examining the distribution of genomic grade according to ER, we found that most ER-negative tumors were associated with a high GGI, whereas ER-positive tumors were made of a mixture of GGI values (25). Thus, although ER status and grade are not completely independent variables, tumor grading can provide additional information for ER-positive tumors. Importantly, we demonstrated that genomic grade was a stronger predictor of clinical outcome than histological grade in these ER-positive tumors.

As described earlier, several microarray studies have classified breast cancer tumors based on gene expression profiles (1–5), and each of these studies has reported different subgroups within the ER-positive group. When applying the GGI to these newly identified molecular subtypes from data sets of Sorlie and Sotiriou et al. (2–4), we found that almost all ER-positive tumors previously classified as luminal-like A or 1 tumors, those that had the best clinical outcome, were associated with low GGI values, when compared to the other luminal-like subgroups, which had significantly higher GGI values and poorer outcome (26). These findings clearly showed that classification based on genomic grade compared favorably with the molecular classification, emphasizing the role of proliferation-related genes in ER-positive breast cancer tumors.

We then showed in over 650 ER-positive breast cancer tumors that patients whose tumors were assigned to a low genomic grade subtype clearly had a better outcome than patients whose tumors belonged to the high genomic grade subtype (26). Notably, the poor outcome of this high genomic grade subtype seemed unaltered by adjuvant tamoxifen, suggesting that this type of treatment was poorly effective in this clinical setting.

Dai et al. (27) also identified a homogeneous group of genes, consisting almost entirely of cell-cycle genes, which strongly predicted the occurrence of metastases in women with ER-rich breast cancers. Although they found that histological grade correlated with this gene set, they showed that the prediction of clinical outcome based on the gene expression classifier was much more accurate than the one based on histological grade, also suggesting that this parameter could be significantly refined by gene expression profiling.

Oh and his colleagues developed a gene expression predictor for ER and/or progesterone receptor-positive breast cancer patients using an approach based solely on the biological characteristics of the tumors (28). To this end, they first selected genes on the basis of estrogen regulation in MCF-7 cells and used these genes to hierarchically cluster 65 breast cancer tumors into two major groups with different clinical outcome. To further characterize these groups, they applied a supervised analysis, which identified a list of 822 genes associated with the expression of these estrogen-induced genes. Consistent with our findings using the GGI, they observed in all the data sets they evaluated, a high expression of proliferation-related genes in the poor-prognosis group and a clear association between their classification and histological grade.

In conclusion, these studies provide consistent results regarding the prognostic power of proliferation-related genes for patients whose tumors express ER.

CONCLUDING REMARKS

The advent of new high-throughput technologies, together with the sequencing of the human genome, has greatly increased our understanding of breast cancer biology in a short period of time. Currently, there are several molecular gene lists derived from expression profiling studies that claim to have significant prognostic value in breast cancer patients.

Although these studies might have used different approaches, different platforms, and different patient cohorts, most of them do highlight an important role for ER- and proliferation-related genes.

That, ER and histological grade/proliferation are associated with clinical outcome in breast cancer has been known for two decades. However, the methods used to evaluate these parameters have suffered from technical limitations and could not estimate prognosis in an accurate and quantitative manner.

The identification of a gene expression profile associated with histological grade provides evidence that the currently used three-category histological grading system could be replaced by a highly reproducible binary gene expression grading system with improved prognostic power.

Importantly, several studies have also elucidated the relationship between ER and tumor grade by highlighting cell proliferation as the driving mechanism associated with poor outcome in this subset of ER-positive breast cancer patients. These studies strongly suggest that by combining ER and proliferation-status, which is captured by the GGI (25), the genes identified by Dai et al. (27), and the new intrinsic gene list of the Stanford researchers (5), we may end with a very strong predictor of outcome for this particular subset of patients. Also, the results have shown that the predictions that were made based on histological grade were not as strong as those relying on gene expression classifiers, emphasizing the fact that the performance of a well-known prognostic indicator, such as histological grade, can be refined and improved by gene expression profiling.

Although most gene sets that have been described in this chapter provide valuable information for classifying breast cancer tumors and consistently predict clinical outcome, the challenge is now to integrate this genomic information into prognostic models that can easily be applied in a clinical setting. Breast cancer diagnosis and treatment decisions will continue to rely largely on classical, histopathological, and clinical parameters until some crucial issues have been resolved:

These issues include: (*i*) how can we compare and eventually integrate the information from these different signatures that have been identified in order to optimize risk stratification for breast cancer patients?; (*ii*) would a combined approach of clinical and genomic data increase clinical outcome predictions?; and (*iii*) are the technologies applicable in routine clinical situations and are they reproducible?

With regard to the first issue, when we tested the prediction based on the GGI in the TRANSBIG validation series relative to those made by the 70- and 76-gene signatures (10,12), we observed a high concordance between these three predictors (29). Using the 295 cases from van de Vijver et al.; Fan et al. (30), in turn, compared the predictions made by their intrinsic subtype SSP (5), the 70-gene (10) and the wound-response signatures (18), as well as the recurrence score (RS) initially developed by Paik et al. (31) to predict distant recurrence in patients with ER-positive breast tumors that have been treated with tamoxifen. Their results showed a high concordance between the different predictors and, in particular, between their intrinsic subtype SSP, the RS, and the 70-gene signature. Interestingly, these three predictors all contained a significant proportion of proliferation-related genes, underscoring once again the crucial role of these genes in breast cancer behavior.

Nevertheless, Chang's results regarding the combination of their wound-response signature with the 70-gene risk classification provided evidence that different gene sets may add complementary information and therefore independently contribute to the tumor phenotype (20). We might even expect more gene sets identified by the hypothesis-driven approach to add independent information regarding breast cancer prognosis. This points to the second issue we have noted.

In their study, Pittman and her colleagues developed, for example, a first-step comprehensive clinicogenomic modeling framework based on classification trees, in which they combined nodal status with multiple metagenes representing different aspects of breast cancer biology (32). Using this approach, they were able to individualize prediction of clinical outcome, supporting their hypothesis that the combination of all forms of potentially relevant information might be the way to proceed.

One can also imagine combining biomarkers derived from gene expression profiling studies, such as the genomic grade, with traditional factors that retain prognostic power, such as tumor size and nodal status, in order to maximize the use of available information for breast cancer patient management. A possibility could then be to replace the histological grade by the more reproducible genomic grade in the well-established Nottingham Prognostic Index (33), which also considers these two clinical parameters in addition to the histological grade.

With regard to the third important issue, the technologies involved and their clinical applicability, we find that although the cost of conducting microarray experiments is decreasing, the requirement for fresh or snap-frozen tissue may still limit their clinical use. High-throughput, real-time reverse transcriptase–polymerase chain reaction (RT–PCR) can now be performed on sections of formalin-fixed paraffin-embedded tissue (31,34) and since paraffin sections can be obtained from every patient, this technology could be seen as a valuable alternative RNA quantitative method that can be used to help move these molecular predictors from the lab to the clinic.

However, identifying "high-risk" patients who clearly need systemic adjuvant therapy is not good enough: we still do not know which type of therapy will be most efficient for each individual patient. Identifying markers that can reliably predict response to particular drugs remains a great challenge.

To this end, the neoadjuvant approach is very attractive, as it provides an in vivo assessment of treatment sensitivity. Several studies have already used a genome-wide approach to identify gene expression profiles that correlate with chemo- or hormonosensitivity (35–40). Although the first results of the studies support the concept that predictors of the efficacy of anti-cancer agents can be developed, they remain largely suboptimal. Indeed, small sample sizes have been used to build and validate these gene predictors, putting their robustness into question. Moreover, many studies suffer from methodological limitations. These include the choice of endpoints (clinical vs. pathological response), the choice of the regimen to be studied (e.g., combination chemotherapy vs. to single agent), and the type of population to be evaluated (e.g., the whole breast cancer population vs. to a relevant molecular subgroup, as evaluating a predictor in an inappropriate cohort might lead to underestimation of its performance).

In summary, gene expression studies have great potential for improving breast cancer management and increasing our understanding of the disease biology. There is no doubt that we are at a transition point between empirical and molecular medicine; however, if we want "tailored" breast cancer management to become reality, we need adequate validation of the predictors in prospective clinical trials, such as the MINDACT study.

REFERENCES

1. Perou CM, Sorlie T, Eisen MB, et al. Molecular portraits of human breast tumours. Nature 2000; 406(6797):747–752.
2. Sorlie T, Perou CM, Tibshirani R, et al. Gene expression patterns of breast carcinomas distinguish tumor subclasses with clinical implications. Proc Natl Acad Sci USA 2001; 98(19):10869–10874.
3. Sorlie T, Tibshirani R, Parker J, et al. Repeated observation of breast tumor subtypes in independent gene expression data sets. Proc Natl Acad Sci USA 2003; 100(14):8418–8423.
4. Sotiriou C, Neo SY, McShane LM, et al. Breast cancer classification and prognosis based on gene expression profiles from a population-based study. Proc Natl Acad Sci USA 2003; 100(18):10393–10398.
5. Hu Z, Fan C, Oh DS, et al. The molecular portraits of breast tumors are conserved across microarray platforms. BMC Genom 2006; 7(1):96.
6. Eifel P, Axelson JA, Costa J, et al. National Institutes of Health Consensus Development Conference Statement: adjuvant therapy for breast cancer, November 1–3, 2000. J Natl Cancer Inst 2001; 93(13):979–989.
7. Goldhirsch A, Wood WC, Gelber RD, et al. Meeting highlights: updated international expert consensus on the primary therapy of early breast cancer. J Clin Oncol 2003; 21(17):3357–3365.
8. Goldhirsch A, Glick JH, Gelber RD, et al. Meeting highlights: international expert consensus on the primary therapy of early breast cancer 2005. Ann Oncol 2005; 16(10):1569–1583.
9. Liu ET. Mechanism-derived gene expression signatures and predictive biomarkers in clinical oncology. Proc Natl Acad Sci USA 2005; 102(10):3531–3532.
10. van't Veer LJ, Dai H, van de Vijver MJ, et al. Gene expression profiling predicts clinical outcome of breast cancer. Nature 2002; 415(6871):530–536.
11. van de Vijver MJ, He YD, van't Veer LJ, et al. A gene-expression signature as a predictor of survival in breast cancer. N Engl J Med 2002; 347(25):1999–2009.
12. Wang Y, Klijn JG, Zhang Y, et al. Gene-expression profiles to predict distant metastasis of lymph-node-negative primary breast cancer. Lancet 2005; 365(9460):671–679.
13. Foekens JA, Atkins D, Zhang Y, et al. Multicenter validation of a gene expression-based prognostic signature in lymph node-negative primary breast cancer. J Clin Oncol 2006; 24(11):1665–1671.
14. Buyse M, Loi S, van't Veer L, et al. Validation and clinical utility of a 70-gene prognostic signature for women with node-negative breast cancer. J Natl Cancer Inst 2006; 98(4):262–272.
15. Desmedt C, Piette F, Cardoso F, et al. TRANSBIG multi-centre independent validation of the Rotterdam 76-gene prognostic signature for patients with node-negative (N-) breast cancer (BC). Late Breaking News Abstract: Fifth European Breast Cancer Conference, Nice, France, March 21–24, 2006.
16. Klein CA, Blankenstein TJ, Schmidt-Kittler O, et al. Genetic heterogeneity of single disseminated tumour cells in minimal residual cancer. Lancet 2002; 360(9334):683–689.
17. Schmidt-Kittler O, Ragg T, Daskalakis A, et al. From latent disseminated cells to overt metastasis: genetic analysis of systemic breast cancer progression. Proc Natl Acad Sci USA 2003; 100(13):7737–7742.
18. Chang HY, Sneddon JB, Alizadeh AA, et al. Gene expression signature of fibroblast serum response predicts human cancer progression: similarities between tumors and wounds. PLoS Biol 2004; 2(2):E7.

19. Chang HY, Chi JT, Dudoit S, et al. Diversity, topographic differentiation, and positional memory in human fibroblasts. Proc Natl Acad Sci USA 2002; 99(20):12877–12882.

20. Chang HY, Nuyten DS, Sneddon JB, et al. Robustness, scalability, and integration of a wound-response gene expression signature in predicting breast cancer survival. Proc Natl Acad Sci USA 2005; 102(10):3738–3743.

21. Lacroix M, Toillon RA, Leclercq G. Stable "portrait" of breast tumors during progression: data from biology, pathology and genetics. Endocr Relat Cancer 2004; 11(3):497–522.

22. Roylance R, Gorman P, Harris W, et al. Comparative genomic hybridization of breast tumors stratified by histological grade reveals new insights into the biological progression of breast cancer. Cancer Res 1999; 59(7):1433–1436.

23. Warnberg F, Nordgren H, Bergkvist L, et al. Tumour markers in breast carcinoma correlate with grade rather than with invasiveness. Br J Cancer 2001; 85(6):869–874.

24. Elston CW, Ellis IO. Pathological prognostic factors in breast cancer. I. The value of histological grade in breast cancer: experience from a large study with long-term follow-up. Histopathology 1991; 19:403–410; 2002; 41(3A):151.

25. Sotiriou C, Wirapati P, Loi S, et al. Gene expression profiling in breast cancer: understanding the molecular basis of histologic grade to improve prognosis. J Natl Cancer Inst 2006; 98(4):262–272.

26. Loi S, Haibe-Kains B, Desmedt C, et al. Definition of clinically distinct subtypes within estrogen receptor positive breast carcinomas. J Clin Oncol. In press.

27. Dai H, van't Veer L, Lamb J, et al. A cell proliferation signature is a marker of extremely poor outcome in a subpopulation of breast cancer patients. Cancer Res 2005; 65(10):4059–4066.

28. Oh DS, Troester MA, Usary J, et al. Estrogen-regulated genes predict survival in hormone receptor-positive breast cancers. J Clin Oncol 2006; 24(11):1656–1664.

29. Sotiriou C, Wirapati P, Loi S, et al. Is genomic grade killing histological grading? Oral Presentation Fifth European Breast Cancer Conference, Nice, France, March 21–24, 2006.

30. Fan C, Oh DS, Wessels L, et al. Different gene expression-based predictors for breast cancer patients are concordant. N Engl J Med 2006; 355(6):560–569.

31. Paik S, Shak S, Tang G, et al. A multigene assay to predict recurrence of tamoxifen-treated, node-negative breast cancer. N Engl J Med 2004; 351(27):2817–2826.

32. Pittman J, Huang E, Dressman H, et al. Integrated modeling of clinical and gene expression information for personalized prediction of disease outcomes. Proc Natl Acad Sci USA 2004; 101(22):8431–8436.

33. Galea MH, Blamey RW, Elston CE et al. The Nottingham Prognostic Index in primary breast cancer. Breast Cancer Res Treat 1992; 22(3):207–219.

34. Cronin M, Pho M, Dutta D, et al. Measurement of gene expression in archival paraffin-embedded tissues: development and performance of a 92-gene reverse transcriptase-polymerase chain reaction assay. Am J Pathol 2004; 164(1):35–42.

35. Ayers M, Symmans WF, Stec J, et al. Gene expression profiles predict complete pathologic response to neoadjuvant paclitaxel and fluorouracil, doxorubicin, and cyclophosphamide chemotherapy in breast cancer. J Clin Oncol 2004; 22(12):2284–2293.

36. Chang JC, Wooten EC, Tsimelzon A, et al. Gene expression profiling for the prediction of therapeutic response to docetaxel in patients with breast cancer. Lancet 2003; 362(9381):362–369.

37. Chang JC, Wooten EC, Tsimelzon A, et al. Patterns of resistance and incomplete response to docetaxel by gene expression profiling in breast cancer patients. J Clin Oncol 2005; 23(6):1169–1177.

38. Cleator S, Tsimelzon A, Ashworth A, et al. Gene expression patterns for doxorubicin (Adriamycin) and cyclophosphamide (Cytoxan) (AC) response and resistance. Breast Cancer Res Treat 2006; 95(3):229–233.

39. Jansen MP, Foekens JA, van Staveren IL, et al. Molecular classification of tamoxifen-resistant breast carcinomas by gene expression profiling. J Clin Oncol 2005; 23(4):732–740.

40. Ma XJ, Wang Z, Ryan PD et al. A two-gene expression ratio predicts clinical outcome in breast cancer patients treated with tamoxifen. Cancer Cell 2004; 5:607–616.

12 Gene Expression Profile Assays as Predictors of Distant Recurrence-Free Survival in Early-Stage Breast Cancer

Nicole M. Kuderer
Department of Medicine, University of Rochester School of Medicine and Dentistry and the James P. Wilmot Cancer Center, Rochester, New York, U.S.A.

Gary H. Lyman
Department of Medicine, University of Rochester School of Medicine and Dentistry and the James P. Wilmot Cancer Center, University of Rochester Medical Center–Strong Memorial Hospital, Rochester, New York, U.S.A.

INTRODUCTION

The main prognostic factors for early-stage breast cancer (ESBC) include tumor size, nodal status, hormone receptor status, HER2/neu status, histology, and tumor grade. While these and other prognostic factors have been incorporated into treatment guidelines, the remaining prognostic uncertainty means that some patients destined to recur do not receive adjuvant therapy and others are unnecessarily treated experiencing only unnecessary side effects. Clearly better prognostic tools are needed to guide treatment decisions in patients with ESBC (1). New, high-performance screening techniques using DNA microarrays have permitted the analysis of patterns of gene expression in thousands of genes simultaneously. Several investigators have reported efforts to define gene expression signatures based on their ability to predict the risk of disease recurrence and guide the use of adjuvant systemic therapy in ESBC. Before the role of such assays in actual clinical practice can be fully understood, a careful evaluation and validation of test performance in a variety of settings is essential. Such an evaluation ideally precedes the wide scale dissemination and utilization of new diagnostic and prognostic technologies.

The analysis reported here is part of an ongoing effort to systematically review the test performance of various classes of gene expression signatures in women with ESBC and to explore any source of heterogeneity observed.

The enormous cost, and duration of observation required for prospective controlled clinical trials of long-term outcomes often prompts interim observational studies to evaluate the performance characteristics of prognostic assays compared to an intermediate gold standard. While such studies are of limited scope, they permit the assessment of specific aspects of test performance in various populations and require much less time and fewer resources to conduct. The availability of archived clinical material and the development of assays that can be performed on such fixed specimens have further enhanced timely and efficient validation in groups of patients with information on long-term clinical outcomes.

METHODS
Data Acquisition
A systematic review of the all-language published literature on gene expression profile studies in patients with ESBC was undertaken using the following data sources: MEDLINE®, EMBASE®, The Cochrane Library, DARE (Database of Abstract of Reviews of Effectiveness), and a review of references in identified articles. Search terms included gene expression profiles or profiling, gene signatures, gene expression chips, microarrays, and breast neoplasm or cancer. The study population had to be an original study group with duplicate articles based on the same group of patients excluded. Follow-up studies in which a subset of previously reported patients were reported, only the most recent article containing the most up-to-date results was reported. Eleven independent cohorts of patients with ESBC were identified in which the relationship between a gene expression signature and distant recurrence-free survival was reported. The primary outcome of interest was distant recurrence-free survival based on gene expression risk category. Data extraction was undertaken by two independent investigators in a blinded fashion with any unresolved issues settled by a third independent investigator.

Statistical Analysis
Primary Outcomes
The primary outcome of interest was distant recurrence-free survival. Patients were stratified according to the gene expression profile risk grouping into high- or low-risk. Measures of test performance consisted of sensitivity, specificity, positive and negative predictive value, likelihood ratio, the diagnostic odds ratio, and the receiver-operating characteristic (ROC) curve. Sensitivity is defined as the proportion of patients with subsequent disease recurrence classified as high risk by the gene signature, while specificity is the proportion of patients without disease recurrence classified as low risk. Sensitivity and specificity will vary as the threshold or cutpoint defining risk is varied. A cutpoint associated with greater sensitivity will result in a loss of specificity and vice versa. The predictive value positive is defined as the probability of disease recurrence in those classified as high-risk, whereas the predictive value negative is the probability of no disease recurrence in those classified as low-risk. The predictive value depends both on model performance and the risk of distant recurrence or death. The likelihood ratio represents the probability of the assay result in someone with recurrence divided by the probability in someone without recurrence and is a useful summary measure for describing the discriminatory ability of high- or low-risk assay results. The diagnostic odds ratio is a useful measure of overall assay prognostic discrimination and can be thought of as the ratio of the likelihood ratio positive and likelihood ratio negative. The ROC curve plots the true positive rate (sensitivity) and the false positive rate $(1 - $ specificity$)$ from different studies. Overall test discrimination is associated with the area under the ROC curve corresponding to the c-statistic for dichotomous measures.

Descriptive Statistics
The distributions of all outcomes were evaluated and summary measures of central tendency and variability were estimated. Measures of central tendency included the overall proportions, mean, median, and variance weighted summary measures based on the method of Mantel and Haenszel. Bivariate correlations between continuous measures were based either on the Pearson coefficient as a measure of linear correlation for data close to normal in distribution or the Spearman's rho

as a nonparametric measure of correlation. Tests for linearity were derived from the sum of squares, degrees of freedom, and mean square associated with linear and nonlinear components based on ANOVA. Categorical measures were compared using a χ^2 test. The relationship of primary outcomes to study size, proportion with positive lymph nodes, technique used, and study quality was evaluated.

Meta-Analysis
Study-by-study heterogeneity was assessed for each test performance measure based on the Q-statistic (2). The hypothesis that the studies are all drawn from a population of studies with the same effect size is rejected if the Q-statistic exceeds the upper 100 $(1 - a)$ percentile of the χ^2 distribution. An inconsistency index (I^2) was estimated by the method of Altman as $(H^2 - 1)/H^2$ where $H^2 = Q/(k - 1)$ and k the degrees of freedom (3). The inconsistency index (I^2) was estimated reflecting the proportion of variation in study estimates due to between study heterogeneity rather than random variation. Due to the significant heterogeneity between studies, weighted summary outcome estimates were based on a random effects model as proposed by DerSimonian and Laird (4). Under a random effects model, the studies are assumed to be from different populations with different true effect sizes. With this conservative approach, the true measure may differ between studies due to differences in patient populations, treatment variation, or because outcome measures differ from one study to the next. Therefore, two sources of variation are assumed consisting of random error and variation due to real differences between the studies. As a result, the standard error of the outcome measure estimates will approach zero as the sample size within studies increases, while the differences in the true effect sizes between studies will persist.

Hypothesis testing on summary effect estimates was based on a z-statistic with estimates of standard error and 95% confidence interval (CI) provided for all individual studies as well as the summary overall effect estimate. Results are presented as forest plots with effect estimates and 95% confidence limits (CLs) presented for each individual study and a summary measure and CLs across all studies. Evidence for a publication bias in studies included in the meta-analysis is evaluated using a funnel plot of the diagnostic odds ratio and its precision (1/standard error).

RESULTS
Summary of Included Studies
Of the 453 studies, in the published or presented literature, identified between 1990 and 2005, 11 were found to represent separate study populations of ESBC patients with validation based on distant recurrence or distant recurrence-free survival (5–14). Table 1 summarizes the 11 validation cohorts included in this systematic review. The 11 series included 1520 patients (range 20–668) of which 824 (54%) patients were classified as high-risk based on the gene assay and 354 (23%) experienced distant breast cancer recurrence during the period of observation. The reported recurrence rates were 35% (95% CI: 26–42) among gene expression profile high-risk patients and 9% (95% CI: 7–12) among low-risk patients. Median follow-up on patients ranged from 2 to 14 years. No adjuvant treatment was utilized in two studies, limited to chemotherapy in one and tamoxifen in one, whereas it was not restricted in three and not specified in the remaining four studies. Six cohorts were evaluated utilizing cross-validation techniques while five were studied in independent cohorts of patients. As shown in

TABLE 1 Gene Expression Profile Assays in Early-Stage Breast Cancer Study Characteristics

Study	Country	Patients	FU[a]	LN status	ER	Treatment
Ahr-1	Germany	27	2.0	Positive	Mixed	Unknown
Ahr-2	Germany	20	2.0	Negative	Mixed	Unknown
Bertucci	France	55	5.0	Both	Mixed	Chemotherapy
Huang	USA	52	3.0	Both	Mixed	Unknown
Iwao	Japan	119	4.5	Both	Mixed	Unknown
Paik	USA	668	14.0	Negative	Positive	Tamoxifen
Esteva	USA	149	10.0	Negative	Mixed	None
van De Vijver-1	The Netherlands	78	7.8	Negative	Mixed	Mixed
van De Vijver-2	The Netherlands	67	7.8	Negative	Mixed	Mixed
van De Vijver-3	The Netherlands	114	7.8	Positive	Mixed	Mixed
Wang	The Netherlands	171	5.0	Negative	Mixed	None

[a]Follow-up in years.
Abbreviations: ER, estrogen receptor; LN, lymph node.

Table 1, reported series included six limited to lymph node negative patients, two restricted to node positive patients, and three with both node positive and negative patients. Only one series limited the study to hormone receptor positive women (11).

Test Performance Characteristics
Summary Measures
Summary test performance characteristics for distant disease recurrence-free survival are shown in Table 2 including the overall rates pooling all studies as well as the average sensitivity, specificity, likelihood ratio positive and negative, the diagnostic odds ratio, and the positive and negative predictive values across studies. Among assay performance measures, significant heterogeneity was observed for sensitivity ($P = 0.0082$), specificity ($P < 0.0001$), positive predictive value ($P < 0.0001$), and the diagnostic odds ratio ($P = 0.0011$) but not for the negative predictive value ($P = 0.2112$), likelihood ratio positive ($P = 0.2632$), or the likelihood ratio negative ($P = 0.1795$).

Sensitivity and Specificity
Weighted summary assay sensitivity and specificity were estimated at 82.4% (95% CI 76.1–88.7) and 53.3% (95% CI 43.9–62.7), respectively. The corresponding overall proportion of patients with recurrence classified as low-risk (false negative rate) was 17.8% (95% CI 14.2–22.1), while the proportion of patients with no recurrence but classified as high-risk (false positive) was 46.1% (95% CI 43.2–49.0).

TABLE 2 Gene Expression Profile Assays in Early-Stage Breast Cancer Summary Performance Measures

Measure	Mean	Overall (95% CLs)
Sensitivity	84.2%	82% (78,86)
Specificity	57.4%	54% (51,57)
Likelihood ratio positive	3.45	1.78 (1.65,1.932)
Likelihood ratio negative	0.32	0.35 (0.26,0.47)
Diagnostic odds ratio	14.98	6.02 (3.02,11.97)
Predictive value positive	45.6%	43% (32,53)
Predictive value negative	89.0%	90% (87,93)

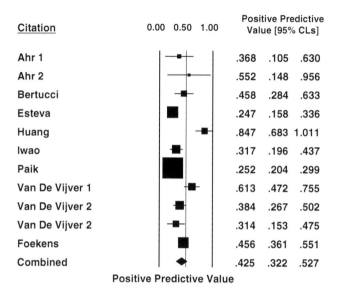

FIGURE 1 Forest plot of the positive predictive value of gene expression profile signatures ±95% CLs in ESBC estimated by the Mantel–Haenszel method for each study. The weighted combined positive predictive value ± 95% CLs based on a random effects model is shown at the bottom.

Predictive Value

Figures 1 and 2 present forest plots with individual study and weighted summary measures for assay positive and negative predictive values demonstrating weighted summary estimates of 42.5% (95% CI 32.2–52.7) and 89.8% (95% CI

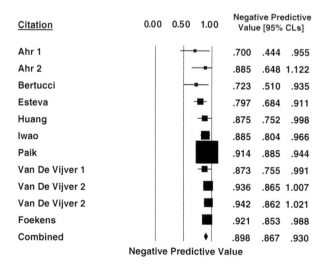

FIGURE 2 Forest plot of the negative predictive value of gene expression profile signatures ±95% CLs in ESBC estimated by the Mantel–Haenszel method for each study. The weighted combined negative predictive value ±95% CLs based on a random effects model is shown at the bottom.

86.7–93.0), respectively. The inconsistency index is 87% and 24% for the positive and negative predictive values, respectively. The overall estimate of distant recurrence risk in those with low-risk assays (1 − predictive value negative) is 9.2% (95% CI 7.2–11.6). Likewise, the overall estimate of no distant recurrence in those with high-risk assays is 64.7% (95% CI 61.4–67.9). As anticipated, the positive predictive value is directly proportional to the overall risk of recurrence in the study population.

Diagnostic Odds Ratio
Weighted summary estimates of 1.78 (95% CI 1.47–2.16) and 0.35 (95% CI 0.26–0.47) were calculated for assay likelihood ratio positive and negative, respectively. The weighted summary estimate of the diagnostic odds ratio as a measure of overall test discrimination was 6.44 (95% CI 3.42, 12.08). The estimated area under the ROC curve (±standard error) was 0.8611 ± 0.0495.

Sources of Heterogeneity
No significant relationship was observed between the measures of assay performance considered and lymph node status, hormone receptor status, or type of adjuvant treatment. Assay performance measures were generally weaker in studies with independent validation but only reached statistical significance for predictive value positive with medians of 54% and 32% for crossover and independent validation studies, respectively ($P = 0.045$). Significant correlation was observed between the number of genes in the signature studied and assay sensitivity ($r_{sp} = 0.673$; $P = 0.047$) and diagnostic odds ratio ($r_{sp} = 0.648$; $P = 0.043$). The association between the number of genes in the signature of each study and the diagnostic odds ratio as a measure of overall model discrimination is shown in Figure 3.

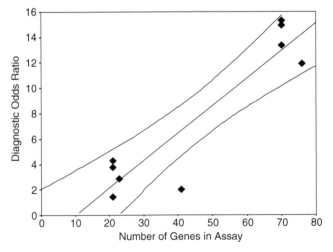

FIGURE 3 Graph of the diagnostic odds ratio and the number of genes in the assay signature from each study of patients with early-stage breast cancer. The filled line is based on linear regression on the mean ±95% CLs.

DISCUSSION

Gene expression profile assays based on microarray analysis show early promise for predicting recurrence-free survival in patients with ESBC. However, the use of these assays in therapeutic decision-making must consider both the limitations of assay test performance and the specific patient population being evaluated (15–17). Systematic reviews of prognostic studies may contribute to a better understanding of these techniques by summarizing the results of test accuracy from several different investigations, identifying reasons for variation in the results of individual studies, and potentially improving the quality of future studies through a delineation of the methodological inadequacies of previous reports. Finally, such reviews may be capable of generating new hypotheses that may be tested in future definitive studies.

A systematic review of reported studies of gene expression assays in women with ESBC is presented here. The gene expression assays included in the analysis were limited to those providing validation in women with ESBC based on distant recurrence-free survival. A formal meta-analysis of test performance characteristics observed for these assays and outcomes was conducted.

The variability of assay prognostic performance characteristics may relate to both random error (chance) and to systematic differences or heterogeneity between studies. Most of the validation studies reported here were small with more than half including less than 100 patients. Since assay performance measures are more accurately estimated in larger studies, such studies deserve particular attention. The methodology employed in this systematic review, in fact, weighs the individual studies inversely in proportion to their contribution to the variance and, therefore, larger studies will generally contribute more to the summary estimates. Substantial heterogeneity was also observed across studies for most performance measures. Weighted pooled performance estimates were therefore based on a random effects model and emphasis was placed on the ROC analysis. While assay performance varied considerably across reports, it was limited to some degree in all studies. Causes of study-by-study variation include the use of different gene signatures and risk score cutpoints. In addition, the inclusion of studies based on cross-validation may overestimate the accuracy of an assay while independent validation offers the truest estimate of how an assay actually performs (15,16). Summary estimates of prognostic performance in this review were found to be less in studies with independent validation, as anticipated. However, these differences were not statistically significant.

Systematic reviews of prognostic studies, like those of therapeutic trials, are dependent upon the quality of the individual studies included in its analysis (18–22). The patient selection process should be fully described and the reference standard outcome explicitly defined and generally accepted. The assay procedure and the definition of high-risk and low-risk results should also be fully described. Ideally, the investigator and interpreter of the test are blinded as to the disease status of the patients and the method of concealment should be detailed. The same uniform assay procedure and outcome evaluation should be employed for all patients. Inconsistent reporting of patient characteristics, assay characteristics, and statistical analysis, increases the inter-study variability, leading to increased variability in the results of the meta-analysis (23,24). Variation in study population and clinical setting as well as the assay utilized can each result in variation in diagnostic accuracy. Additional sources of heterogeneity in assay performance may include the cutpoint or threshold defining high-risk and low-risk patients, measurement differences between observers, and differences in risk of recurrence.

Superior prognostic performance compared to conventional clinical prognostic markers or guidelines has been reported for some gene expression assays (6,11,14). Despite the prognostic information provided by these assays, however, clinicians need to be familiar with their limitations, in order to appropriately utilize them in clinical practice. As reported here, while the sensitivity of the gene assays for predicting recurrence was relatively high in some studies, the specificity for identifying those who remain disease-free was quite low. An assay is most useful for ruling out a future recurrence if it has high sensitivity, whereas it is most useful for confirming the risk of future recurrence if it has high specificity. Therefore, while the negative predictive value ranged from 75% to 100% across studies, the positive predictive value ranged from 25% to 88% or 43% overall. As expected, the predictive value of the gene signatures depends on not only the sensitivity and specificity of assay but also upon the risk of distant recurrence in the population under study. Assays utilized in higher risk women with ESBC will be associated with greater predictive value positive but lower predictive value negative despite a low-risk assay result.

The risk of distant recurrence, the potential effect of treatment on risk as well as the impact of disease and treatment on patient quality of life must all be considered in determining the appropriate role for such assays in clinical care. Although systematic reviews of prognostic accuracy can be quite valuable, particularly early in the evaluation of a new assay, such studies are not capable of addressing all clinically relevant questions. Clearly, large controlled clinical trials represent the gold standard for evaluating any prognostic or therapeutic intervention that might have an impact on important clinical outcomes. However, such trials are handicapped by the great cost, resources, and time required. Clearly, the validity of meta-analyses of assay performance studies as well as controlled clinical trials are both dependent upon the quality of the original studies. In addition, the validity of systematic reviews is dependent upon capturing results from all available studies. This review was based on assay validation studies published in the peer-review literature or recently presented at major meetings.

Systematic evaluations such as that reported here should be useful not only to clinicians in evaluating and potentially incorporating the results of such assays into clinical practice but also to investigators involved in the development and validation of new gene expression signatures. Undoubtedly, the greatest challenge will be to define the potential role of these assays in clinical decision-making considering the clinical, economic, and quality of life impact of disease and treatments guided by the results of such prognostic tools. Current efforts to enhance the value of gene expression assays through incorporation of genes that are not only prognostic but also predictive of response and toxicity of specific therapies should further increase the clinical and quality of life impact as well as the cost-effectiveness of these tests.

Several specific recommendations can be put forth for current and future studies of gene expression signatures in ESBC as well as those related to other malignancies. Investigators should strive for independent validation in a large enough population of patients to provide unbiased and accurate estimates of assay performance. Transparency is needed in study design including the selection of genes for inclusion in the assay and the patient population utilized including clinical prognostic factors and methods of treatment. It is essential that any potential role for these assays be defined in comparison to or in combination with recognized clinical prognostic factors.

REFERENCES

1. Altman DG, Lyman GH. Methodological challenges in the evaluation of prognostic factors in breast cancer. Breast Cancer Res Treat 1998; 52:289–303.
2. Laird NM, Mosteller F. Some statistical methods for combining experimental results. Int J Technol Assess Health Care 1990; 6:5–30.
3. Higgins JP, Thompson SG, Deeks JJ, Altman D. Measuring inconsistency in meta-analyses. Brit Med J 2003; 327:557–560.
4. DerSimonian R, Laird NM. Meta-analysis in clinical trials. Contr Clin Trials 1986; 7:177–188.
5. van't Veer LJ, Dai H, van De Vijver MJ, et al. Gene expression profiling predicts clinical outcome of breast cancer. Nature 2002; 415:530–536.
6. van De Vijver MJ, He YD, van't Veer LJ, et al. A gene-expression signature as a predictor of survival in breast cancer. N Engl J Med 2002; 347:1999–2009.
7. Ahr A, Karn T, Solbach C, et al. Identification of high risk breast-cancer patients by gene expression profiling. Lancet 2002; 359:131–132.
8. Bertucci F, Nasser V, Granjeaud S, et al. Gene expression profiles of poor prognosis primary breast cancer correlate with survival. Hum Mol Genet 2002; 11:863–872.
9. Huang E, Cheng SH, Dressman H, et al. Gene expression predictors of breast cancer outcomes. Lancet 2003; 361:1590–1596.
10. Iwao K, Matoba R, Ueno N, et al. Molecular classification of primary breast tumors possessing distinct prognostic properties. Hum Mol Genet 2002; 11:199–206.
11. Paik S, Shak S, Tang G, et al. A multigene assay to predict recurrence of tamoxifen-treated, node negative breast cancer. N Engl J Med 2004; 351:2817–2826.
12. Esteva FJ, Sahin AA, Coombes L, et al. Multi-gene RT-PCR assay for predicting recurrence in node-negative breast cancer patients that did not receive adjuvant tamoxifen nor chemotherapy. Breast Cancer Res Treat 2004; 88(suppl 1):1–253.
13. Esteva FJ, Sahin AA, Cristofanilli M, et al. Prognostic role of a multi-gene RT-PCR assay in patients with node-negative breast cancer not receiving adjuvant systemic therapy. Clin Cancer Res 2005; 104:676–681.
14. Wang Y, Klijn JGM, Zhang Y, et al. Gene-expression profiles to predict distant metastasis of lymph-node negative primary breast cancer. Lancet 2005; 365:671–679.
15. Simon R, Radmacher MD, Dobbin K, McShane LM. Pitfalls in the use of DNA micro-array data for diagnostic and prognostic classification. J Natl Cancer Inst 2003; 95:14–18.
16. Ntzani EE, Ioannidis JPA. Predictive ability of DNA microarrays for cancer outcomes and correlates: an empirical assessment. Lancet 2003; 362:1439–1444.
17. Simon R. Diagnostic and prognostic prediction using gene expression profiles in high-dimensional microarray data. Brit J Cancer 2003; 89:1599–1604.
18. Lyman GH, Djulbegovic B. The challenge of systematic reviews in cancer screening, diagnostic and staging studies. Cancer Treat Rev 2005; 31:628–639.
19. Deeks JJ. Systematic reviews of evaluations of diagnostic and screening tests. BMJ 2001; 323:157–162.
20. Vamvakas E. Meta-analysis of studies of the diagnostic accuracy of laboratory tests: a review of the concepts and methods. Arch Pathol Lab Med 1998; 122:675–686.
21. Irwig L, Tosteson ANA, Gatsonis C, et al. Guidelines for meta-analysis evaluating diagnostic tests. Ann Intern Med 1994; 120:667–676.
22. Shepes SB, Schechter MT. The assessment of diagnostic tests. J Am Med Assoc 1984; 252(17):2418–2422.
23. Lyman GH, Kuderer NM. The strengths and limitations of meta-analyses based on aggregate patient data. BMC Med Res Methodol 2005; 5(14):1–7.

13 Economic Analysis of Gene Expression Profile Data to Guide Adjuvant Treatment in Women with Early-Stage Breast Cancer

Leon E. Cosler
Department of Pharmacy Practice, Albany College of Pharmacy, Albany, New York, U.S.A.

Gary H. Lyman
Department of Medicine, University of Rochester School of Medicine and Dentistry and the James P. Wilmot Cancer Center, University of Rochester Medical Center–Strong Memorial Hospital, Rochester, New York, U.S.A.

INTRODUCTION

Breast cancer is the second most common type of cancer among women in the United States with more than 200,000 women diagnosed with invasive disease and with approximately 40,000 dying annually from the disease (1). As a result of early detection efforts, nearly half of these women present with lymph node negative hormone receptor positive disease. Current treatment for early-stage breast cancer (ESBC) with adjuvant hormonal therapy and/or chemotherapy is based on clinical and pathological criteria including the presence and number of involved lymph nodes, tumor size and grade, hormone receptor status, and the presence of HER2/*neu* overexpression among others. Treatment decisions may also take into consideration patient age or menopausal status due to the anticipated lower risk of cancer recurrence, and the potential for smaller benefit and greater toxicity with aggressive systemic chemotherapy in older women. These considerations form the basis for clinical practice guidelines for the management of patients with ESBC (2,3). Current guidelines recommend adjuvant systemic chemotherapy and endocrine therapy for most women with lymph node negative, hormone receptor positive, ESBC. Unfortunately, such systemic chemotherapy is associated with considerable cost, proximal morbidity, as well as increasing evidence for serious delayed toxicities including neurocognitive dysfunction and secondary malignancies.

The risk of distant recurrence is generally low among ESBC patients with lymph node negative, hormone receptor positive disease regardless of treatment with adjuvant chemotherapy. However, several randomized controlled trials of adjuvant chemotherapy and meta-analyses have shown the value of adjuvant chemotherapy in reducing the risk of disease recurrence and death in patients who may be at an increased risk (4). These trials have also demonstrated that some patients develop distant recurrences despite having received adjuvant chemotherapy for their ESBC. Currently, national and international consensus guidelines endorse the addition of adjuvant chemotherapy to hormonal therapy in lymph node negative, estrogen receptor positive ESBC patients who are at increased risk for recurrence. The guidelines also recommend hormonal therapy alone in women with a lower risk of recurrence (2,3). Since predicting an individual patient's risk of recurrence based on conventional measures is limited in its accuracy, many patients continue to be treated inappropriately with adjuvant chemotherapy. Recently, gene expression profiles and other molecular techniques have demonstrated value in their ability to more accurately predict the risk of disease recurrence and the potential impact of treatment in order to guide clinical decisions for adjuvant ESBC therapy (5).

A 21-gene expression profile assay has been developed based on reverse transcriptase polymerase chain reaction (RT-PCR) methods permitting the quantification of gene expression in fixed paraffin embedded tissue (6). The profile was derived from 250 cancer-related candidate genes identified from the cancer literature, genomic databases, and microarray data (7–10). The 21-gene expression signature included 16 functional and five reference genes, which provide optimal RT-PCR performance. Based on tissue from 447 women with ESBC including 233 from National Surgical Adjuvant Breast Program (NSABP) B-20, the 21-gene profile was shown to have robust prediction for distant recurrence (11). Using a proprietary formula, a recurrence score (RS; Oncotype DX) ranging from 0 to 100 was derived from each patient's gene tumor expression results. Patients were subsequently categorized into low-risk (RS <18); intermediate-risk (RS = 18–30); and high-risk (RS ≥31) groups. This 21-gene expression profile has been independently validated as a predictive indicator of distant recurrence-free survival (DRFS) in 668 evaluable patients in lymph node negative, receptor positive ESBC receiving tamoxifen on the NSABP B-14 study (12–15). The assay has been shown to be a significant independent prognostic factor for distant recurrence in multivariate analysis after adjustment for age and tumor size with an adjusted hazard ratio of 3.21 (95% CI 2.23, 4.61; $P < 0.00001$) (10).

A cost-utility analysis was conducted using the 21-gene assay in patients classified as having low- or high-risk of distant recurrence based on National Comprehensive Cancer Network (NCCN) clinical guidelines (16) The analysis considered survival, quality of life, and relevant costs from a societal perspective. The results demonstrated that at baseline values, the RS applied to 100 hypothetical patients was predicted to increase survival by 8.6 quality-adjusted life years (QALYs) and reduce overall treatment costs by US $202,828. Using a Monte Carlo simulation model, the RS was cost-saving in more than two-thirds of simulations. The RS was shown to be more accurate as a prognostic tool than the NCCN guidelines for lymph node negative, estrogen receptor positive ESBC, and was cost-effective when applied appropriately (16).

Use of the 21-gene profile has recently undergone additional validation directed towards the response to chemotherapy followed by tamoxifen among 651 patients on NSABP B-20 and 645 patients on NSABP B-14 (17). This research incorporates the additional validation results into an economic prediction model of the 21-gene expression signature for its ability to guide the use of adjuvant chemotherapy and hormonal therapy in patients with lymph node negative, estrogen receptor positive ESBC.

METHODS
Risk Assessment
The initial validation study of the accuracy of the 21-gene expression signature was based on the 2617 eligible lymph node negative, estrogen receptor positive women with ESBC, treated with tamoxifen on NSABP B-14, of whom 688 were evaluable based on the availability of the original tumor samples with sufficient tissue to

provide adequate RNA for RT-PCR analysis (11). The predictive accuracy for DRFS based on response to systemic chemotherapy followed by tamoxifen has also undergone validation in 651 patients randomized on NSABP B-20 and 645 patients on NSABP B-14 (17). No significant differences were found among patients included in these analyses from all subjects randomized to treatment groups for these two trials. Kaplan–Meier methods were applied to the primary outcome of DRFS and secondary measures of relapse-free survival, and overall survival. Patients were censored at the time of the development of contralateral breast cancer, second nonbreast cancer, or death without cancer recurrence. A continuous variable RS was generated by fitting a time-dependent log-hazard ratio model to the data. The 10-year distant recurrence rate was estimated by a Breslow-type estimator as previously described (18). Women with node negative, receptor positive, ESBC with and without adjuvant chemotherapy (NSABP B-20) or tamoxifen alone (NSABP B-14) were classified as high (RS ≥31), intermediate (RS 18–30), or low (RS <18) risk of distant recurrence at 10 years (Fig. 1).

Outcome Measures

The clinical impact of different treatment strategies (i.e., tamoxifen alone vs. systemic chemotherapy followed by tamoxifen) was assessed by estimating life-years saved (LYS) as estimated from NSABP B-20 and B-14. The impact of the treatment strategies on health-related quality of life was derived from published studies of patient preferences or health utilities for different treatment strategies (19,20). These studies are based on a time trade-off method where patients determine the maximum number of years of their life expectancy with disease that they would be willing to give up for an ability to live in full health. This game theory approach is based on the premise that many patients would be willing to give up some length of life for a higher quality (or disease free) survival. A utility index is calculated as the ratio

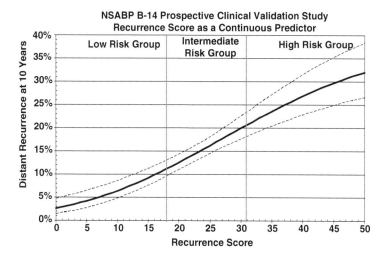

FIGURE 1 A recurrence score (RS) generated as a continuous measure by fitting a time-varying piece-wise log-hazard ratio model to the 10-year distant recurrence rate. Women with node negative, receptor positive, early-stage breast cancer are classified as high (RS ≥31), intermediate (RS 18–30), or low (RS <18) risk of distant recurrence at 10 years. *Source*: From Ref. 11.

of disease-free years divided by the equivalent number of years in the current diseased state. The utility value will range from 0 (worst possible health or death) to
1 (perfect health). Clinical outcomes were then adjusted in the form of the QALY
as a product of the actual life expectancy multiplied by the patient health utility.

The costs of cancer care were obtained from data available from the Centers
for Medicare and Medicaid Services (CMS) and published literature (21). Chemotherapy costs were calculated using drug average wholesale price (AWP) and
other treatment-related direct and indirect costs were not considered. Utility estimates for the quality of life impact of adjuvant breast cancer chemotherapy were
derived from published literature for this disease state (19,20). Costs not considered
in this analysis include additional direct costs associated with drug administration,
professional fees, and laboratory testing along with indirect costs such as transportation and loss of productivity costs and patient out-of-pocket expenses.

Cost-Effectiveness and Cost-Utility

The economic analysis presented here is based upon a clinical decision model to
compare and evaluate the clinical, economical, and quality of life outcomes for
three adjuvant treatment strategies: (*i*) tamoxifen alone; (*ii*) chemotherapy followed
by tamoxifen; or (*iii*) RS-guided therapy using the results of the RS derived from the
21-gene RT-PCR assay, that is, tamoxifen for low-risk patients; chemotherapy and
tamoxifen for intermediate- and high-risk patients (Fig. 2). Baseline probability
and cost-assumptions are provided in Table 1. Cost-effectiveness and cost-utility

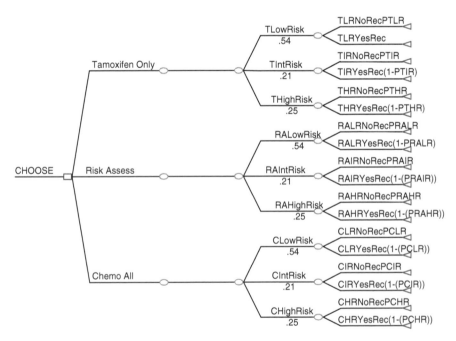

FIGURE 2 Clinical decision model comparing and evaluating the clinical, economic, and quality-of-
life outcomes for three adjuvant treatment strategies: tamoxifen alone, chemotherapy followed by
tamoxifen, or recurrence score (RS)-guided therapy using the results of the RS derived from the
21-gene RT-PCR assay, that is, tamoxifen for low-risk patients, chemotherapy and tamoxifen for
intermediate- and high-risk patients.

TABLE 1 Baseline Values Subjected to Sensitivity Analyses

Group	Description	Baseline value	Range	Distribution type	Source
10-year distant recurrence-free survival					
Low-risk	Tamoxifen	96.3	—	Binomial	Paik
	Chemotherapy +tamoxifen	95.0			
	RS-guided therapy	96.3			
Intermediate-risk	Tamoxifen	82.2			
	Chemotherapy +tamoxifen	89.9			
	RS-guided therapy	89.9			
High-risk	Tamoxifen	61.7			
	Chemotherapy +tamoxifen	88.9			
	RS-guided therapy	88.9			
Proportions					
Low-risk		0.54	—	—	Paik
Intermediate-risk		0.21			
High-risk		0.25			
Direct costs (US $)					
	Adjuvant chemotherapy	10,000	500–25,000	Normal, SD = 2500	CMS, Oestreicher
	Surveillance without recurrence	5000	500–20,000	Normal, SD = 1000	CMS, Oestreicher
	OncotypeDx assay	3460	—	—	Genomic Health
	Treatment of recurrence	50,000	10,000–150,000	Normal, SD = 20,000	CMS, Oestreicher
Time					
	Healthy life expectancy (yrs)	20	5–30	—	NCHS
	Annual mortality rate following recurrence	0.347	—		Paik
Quality-of-life					
	Utility with chemotherapy	1.0	0.5–1.0	—	Earle

Abbreviations: CMS, Centers for Medical and Medicaid Services; RS, recurrence score; SD, standard deviation.

analyses were used to evaluate the treatment strategies as methods reflecting the additional cost of one strategy over another (marginal cost) and the additional clinical benefit (marginal efficacy) or quality adjusted clinical benefit (marginal utility). A cost-effectiveness ratio comparing the marginal cost and the marginal effectiveness (marginal cost-effectiveness) represents the incremental cost per LYS (22–24). A cost-utility ratio measures the tradeoff between cost and benefit expressed in terms of the marginal cost and the marginal utility (marginal cost-utility) defined as the incremental cost per QALY saved. Incremental costs ($), LYS, QALYs, and cost-effectiveness (cost per LYS) were estimated for RS-guided treatment with tamoxifen for low-risk patients and chemotherapy followed by tamoxifen for intermediate- and high-risk patients, compared to either chemotherapy and tamoxifen or tamoxifen alone administered to all patients without the benefit of risk score.

Monte Carlo Simulation

Variation in the estimates of cost and outcomes were assessed using Monte Carlo simulation. Data was randomly sampled from all available distributions for DRFS and estimated costs. The sampling distributions and summary cost, efficacy, and variance estimates were based on 1000 patient replicates.

RESULTS

Risk Stratification

Results of the 651 evaluable patients on NSABP B-20 with corresponding gene expression assays, 64 (9.83%) developed distant recurrence including 31 (13.66%) who were randomized to tamoxifen only therapy and 33 (7.78%) receiving chemotherapy plus tamoxifen. Distant recurrence in the risk score low-, intermediate-, and high-risk patients at 10 years was 3.2%, 9.1%, and 39.5% with tamoxifen alone and 4.4%, 10.9%, and 11.9% for patients receiving chemotherapy plus tamoxifen. The RS-guided therapy is associated with a gain in individual life expectancy of 2.2 years compared to tamoxifen alone for all patients. There was no significant difference in life expectancy at 10 years between the RS-guided therapy and the chemotherapy plus tamoxifen strategies.

Expected Costs

Under baseline cost assumptions (Table 1), the lowest expected total cost of treatment is associated with treatment with tamoxifen alone (US $11,890), whereas the greatest expected cost is that associated with the chemotherapy plus tamoxifen strategy (US $18,418), with the RS-guided therapy associated with an expected cost of US $16,162. Based on all reasonable assumptions about the cost of patient follow-up among patients without recurring disease, tamoxifen is associated with the lowest costs and the RS-guided therapy is always associated with lower costs than the chemotherapy plus tamoxifen strategy.

The expected costs associated with both the chemotherapy plus tamoxifen strategy and the RS-guided therapy strategy increased as the direct cost of the chemotherapy increased but at differing rates. The RS-guided therapy strategy is preferred over the chemotherapy plus tamoxifen strategy when total chemotherapy costs exceed US $5822. While adriamycin and cyclophosphamide given every three weeks without myeloid growth factor support is associated with a lower treatment cost, most of the commonly utilized adjuvant breast cancer regimens are associated with higher costs that favor the utilization of the 21-gene expression signature.

Cost-Effectiveness

The incremental costs associated with the RS-guided therapy and chemotherapy plus tamoxifen strategies are US $4272 and US $6527, respectively, compared to tamoxifen alone. The corresponding overall gain in life expectancy with RS-guided therapy compared to tamoxifen alone is 2.2 years, whereas no significant difference is seen between RS-guided therapy compared to chemotherapy and tamoxifen strategy. When compared to tamoxifen alone, the resulting incremental cost-effectiveness ratio favors the RS-guided therapy strategy (US $1944/LYS). Likewise when compared to the chemotherapy plus tamoxifen approach, the incremental cost-effectiveness ratio (US $3385/LYS) is well within accepted ranges for adopted medical strategies. Declining age-specific life expectancy is associated

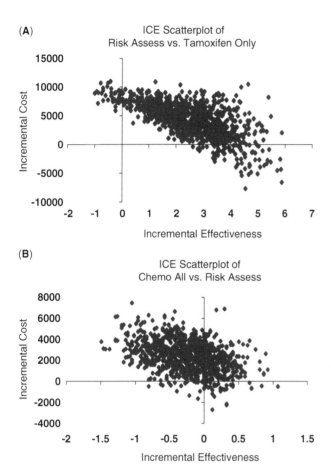

FIGURE 3 Incremental cost-effectiveness scatterplot for (**A**) RS-guided therapy versus tamoxifen alone and (**B**) RS-guided therapy versus chemotherapy and tamoxifen. Incremental effectiveness (LYS) is represented by the horizontal axis and incremental costs (US $) on the vertical axis.

with a reduction in the incremental efficacy in LYS and thus increases the incremental cost-effectiveness ratios for RS-guided therapy when compared to tamoxifen alone (Fig. 3). Alternatively, life expectancy has no significant effect on the incremental cost-effectiveness of RS-guided therapy when compared to chemotherapy plus tamoxifen.

Cost-Utility
The baseline assumptions indicated in Table 1 do not include an adjustment for the impact of chemotherapy on quality-of-life. However, such adjustments have an anticipated effect on the estimated QALYs and, therefore, the cost-utility or cost per QALY gained. Expected QALYs favor the RS-guided therapy strategy over chemotherapy plus tamoxifen strategy for all utility assumptions. The health utility associated with chemotherapy has no impact on the expected QALYs associated with the strategy of tamoxifen alone. When compared to tamoxifen alone, the

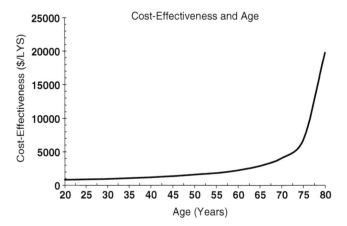

FIGURE 4 Graphical display of incremental cost-effectiveness ratios for recurrence score–guided therapy compared to tamoxifen alone with increasing age in years.

RS-guided therapy results in greater expected QALYs until the health utility associated with chemotherapy falls below 0.82. At a utility of 0.9 associated with adjuvant chemotherapy, RS-guided therapy is associated with both a net cost savings in addition to a gain in individual QALYs of 0.97 QALY when compared to tamoxifen alone and a cost-utility ratio of US $4432/QALY and a gain in 1.71 QALYs when compared to chemotherapy and tamoxifen.

Monte Carlo Simulation
Using data from the 1000 Monte Carlo replicates, the mean Standard Deviation (SD) and median incremental cost-effectiveness ratios were US $2769/LYS (US $20,164) and US $1784/LYS, respectively, for RS-guided therapy compared to tamoxifen alone and US $3856/LYS (US $23,106) and US $4198 for chemotherapy plus tamoxifen compared to RS-guided therapy. As shown in Figure 4A, incremental cost-effectiveness ratios for the relationship between RS-guided therapy and tamoxifen alone are primarily represented by an increase in LYS while simultaneously associated with an increase in cost. As shown in Figure 4B, incremental cost-effectiveness ratios for the relationship between RS-guided therapy and the chemotherapy plus tamoxifen strategy demonstrate that the RS-guided therapy reduces estimated total treatment costs in 70% of the randomly drawn samples in Monte Carlo analysis with and an overall benefit in terms of life expectancy.

DISCUSSION

When compared to tamoxifen alone, treatment decisions guided by a 21-gene profile are associated with greater efficacy as well as cost-effectiveness ratios, which are well within accepted ranges for technology adoption. RS-guided therapy are also associated with increased efficacy with substantially lower toxicity and treatment costs compared to chemotherapy plus tamoxifen for all patients. The efficacy of adjuvant systemic therapy in ESBC has been repeatedly demonstrated in multiple large randomized controlled trials and the extensive review of those trials.

However, systemic chemotherapy is associated with both short- and long-term toxicities of significant concern. As a result, many patients who are already disease-free, receive potentially toxic adjuvant chemotherapy, whereas some who would have otherwise benefited from chemotherapy do not receive potentially curative adjuvant therapy. Current clinical guidelines recommend the use of adjuvant chemotherapy in addition to hormonal therapy in all but the lowest risk categories of lymph node negative, estrogen receptor positive women with ESBC (2,3). The 21-gene expression signature RS for distant disease-recurrence derived from a proprietary algorithm applied to the results of the 21-gene expression signature was initially validated in 668 evaluable lymph node negative, estrogen receptor positive, ESBC patients treated with tamoxifen on NSABP B-14 (11). More recently, the predictive accuracy of the assay has also been validated based on patients' response to chemotherapy plus tamoxifen among 651 patients on NSABP B-20 and 645 patients on NSABP B-14 (17). This research was undertaken to further evaluate the economic impact of the 21-gene signature profile when used to guide common clinical decisions concerning the use of adjuvant chemotherapy and hormonal therapy in patients with lymph node negative, estrogen receptor positive ESBC. The economic impact of the gene expression profile signature to guide the type of adjuvant systemic therapy was compared with commonly employed treatment strategies of tamoxifen alone or chemotherapy plus tamoxifen.

Using baseline cost assumptions, the lowest expected cost was found to be associated with tamoxifen alone, whereas the RS-guided therapy strategy was associated with lower expected costs than the chemotherapy strategy. The estimated incremental costs with RS-guided therapy and chemotherapy compared to tamoxifen alone were US \$4272 and US \$6527, respectively, with an estimated average cost savings of greater than US \$2000. The estimated incremental cost per LYS favored RS-guided therapy over the chemotherapy plus tamoxifen strategy with a cost savings of over US \$1000 per LYS with RS-guided therapy. The RS-guided therapy strategy was found to be more costly only for low-cost chemotherapy regimens such as adriamycin/cyclophosphamide (AC) every three weeks without additional supportive care, whereas a net cost savings from US \$500 to US \$10,000 is estimated with RS-guided therapy for other commonly employed adjuvant chemotherapy regimens. Consideration of additional direct costs associated with adjuvant chemotherapy including drug administration, professional fees, and laboratory testing suggest that the above cost savings are actually minimum estimates. Indirect costs such as those associated with transportation and loss of productivity as well as out-of-pocket expenses suggests further potential savings from a societal perspective with the RS-guided therapy strategy.

The impact of quality-of-life on patients receiving cancer chemotherapy has received considerable attention (25–29). Our research demonstrates that the greater the impact of chemotherapy on quality-of-life, the greater the incremental cost-utility favoring RS-guided therapy compared to widespread use of chemotherapy. Likewise, RS-guided therapy was associated with superior cost-utility when compared to tamoxifen alone when the patient reported utility for chemotherapy exceeded 0.82.

In summary, when treating women with lymph node negative, estrogen receptor positive ESBC, the RS-guided therapy appears to be associated with lower expected treatment cost per LYS or QALY compared to empiric chemotherapy for all reasonable model treatment assumptions. There is greater cost-effectiveness with the RS-guided therapy strategy for more toxic and more costly chemotherapy regimens although it may increase the treatment costs associated with a low drug cost regimen such as AC administered every three weeks without growth factor support. Favorable cost-utility ratios favoring RS-guided therapy were found for most reasonable assumptions of patient preferences for chemotherapy. However, further evaluation is needed of the clinical utility of gene expression profiles used to estimate both disease prognosis and treatment response prediction in women with ESBC (30–33). However, their use in targeting systemic chemotherapy and hormonal therapy toward a large proportion of ESBC patients at greatest risk and most likely to benefit from adjuvant therapy appears to have the potential to provide considerable cost savings or prolongation of survival with acceptable cost-effectiveness ratios compared to other commonly employed adjuvant treatment strategies.

REFERENCES

1. Jemal A, Siegel R, Ward E, et al. Cancer statistics 2006. Ca-A J Clin 2006; 56:106–130.
2. Goldhirsch A, Wood WC, Gelber RD, et al. Meeting highlights: updated international expert consensus on the primary therapy of early breast cancer. J Clin Oncol 2003; 21:3357–3365.
3. NCCN guidelines for breast cancer. NCCN Task Force Report: adjuvant therapy for breast cancer. J Natl Compr Canc Netw 2006; 4(suppl 1):S1–26. http://www.nccn.org/professionals/physician_gls/PDF/breast.pdf
4. Early Breast Cancer Trialists Collaborative Group (EBCTCG). Effects of chemotherapy and hormonal therapy for early breast cancer on recurrence and 15-year survival: an overview of the randomised trials. Lancet 2005; 365(9472):1687–1717.
5. Cleator S, Ashworth A. Molecular profiling of breast cancer: clinical implications. Br J Cancer 2004; 90:1120–1124.
6. Cronin M, Pho M, Dutta D, et al. Measurement of gene expression in archival paraffin-embedded tissues. Development and performance of a 92-gene reverse transcriptase-polymerase chain reaction assay. Am J Pathol 2004; 164:35–42.
7. van't Veer LJ, Dai H, van de Vijer MJ, et al. Gene expression profiling predicts clinical outcome of breast cancer. Nature 2002; 415:530–535.
8. Sorlie T, Perou CM, Tibshirani R, et al. Gene expression patterns of breast carcinomas distinguish tumor subclasses with clinical implications. Proc Natl Acad Sci USA 2001; 98:10869–10874.
9. Ramaswamy S, Ross KN, Lander ES, Golub TR. A molecular signature of metastseis in primary solid tumors. Nat Genet 2003; 33:49–54.
10. Gruvberger S, Ringner M, Chen Y, et al. Estrogen receptor status in breast cancer is associated with remarkably distinct gene expression patterns. Cancer Res 2001; 61:5979–5984.
11. Paik S, Shak S, Tang G, et al. A multi-gene assay to predict recurrence of tamoxifen-treated, node-negative breast cancer. N Engl J Med 2004; 351:2817–2826.
12. Fisher B, Jeong J-H, Bryant J, et al. Treatment of lymph-node-negative, oestrogen-receptor-positive breast cancer: long-term findings from National Surgical Adjuvant Breast and Bowel Project Randomized Clinical Trials. Lancet 2004; 364:858–868.
13. Fisher B, Dignam J, Bryant J, et al. Five versus more than five years of tamoxifen therapy for breast cancer patients with negative lymph nodes and estrogen receptor-positive tumors. J Natl Cancer Inst 1996; 88:1529–1542.
14. Fisher B, Dignam J, Bryant J, Wolmark N. Five versus more than five years of tamoxifen for lymph node-negative breast cancer: updated findings from the National Surgical Adjuvant Breast and Bowel Project B-14 Randomized Trial. J Natl Cancer Inst 2001; 93:684–690.
15. Fisher B, Dignam J, Wolmark N, et al. Tamoxifen and chemotherapy for lymph node-negative, estrogen receptor-positive breast cancer. J Natl Cancer Inst 1997; 89:1673–1682.

16. Hornberger J, Cosler LE, Lyman GH. Economic analysis of targeting chemotherapy using a 21-gene RT-PCR assay in lymph-node-negative, estrogen-receptor-positive, early-stage breast cancer. Am J Manage Care 2005; 11:313–324.

17. Soonmyung Paik, Gong Tang, Steven Shak, et al. Gene expression and benefit of chemotherapy in women with node-negative, estrogen receptor-positive breast cancer. J Clin Oncol 2006; 24:3726–3734.

18. Valenta Z, Weissfeld L. Estimation of the survival function for Gray's piecewise-constant time-varying coefficients model. Stat Med 2002; 21:717–727.

19. Earle, C, Chapman R, Baker C, et al. Systematic overview of cost-utility assessment in oncology. J Clin Oncol 2000; 18:3302–3317.

20. Bruera E, Willey JS, Palmer JL, Rosales M. Treatment decisions for breast carcinoma: patient preferences and physician perceptions. Cancer 2002; 94:2076–2080.

21. Oestreicher N, Ramsey SED, McCune JS, Linden HM, Veenstra DL. The cost of adjuvant chemotherapy in patients with early-stage breast carcinoma. Cancer 2005; 104: 2054–2062.

22. Detsky AS, Naglie IG. A clinician's guide to cost-effectiveness analysis. Ann Intern Med 1990; 113:147–154.

23. Russell LB, Gold MR, Siegel JE, Daniels N, Weinstein MC. The role of the cost-effectiveness analysis in health and medicine. J Am Med Assoc 1996; 276:1172–1177.

24. Lyman GH, Djulbegovic B. Understanding economic analyses. Evidence-Based Oncol 2001; 2:2–5.

25. Broeckel JA, Jacobsen PB, Balducci L, Horton J, Lyman GH. Quality of life after adjuvant chemotherapy for breast cancer. Breast Cancer Res Treat 2000; 62:142–150.

26. Cole BF, Gelber RD, Gelber S, Coates AS, Goldhirsch A. Polychemotherapy for early breast cancer: an overview of the randomised clinical trials with quality-adjusted survival analysis. Lancet 2001; 358:277–286.

27. Land SR, Kopec JA, Yothers G, et al. Health-related quality of life in axillary node-negative, estrogen receptor-negative breast cancer patients undergoing AC versus CMF chemotherapy: findings from the National Surgical Adjuvant Breast and Bowel Project B-23. Breast Cancer Res Treat 2004; 86:153–164.

28. Bernhard J, Zahrieh D, Coates AS, et al. Quantifying trade-offs: quality of life and quality-adjusted survival in a randomized trial of chemotherapy in postmenopausal patients with lymph node-negative breast cancer. Br J Cancer 2004; 91:1893–1901.

29. Efficace F, Therasse P, Piccart MJ, et al. Health-related quality of life parameters as prognostic factors in a nonmetastatic breast cancer population: an international multicenter study. J Clin Oncol 2004; 22:3381–3388.

30. Simon R. Diagnostic and prognostic prediction using gene expression profiles in high-dimensional microarray data. Br J Cancer 2003; 89:1599–1604.

31. Chang JC, Wooten EC, Tsimelzon A, et al. Gene expression profiling for the prediction of therapeutic response to docetaxel in patients with breast cancer. Lancet 2003; 362: 362–369.

32. Iwao-Koizumi K, Matoba R, Ueno N, et al. Prediction of docetaxel response in human breast cancer by gene expression profiling. J Clin Oncol 2005; 23:422–431.

33. Jansen MPHM, Foekens JA, van Staveren IL, et al. Molecular classification of tamoxifen-resistant breast carcinomas by gene expression profiling. J Clin Oncol 2005; 23:732–740.

Aromatase Inhibitors for Breast Cancer Treatment and Prevention

Erica L. Mayer and Eric P. Winer

Dana-Farber Cancer Institute, Harvard Medical School, Boston, Massachusetts, U.S.A.

INTRODUCTION

Hormonal manipulation is a mainstay of breast cancer treatment. Over the past 30 years, tamoxifen, a selective estrogen agonist/antagonist, has been shown to be effective in preventing breast cancer and in treating early-stage and metastatic disease (1–3). Tamoxifen is active in both premenopausal and postmenopausal patients, but the benefits are restricted to patients whose tumors express hormone receptors, and a percentage of women treated with tamoxifen will ultimately develop recurrent disease. In addition, tamoxifen treatment can have serious, though rare adverse effects, including venous thromboembolic disease, cerebrovascular disease, and endometrial carcinoma. Aromatase inhibition, an alternative hormonal therapy targeting breast cancer cells through estrogen depletion, provides an effective and possibly superior option for postmenopausal women.

MECHANISM OF AROMATASE INHIBITION

Aromatase, a cytochrome P450-dependent enzyme, converts adrenal androgens into estrogens and accounts for most of the estrogen produced in postmenopausal women. Inhibition of aromatase depletes available estrogen, thus preventing estrogen-specific stimulation of the growth of breast cancer cells. The first aromatase inhibitor (AI) that was developed, aminoglutethimide, has clinical activity against breast cancer, but its use is limited by side effects from concomitant adrenal suppression. Second-generation agents have increased specificity for aromatase with improved tolerability. The third-generation AIs, including the non-steroidal agents anastrozole and letrozole and the steroidal agent exemestane, provide potent and highly selective aromatase inhibition. The non-steroidal agents function through reversible inhibition of the aromatase enzyme, whereas the steroidal agent forms irreversible bonds. AIs are contraindicated in premenopausal women because the small decrease in systemic estrogen levels through inhibition of peripheral aromatization may paradoxically stimulate ovarian estrogen production and negate any anti-breast cancer effects.

Use of third-generation AIs lowers total body aromatization and plasma estradiol levels by more than 95% (4,5). Some variation in the action of the third-generation AIs has been noted. Data from small studies suggest that letrozole has superior potency than the other agents, with a greater overall decrease in estrogen after short-term exposure (6). Furthermore, differences in cytochrome P450 inhibition between the steroidal and non-steroidal AIs may lead to variation in the risk of drug interactions (7). In general, however, all three agents have been shown to be both potent and selective.

INITIAL USE OF AROMATASE INHIBITORS IN METASTATIC BREAST CANCER

Third-generation AIs were first evaluated in the management of metastatic breast cancer. Initial clinical trials, comparing anastrozole, letrozole, or exemestane with megesterol acetate as second-line therapy, showed that the AIs had equivalent or improved efficacy, with a favorable side effect profile (8–11). A meta-analysis of data from these studies demonstrated a survival advantage for the AIs, with a relative risk of death of 0.79 (95% CI, 0.69–0.91) (12).

In the first-line metastatic setting, several large randomized trials have compared the various AIs with tamoxifen. A combined analysis of two studies comparing anastrozole with tamoxifen showed a significantly improved time to progression (TTP) among the women who received anastrozole, with less frequent thromboembolic events and vaginal bleeding (13–15). A mature survival analysis at 44 months showed no advantage of anastrozole over tamoxifen but confirmed the favorable tolerability profiles of both agents (16). First-line treatment with letrozole, as compared with tamoxifen, is also associated with an improved response rate and TTP (17). In a randomized, un-blinded trial comparing letrozole with anastrozole, no differences in TTP, clinical benefit, or overall survival (OS) were observed (18). In addition, as compared with tamoxifen, exemestane is also associated with superior progression-free survival in the first-line setting (19). On the basis of these findings, AIs have a well-established role as first- and second-line treatment for metastatic breast cancer.

EVOLVING ROLE OF AROMATASE INHIBITORS IN ADJUVANT THERAPY

Given the success of treatment with AIs in the metastatic setting, multiple large trials have investigated the use of these agents as adjuvant therapy. Data from six trials, involving a total of approximately 30,000 patients, have been reported. These trials evaluated both upfront initiation of AI monotherapy and sequential administration of tamoxifen followed by an AI. Most subjects enrolled were hormone receptor (HR)-positive, with equal representation of both node-negative and node-positive disease. The primary endpoint in all the studies was disease-free or event-free survival, although the precise definition of the endpoint varied. The results of these adjuvant trials have changed the landscape of hormonal therapy and altered recommendations for adjuvant treatment.

INITIAL HORMONAL THERAPY

Two studies have compared upfront AI therapy with standard tamoxifen therapy. The Arimidex, Tamoxifen, Alone or in Combination (ATAC) study was a randomized, double-blind trial designed to compare tamoxifen with anastrozole as initial adjuvant hormonal treatment in 6214 postmenopausal women. An additional combination therapy arm containing 3152 patients was un-blinded at the time of the first interim analysis because of the lack of benefit as compared with the control tamoxifen arm. In the overall study population, 84% of the subjects were HR-positive, and 64% had tumors that were 2 cm or less. At a median follow-up of

68 months, disease-free survival (DFS) was significantly better in the anastrozole group than in the tamoxifen group (hazard ratio, 0.87; 95% CI, 0.78–0.97; $P = 0.005$), with an absolute difference of 3.3% in the recurrence rate at six years. Time to recurrence was also significantly improved with initial use of anastrozole (hazard ratio, 0.74; 95% CI, 0.64–0.87; $P = 0.0002$). The absolute difference in rates of recurrence continued to diverge even after completion of therapy, suggesting the presence of a carryover effect (20). However, prolonged follow-up has not identified a survival advantage with anastrozole over tamoxifen.

The Breast International Group 1–98 (BIG 1-98) study randomized 8010 postmenopausal women who had undergone resection of HR-positive tumors to one of four regimens: five years of tamoxifen, five years of letrozole, initial use of tamoxifen with a switch to letrozole after two years, and initial use of letrozole with a switch to tamoxifen after two years. As with ATAC, almost all patients were postmenopausal at the time of diagnosis; 41% of the women were node-positive and 64% had tumors that were less than 2 cm. Results from the first protocol-specified analysis of initial treatment with tamoxifen versus letrozole for patients in all four arms were released after a median follow-up of 25.8 months. This analysis demonstrated improved DFS in the letrozole group (hazard ratio, 0.81; 95% CI, 0.7–0.93; $P = 0.003$), with lower rates of distant recurrence and contralateral disease as well. The improvement in DFS translated into an estimated absolute benefit of 2.6% at five years. Although there were fewer deaths in the letrozole group, no statistically significant difference in OS was seen between the two groups (21). Mature results, including data from the crossover arms, are expected by 2008.

SEQUENTIAL HORMONAL THERAPY

Four reported studies have evaluated the benefit of a crossover to AI therapy after two to five years of tamoxifen. The Intergroup Exemestane Study (IES) randomized 4742 postmenopausal women who were disease-free after two to three years of tamoxifen to either exemestane or continued treatment with tamoxifen, for a total of five years. At a median follow-up of 30.6 months, a significant improvement in DFS was noted in the exemestane group (hazard ratio, 0.68; 95% CI, 0.56–0.82; $P < 0.001$), including a decrease in the risk of distant relapse (22). At 56 months median follow-up, an intention-to-treat analysis as well as an analysis restricted to estrogen receptor (ER)-positive or unknown patients showed sustained improvement in DFS in the exemestane group (intention-to-treat analysis: hazard ratio, 0.76; 95% CI, 0.66–0.88; $P = 0.0001$; ER-positive/unknown group: hazard ratio, 0.75; 95% CI, 0.65–0.87; $P = 0.0001$). In addition, the analysis restricted to the patients with positive or unknown ER status showed a significant benefit in OS (hazard ratio, 0.83; 95% CI, 0.69–1.00; $P = 0.05$). A carry-over effect, as observed in ATAC, has not been observed in IES (23).

Similarly, the smaller Italian Anastrozole Trial (ITA) randomized 426 node-positive postmenopausal women who had successfully undergone two to three years of tamoxifen therapy to either open-label anastrozole or continued treatment with tamoxifen to complete a five-year course. At a median follow-up of 24 months, the sequential treatment arm had a significantly lower rate of recurrence (hazard ratio, 0.36; 95% CI, 0.17–0.75; $P = 0.006$), with a 5.8% absolute improvement in DFS; OS was not assessed (24).

Two multicenter randomized studies of sequential therapy, the Austrian Breast and Colorectal Cancer Study Group trial 8 (ABCSG-8) and the German

Arimidex–Nolvadex (ARNO) 95 trial, have been analyzed together. In the combined analysis, a total of 3224 patients were randomized to treatment with anastrozole after completion of two years of tamoxifen or to continued treatment with tamoxifen to complete a five-year course. Although ABCSG-8 enrolled patients at the time of initiation of tamoxifen, capturing events both before and after initiation of AI, only events that occurred after crossover were included in the combined analysis. With a median follow-up of 28 months, a benefit in event-free survival was observed in the anastrazole arm (hazard ratio, 0.60; 95% CI, 0.44–0.81; $P = 0.0009$), including a significant decrease in distant recurrence, translating into an absolute benefit of 3.1% (25). A meta-analysis of the ABCSG-8, ARNO-95, and ITA trials has demonstrated a significant benefit in OS for the crossover population, with 66 deaths (3.3%) in the anastrozole arm versus 90 deaths (4.5%) in the tamoxifen arm (hazard ratio, 0.71; $P = 0.038$) (26). Analysis of extended follow-up data from ARNO-95, at a median follow-up of 30.1 months, showed a continued benefit in DFS (hazard ratio, 0.66; 95% CI, 0.44–1.00; $P = 0.05$), with a significant benefit in OS as well (hazard ratio, 0.53; 95% CI, 0.28–0.99; $P = 0.04$) (27).

EXTENDED ADJUVANT HORMONAL THERAPY

MA.17 evaluated both the sequencing of hormonal therapy and the role of extended hormonal therapy. In this study, 5187 women who had completed five years of adjuvant tamoxifen therapy without recurrence were randomized to either letrozole or placebo for a period of five years. Approximately, 85% of the subjects were postmenopausal at the initiation of tamoxifen treatment, and all were postmenopausal at the time of randomization. After a planned interim analysis occurring at a median follow-up of 30 months, the trial was un-blinded, and the data were analyzed. DFS was significantly improved in the letrozole group (hazard ratio, 0.57; 95% CI, 0.43–0.75; $P < 0.001$), with an absolute improvement of 6%. There were reductions in the risks of locoregional events, contralateral primary breast cancer, and distant recurrences. Although an advantage in OS was not seen in the study as a whole, the subset of node-positive patients treated with letrozole had improved survival (hazard ratio, 0.61; 95% CI, 0.38–0.98; $P = 0.04$) (28,29). A non-randomized analysis of data from the 1601 women in the placebo arm who crossed over to letrozole at the time of study unblinding showed that DFS, distant DFS, the risk of contralateral breast cancer, and OS were all improved, as compared with the outcomes in the subgroup of women who did not crossover to letrozole (30).

PREMENOPAUSAL WOMEN

The role of adjuvant AI therapy in premenopausal women undergoing ovarian suppression is not known. Two international randomized trials coordinated by the International Breast Cancer Study Group—the Suppression of Ovarian Function Trial (SOFT) and the Tamoxifen and Exemestane Trial (TEXT)—are examining this question. These trials are comparing ovarian suppression plus tamoxifen with ovarian suppression plus exemestane; in addition to the two combination regimens, SOFT has a third arm of tamoxifen alone. Patients can be enrolled either at the initiation of adjuvant therapy or after completion of chemotherapy, if they are still premenopausal.

The role of AIs in the adjuvant treatment of women who become postmenopausal while receiving either chemotherapy or initial treatment with tamoxifen is also unclear. Although some women with chemotherapy-induced amenorrhea were included in the adjuvant AI studies, apart from MA.17, the proportion was very small, making it difficult to extrapolate results to this specific population. Furthermore, amenorrhea following chemotherapy can be transient, and ovarian function may return months to years later, often not accompanied by a return of menses (31–33). In general, it is prudent to begin tamoxifen therapy in all women who were premenopausal at the time of diagnosis, regardless of their apparent menopausal status after chemotherapy. If one is going to consider a switching strategy after fewer than five years of tamoxifen, menopausal status should be ascertained biochemically when the patient discontinues tamoxifen and periodically thereafter.

UNANSWERED QUESTIONS

Despite the wealth of new data regarding the role of AIs in the adjuvant setting, many questions remain about the choice of agent and timing of administration. Proponents of upfront aromatase inhibition propose that much of the benefit from AIs is seen in the first few years of treatment, suggesting that AIs may be highly effective in suppressing early recurrences (34). It can be argued that a crossover approach, which typically employs two to three years of tamoxifen before administering the AI, misses a modest but important early benefit. However, proponents of the sequential pattern point out that during the first two to three years, the absolute difference in the rate of events between women taking tamoxifen and those on AIs is small (approximately 1.5%), and it appears to be overcome in years three to five by the favorable hazard ratio associated with the switch to AI as compared with continued treatment with tamoxifen. It has also been postulated that initial treatment with tamoxifen may have a priming effect and thereby make AI therapy particularly effective. Furthermore, supporters of the sequential strategy also argue that giving extended adjuvant therapy (beyond five years) requires starting with tamoxifen and then switching to an AI, since there are currently no data supporting either more than five years of AI therapy or the use of tamoxifen or another hormonal intervention after an AI. Critics of sequential studies counter that bias may arise from the enrollment of women who have survived the initial two years of tamoxifen therapy without relapse. However, the ABCSG-8 study enrolled patients at the time of primary surgery, and an analysis, including the first two years of events with tamoxifen showed a benefit in event-free survival for the AI group (hazard ratio, 0.68; 95% CI, 0.49–0.91; $P = 0.02$) (35).

Statistical models have been created in an attempt to determine the preferred method of administration of hormonal therapies (34,36). In its latest update, the American Society of Clinical Oncology's Technology Assessment Panel concluded that postmenopausal women without contraindications to AI therapy should receive an AI at some time during the adjuvant period. However the "best" adjuvant use of an AI—upfront or sequential and for two, five, or more than five years—remains unclear. Physicians are advised to weigh the risks and benefits of the various treatment options and design a treatment plan for each individual patient (37). Ultimately, the BIG 1-98 data will provide the most critical information related to the use of upfront versus crossover approaches. However, given the heterogeneity in HR-positive tumors and variations in host factors (e.g., drug metabolism), it is quite possible that a single approach will not be "best" for all patients.

The appropriate duration of AI therapy is also unclear. In the current trial, the maximum duration of therapy has been five years. Previous studies of tamoxifen in which therapy was extended beyond five years showed no benefit of a longer duration in either DFS or OS (38). An extension study of MA.17, in which patients are randomized at the completion of five years of letrozole therapy to either a further five years of therapy or placebo, will investigate this question.

ADVERSE EFFECTS OF AROMATASE INHIBITORS

Adjuvant hormonal therapy exposes otherwise healthy women to prolonged drug therapy, and determination of safety is therefore crucial. All of the adjuvant studies have closely examined the frequency of adverse effects of AIs, but only MA.17 has compared adverse effects in the AI group with those in the placebo group. AIs are consistently associated with several short-term side-effects, including vasomotor instability and vaginal changes (21,28,39). In ATAC, the rate of withdrawal from treatment because of adverse effects was lower with AIs than with tamoxifen (11.1% vs. 14.3%, $P = 0.0002$) (20), suggesting that AIs may be better tolerated. Furthermore, an analysis in MA.17 has shown no decrement in quality of life among women taking letrozole as compared with those taking placebo (40). The rates of endometrial cancer and venous thromboembolic events in the AI-treated population remain consistently equal to or lower than those among women receiving tamoxifen (21,39). Currently, there are no comparative data on the frequency of adverse effects among the three AIs. MA.27, in which patients are randomized to treatment with anastrozole or exemestane, may begin to address this question. Several class-specific adverse effects of AIs deserve further exploration.

BONE EFFECTS

Since AIs, unlike tamoxifen, do not have a bone-protective effect and may increase bone loss in postmenopausal women, significant attention has focused on adverse bone outcomes in the major clinical trials. Both IES and MA.17 examined the incidence of new osteoporosis and found that it was increased among women receiving AIs, although the difference did not reach statistical significance (22,28). The rate of fracture has been examined as well. In ATAC, the study with the longest follow-up, the annual rate of fracture for anastrozole was 2.2, as compared with 1.56 for tamoxifen (hazard ratio, 1.44; 95% CI, 1.21–1.68; $P < 0.0001$), with a cumulative rate at six years of 11.0% versus 7.7% (20). The findings were similar in BIG 1-98 and ABCSG-8/ARNO-95. In addition, myalgias and arthralgias of the small joints are relatively common among women taking AIs. In the ATAC trial, 36% of women taking anastrozole, as compared with 23% of those taking tamoxifen, had myalgias or arthralgias ($P < 0.0001$). The cause of this symptom is not completely understood but may be related to estrogen deprivation (41).

CARDIOVASCULAR EFFECTS

Several studies have reported an increase in cardiovascular-related toxicity in patients treated with adjuvant AIs. In BIG 1-98, more grade three to five cardiac events were noted in the letrozole arm than in the tamoxifen arm (2.1% vs. 1.1%, $P < 0.001$), including deaths from cardiac events (13 vs. 6) and deaths from vascular events (7 vs. 1). A numerically greater number of non-breast cancer deaths was also observed in this study (3.1% vs. 1.8%, $P = 0.08$) (21). In IES, both the number of myocardial infarctions and the number of deaths from cardiac or vascular causes were greater in the group that switched to exemestane than in the group that continued to receive tamoxifen (13 vs. 6 myocardial infarctions and 28 vs. 19 deaths) (22). In ATAC, a slight increase in the number of cardiac events was observed in the anastrozole arm (127 vs. 104), but there was no increase in deaths from cardiovascular causes overall (20). However, in other adjuvant trials of AIs, including MA.17 and ABCSG-8/ARNO-95, no increase in cardiovascular-related events or deaths was reported.

The reason for the increase in cardiac events and mortality with AI therapy is unknown. It may reflect a statistical aberration or differential effects of hormonal therapy on the lipid profile. Prospective evaluations of changes in lipid profiles in patients receiving tamoxifen consistently suggest a beneficial effect with no increase in the risk of myocardial infarction (42). AI therapy appears to provide no cardioprotection and may possibly worsen lipid profiles, perhaps predisposing women to atherosclerotic disease (43–45). This hypothesis is supported by BIG 1-98, which reported stable cholesterol values in the letrozole group (rate of hypercholesterolemia, 43.6%) and values that decreased by 14% from baseline in the tamoxifen group (rate of hypercholesterolemia, 19.2%) (21). Furthermore, in MA.17, there were no increases in hyperlipidemia or cardiac-related deaths in the letrozole arm as compared with the placebo arm (46). This finding suggests that a modest cardioprotective effect of tamoxifen may account for the apparent cardiac toxicity of AIs in the randomized trials comparing tamoxifen with AIs. Decreased mortality from coronary heart disease has also been observed in a retrospective analysis of a trial of adjuvant tamoxifen therapy (47). Overall, however, despite these provocative data, none of the observations from the AI trials have demonstrated statistical significance and may represent chance findings. Data from the ongoing breast cancer prevention studies using AIs may clarify the relationship between AIs and cardiac disease.

PREOPERATIVE AROMATASE INHIBITOR THERAPY

Evaluation of therapies in the preoperative setting offers several advantages, including a rapid time to assess the response, a small sample size, and a facile method to obtain and evaluate tissue exposed to drug, possibly generating surrogate outcome endpoints. There have been several studies of AIs in the preoperative setting. First, Eiermann et al. evaluated four months of preoperative letrozole as compared with tamoxifen in 337 postmenopausal patients with HR-positive breast cancer. The clinical response rate was higher for letrozole than for tamoxifen (55% vs. 36%, $P < 0.001$), with a corresponding improvement in the rate of breast-conserving therapy (48). Subset analysis in this study also suggested tamoxifen resistance in tumors that were positive for HER2 and/or epidermal growth factor receptor (EGFR), which was overcome by the AI (49). A subsequent trial, the Immediate Preoperative Anastrozole, Tamoxifen, or Combined with Tamoxifen (IMPACT) study, was designed to assess whether similar results could be achieved with anastrozole. In this study, 330 women with operable or locally advanced ER-positive tumors were randomized to a 12-week course of preoperative anastrozole, tamoxifen, or both. In contrast to the letrozole study, no significant differences in overall clinical response were seen among the three groups (50). Possible explanations for this result are the small group size, small tumor size, and variability in ER positivity (51).

Neoadjuvant AI therapy is an acceptable option for patients with large or locally advanced HR-positive primary tumors who are not candidates for chemotherapy. Ongoing trials of neoadjuvant endocrine therapy include the phase III American College of Surgeons Oncology Group (ACOSOG) Z-1031 trial, which is comparing the three third-generation AIs, and a phase II neoadjuvant letrozole trial, coordinated through the National Cancer Institute, which is evaluating the predictive ability of gene expression array analysis.

PREVENTION

Data on the activity of AIs as preventive agents has been gathered largely through secondary analysis of the adjuvant data. Several of the adjuvant trials have examined the frequency of contralateral breast cancers, with provocative results, despite the small number of total events. These analyses suggest that AIs may have an active role in the prevention of breast cancer. Among women with HR-positive tumors who were enrolled in the ATAC trial, contralateral breast cancers in the anastrozole group were reduced by 53%, as compared with the tamoxifen group (21 vs. 48 events; hazard ratio, 0.47; 95% CI, 0.29–0.75; $P = 0.001$) (20). Similarly, in the IES study, AI therapy was associated with a significant reduction in the risk of contralateral breast cancer (hazard ratio, 0.44; 95% CI, 0.20–0.98; $P = 0.04$).

Prospective studies are also evaluating the role of AIs in breast cancer prevention. MAP3, a trial from the National Cancer Institute of Canada, is randomizing 4500 women at risk for breast cancer to five years of exemestane or placebo. In addition, a study coordinated through the Dana-Farber Cancer Institute is evaluating a five-year regimen of letrozole in 110 women at increased risk of breast cancer, on the basis of serum estradiol levels.

FUTURE DIRECTIONS

Contemporary breast cancer management attempts to select therapies and predict outcomes more accurately through better characterization of tumors. Recent data from gene expression microarray analyses have delineated subtypes of breast cancer with distinctive behavior, including two luminal ER-positive subgroups, a HER2 (erB2)-positive subgroup, and a "basal-like" subgroup, typically ER-negative and HER2-negative (52,53). Both therapeutic options and prognoses differ among these groups, because hormonal therapy and trastuzumab are useful only for tumors expressing the correct receptors, and inferior outcomes are often seen for HER2-positive and basal-like tumors.

Precise tumor characterization may also identify subgroups of patients who are more appropriate candidates for AI therapy, specifically the HR-positive subpopulation with relative tamoxifen resistance. Initial retrospective analyses of hormonal studies in the metastatic population suggested that patients with tumors that were positive for ER and negative for progesterone receptor (PR) had a significantly decreased response to tamoxifen, as compared with the ER-positive/PR-positive patients (54,55). In the adjuvant setting, analysis of outcomes from a database of over 12,000 patients with centrally confirmed positive hormonal status treated with endocrine therapy only (tamoxifen in nearly all cases) has also shown inferior DFS and OS in the ER-positive/PR-negative group, as compared with the ER-positive/PR-positive group (56). These findings, which suggest that loss of PR predicts resistance to tamoxifen, were initially ascribed to variability in the functionality of the ER pathway.

Preclinical research has suggested an alternative hypothesis involving tumor cell crosstalk between the ER and growth factor pathways, including those under the influence of the HER family of proteins. Over-expression or amplification of HER2 has been associated with decreased levels of both ER and PR expression, with more marked decreases in PR than in ER (57). High levels of other growth factor receptors, such as insulin-like growth factor I receptor (IGF-IR) and EGFR, have also been associated with low PR expression independently of ER expression, a finding thought to be mediated by the PI3 kinase/Akt pathway (58). Tissue microarray analysis in a cohort of tamoxifen-treated patients showed that the HER2-positive, EGFR-positive, and PR-negative group had an increased chance of disease relapse, particularly within the first three years of tamoxifen treatment (59). Thus, decreased PR expression appears to be associated with increased growth factor signaling in tumor cells, and possibly with a more aggressive phenotype. It has also been observed that in tumors with more active growth factor signaling, such as those with over-expression of HER2 or EGFR, alternative activation of ER can occur through membrane-initiated steroid signaling (MISS). In contrast to the usual nuclear-initiated signaling, tamoxifen-induced MISS can lead to agonist, rather than antagonist, effects, paradoxically promoting tumor stimulation and growth (60). These in vitro observations may explain the prior clinical observations of tamoxifen resistance in ER-positive/PR-negative cohorts.

AIs offer an alternative treatment option for the subset of tumors with possible tamoxifen-resistance. In the laboratory, estrogen deprivation such as that induced by AIs in vivo inhibits the growth of HER2-positive MCF-7 tumors, which have known de novo resistance to tamoxifen (61). Observations from clinical trials may support this hypothesis. An unplanned subgroup analysis of data from ATAC has suggested a greater benefit of anastrozole in terms of time to recurrence in the ER-positive/PR-negative group than in the ER-positive/PR-positive group (hazard ratio, 0.43 vs. 0.84; $P = 0.0001$), with much of the difference due to an increased rate of recurrence among the ER-positive/PR-negative patients who received tamoxifen (62). In the preoperative setting, letrozole had greater activity than tamoxifen in the subset of tumors that were positive for HER2 and/or EGFR than in those that were negative for both ($P = 0.02$). Letrozole was also more active than tamoxifen in the treatment of HER2-positive/EGFR-positive tumors, with an odds ratio for response rate of 28 ($P = 0.004$). Analysis restricted to HR-positive patients suggested that the HER2-positive/EGFR-positive tumors were more resistant to tamoxifen than were the HER2-negative/EGFR-negative tumors (49). In the IMPACT preoperative study, there was an increased response to anastrozole in the HER2-positive population, although the difference was not statistically significant (50). These observations are certainly hypothesis-generating; however, they have not been confirmed through centralized review of BIG 1-98 (21,63) or in the sequential AI switching studies, although a numerical trend towards a benefit was seen in ABCSG-8/ARNO-95 (25,64,65). Despite this lack of conclusive data, upfront treatment with an AI rather than tamoxifen may be considered for HER-positive, EGFR-positive, and/or PR-negative tumors that are more likely to be resistant to tamoxifen.

Gene expression array technology will likely play a central role in future efforts to predict a tumor's response to hormonal therapy. Microarray analysis of breast cancer cell lines before and after treatment with AIs and tamoxifen has demonstrated that AI-treated cells have a consistent response profile, regardless of the specific agent used, that differs from the response profile of the tamoxifen-treated cells (66). Loi et al. (67) performed microarray analyses in patients with HR-positive, early-stage tumors treated with tamoxifen. Differential expression of 50 genes divided the cohort into two groups: patients who had disease that appeared to be resistant to tamoxifen, with a median time to distant relapse of 2.4 years, and those who had tamoxifen-sensitive disease, with a median time to relapse of seven years. On multivariate analysis, this tool provided independent prognostic information when compared with traditional histological predictors, such as size, grade, and immunohistochemical (IHC) status. Pretreatment identification of patients with a poor prognosis on the basis of microarray analysis might point to the use of upfront AI therapy rather than tamoxifen. In addition, microarray analyses of specimens from biopsies performed at baseline and during neoadjuvant endocrine therapy in 52 patients have demonstrated differential gene signatures that correlated with the subsequent clinical response to endocrine treatment (68).

Alternatively, an emerging understanding of hormonal agent metabolism suggests that the selection of appropriate therapy can be based on CYP2D6 genotype. Retrospective evaluation of 190 subjects from a North Central Cancer Treatment Group (NCCTG) study suggested that patients with poor metabolism of tamoxifen have a worse prognosis and could benefit from an alternative hormonal therapy such as an AI (69). This idea will be examined in an NCCTG/Intergroup study in which adjuvant hormonal therapy is partially selected on the basis of the CYP2D6 genotype.

Additional emerging avenues of investigation will also enrich our understanding of AI activity. Methods of forecasting toxicity before initiating treatment, such as using genotypic positivity for a factor V Leiden mutation to predict an increased risk of venous thromboembolic disease from tamoxifen, may facilitate the selection of appropriate hormonal therapy (70). In addition, estrogens appear to have a role in the control of angiogenesis, the process of new blood vessel growth modulated by the vascular endothelial growth factor (VEGF) receptor (71). Clinical observations suggest that tumors rich in VEGF or its receptor may be resistant to tamoxifen, thus providing another possible indication for AI therapy (72,73). On the basis of encouraging findings in a phase II trial of therapy with letrozole and bevacizumab (74), the CALGB will initiate a phase III study comparing this combination with AI monotherapy in the metastatic setting.

CONCLUSIONS

AIs are highly active against breast cancer. They have an established role in the treatment of metastatic disease and a rapidly evolving role in adjuvant management. Ongoing investigations may confirm additional strategies for AI use in premenopausal women with breast cancer and in women at risk for the disease.

Despite extensive prior work, many questions still remain about the proper use of AIs, including the timing and duration of administration, management of side-effects, and whether class differences exist among the agents. Results from ongoing studies, such as BIG1-98, SOFT/TEXT, and MAP3, may answer some of these questions. Developments in the laboratory may also elucidate the subgroup of patients for whom AI therapy is optimal, on the basis of IHC studies or gene expression microarrays. Future investigations should prospectively evaluate markers of AI sensitivity so that this powerful and effective treatment can be harnessed most efficiently to benefit patients with breast cancer.

REFERENCES

1. Fisher B, Costantino JP, Wickerham DL, et al. Tamoxifen for the prevention of breast cancer: current status of the National Surgical Adjuvant Breast and Bowel Project P-1 study. J Natl Cancer Inst 2005; 97(22):1652–1662.
2. Effects of chemotherapy and hormonal therapy for early breast cancer on recurrence and 15-year survival: an overview of the randomised trials. Lancet 2005; 365(9472): 1687–1717.
3. Muss HB, Case LD, Atkins JN, et al. Tamoxifen versus high-dose oral medroxyprogesterone acetate as initial endocrine therapy for patients with metastatic breast cancer: a Piedmont Oncology Association study. J Clin Oncol 1994;12(8):1630–1638.
4. Geisler J, King N, Anker G, et al. In vivo inhibition of aromatization by exemestane, a novel irreversible aromatase inhibitor, in postmenopausal breast cancer patients. Clin Cancer Res 1998; 4(9):2089–2093.
5. Geisler J, Lonning PE. Endocrine effects of aromatase inhibitors and inactivators in vivo: review of data and method limitations. J Steroid Biochem Mol Biol 2005; 95(1–5):75–81.
6. Geisler J, Haynes B, Anker G, Dowsett M, Lonning PE. Influence of letrozole and anastrozole on total body aromatization and plasma estrogen levels in postmenopausal breast cancer patients evaluated in a randomized, cross-over study. J Clin Oncol 2002; 20(3):751–757.
7. Buzdar AU, Robertson JF, Eiermann W, Nabholtz JM. An overview of the pharmacology and pharmacokinetics of the newer generation aromatase inhibitors anastrozole, letrozole, and exemestane. Cancer 2002; 95(9):2006–2016.
8. Buzdar A, Jonat W, Howell A, et al. Anastrozole, a potent and selective aromatase inhibitor, versus megestrol acetate in postmenopausal women with advanced breast cancer: results of overview analysis of two phase III trials. Arimidex Study Group. J Clin Oncol 1996; 14(7):2000–2011.
9. Dombernowsky P, Smith I, Falkson G, et al. Letrozole, a new oral aromatase inhibitor for advanced breast cancer: double-blind randomized trial showing a dose effect and improved efficacy and tolerability compared with megestrol acetate. J Clin Oncol 1998; 16(2):453–461.
10. Buzdar A, Douma J, Davidson N, et al. Phase III, multicenter, double-blind, randomized study of letrozole, an aromatase inhibitor, for advanced breast cancer versus megestrol acetate. J Clin Oncol 2001; 19(14):3357–3366.
11. Kaufmann M, Bajetta E, Dirix LY, et al. Exemestane is superior to megestrol acetate after tamoxifen failure in postmenopausal women with advanced breast cancer: results of a phase III randomized double-blind trial. The Exemestane Study Group. J Clin Oncol 2000; 18(7):1399–1411.
12. Messori A, Cattel F, Trippoli S, Vaiani M. Survival in patients with metastatic breast cancer: analysis of randomized studies comparing oral aromatase inhibitors versus megestrol. Anticancer Drugs 2000; 11(9):701–706.
13. Nabholtz JM, Buzdar A, Pollak M, et al. Anastrozole is superior to tamoxifen as first-line therapy for advanced breast cancer in postmenopausal women: results of a North American multicenter randomized trial. Arimidex Study Group. J Clin Oncol 2000; 18(22):3758–3767.
14. Bonneterre J, Thurlimann B, Robertson JF, et al. Anastrozole versus tamoxifen as first-line therapy for advanced breast cancer in 668 postmenopausal women: results of the Tamoxifen or Arimidex Randomized Group Efficacy and Tolerability study. J Clin Oncol 2000; 18(22):3748–3757.
15. Bonneterre J, Buzdar A, Nabholtz JM, et al. Anastrozole is superior to tamoxifen as first-line therapy in hormone receptor positive advanced breast carcinoma. Cancer 2001; 92(9):2247–2258.

16. Nabholtz JM, Bonneterre J, Buzdar A, Robertson JF, Thurlimann B. Anastrozole (Arimidex) versus tamoxifen as first-line therapy for advanced breast cancer in postmenopausal women: survival analysis and updated safety results. Eur J Cancer 2003; 39(12):1684–1689.

17. Mouridsen H, Gershanovich M, Sun Y, et al. Phase III study of letrozole versus tamoxifen as first-line therapy of advanced breast cancer in postmenopausal women: analysis of survival and update of efficacy from the International Letrozole Breast Cancer Group. J Clin Oncol 2003; 21(11):2101–2109.

18. Rose C, Vtoraya O, Pluzanska A, et al. An open randomised trial of second-line endocrine therapy in advanced breast cancer. comparison of the aromatase inhibitors letrozole and anastrozole. Eur J Cancer 2003; 39(16):2318–2327.

19. Paridaens R, Therasse P, Dirix L, et al. First line hormonal treatment (HT) for metastatic breast cancer (MBC) with exemestane (E) or tamoxifen (T) in postmenopausal patients (pts)—a randomized phase III trial of the EORTC Breast Group. Proc Am Soc Clin Oncol 2004; 22:S14.

20. Howell A, Cuzick J, Baum M, et al. Results of the ATAC (Arimidex, Tamoxifen, Alone or in Combination) trial after completion of 5 years' adjuvant treatment for breast cancer. Lancet 2005; 365(9453):60–62.

21. Thurlimann B, Keshaviah A, Coates AS, et al. A comparison of letrozole and tamoxifen in postmenopausal women with early breast cancer. N Engl J Med 2005; 353(26): 2747–2757.

22. Coombes RC, Hall E, Snowdon CF, Bliss JM. The Intergroup Exemestane Study: a randomized trial in postmenopausal patients with early breast cancer who remain disease-free after two to three years of tamoxifen-updated survival analysis. Breast Cancer Res Treat 2004; 88(suppl 1):S6.

23. Coombes RC, Paridaens R, Jassem J, et al. First mature analysis of the Intergroup Exemestane Study. J Clin Oncol 2006; 24(18S):LBA527.

24. Boccardo F, Rubagotti A, Puntoni M, et al. Switching to anastrozole versus continued tamoxifen treatment of early breast cancer: preliminary results of the Italian Tamoxifen Anastrozole Trial. J Clin Oncol 2005; 23(22):5138–5147.

25. Jakesz R, Jonat W, Gnant M, et al. Switching of postmenopausal women with endocrine-responsive early breast cancer to anastrozole after 2 years' adjuvant tamoxifen: combined results of ABCSG trial 8 and ARNO 95 trial. Lancet 2005; 366(9484): 455–462.

26. Jonat W, Gnant M, Boccardo F, Kaufmann M, Rubagotti A, Jakesz R. Switching from adjuvant tamoxifen to anastrozole in postmenopausal women with hormone-responsive early breast cancer: a meta-analysis of the ARNO 95 Trial, ABCSG Trial 8, and the ITA Trial. Breast Cancer Res Treat 2005; 94:S11.

27. Kaufmann M, Jonat W, Hilfrich J, et al. Survival benefit of switching to anastrozole after 2 years' treatment with tamoxifen versus continued tamoxifen therapy: the ARNO 95 study. J Clin Oncol 2006; 24(18S):547.

28. Goss PE, Ingle JN, Martino S, et al. A randomized trial of letrozole in postmenopausal women after five years of tamoxifen therapy for early-stage breast cancer. N Engl J Med 2003; 349(19):1793–1802.

29. Goss PE, Ingle JN, Martino S, et al. Randomized trial of letrozole following tamoxifen as extended adjuvant therapy in receptor-positive breast cancer: updated findings from NCIC CTG MA.17. J Natl Cancer Inst 2005; 97(17):1262–1271.

30. Goss P, Ingle J, Palmer M, Shepherd L, Tu D. Updated analysis of NCIC CTG MA.17 (letrozole vs. placebo to letrozole vs. placebo) post unblinding. Breast Cancer Res Treat 2005; 94:S10.

31. Braverman AS, Sawhney H, Tendler A, Patel N, Rao S. Pre-menopausal serum estradiol (E2) levels may persist after chemotherapy (CT)-induced amenorrhea in breast cancer (BC). Proc Am Soc Clin Oncol 2002; A164.

32. Burstein HJ, Mayer EL, Partridge AP, et al. Inadvertent use of aromatase inhibitors in breast cancer patients with residual ovarian function: cases and lessons. Clin Breast Cancer 2006; 7(2):158–161.

33. Smith IE, Dowsett M, Yap YS, et al. Adjuvant aromatase inhibitors for early breast cancer after chemotherapy-induced amenorrhoea: caution and suggested guidelines. J Clin Oncol 2006; 24(16):2444–2447.

34. Buzdar AU, Cuzick J. Anastrozole as an adjuvant endocrine treatment for postmenopausal patients with breast cancer: emerging data. Clin Cancer Res 2006; 12(3): 1037s–1048s.
35. Jakesz R, Gnant M, Greil R, et al. The benefits of sequencing adjuvant tamoxifen and anastrozole in postmenopausal women with hormone-responsive early breast cancer: 5 year-analysis of ABCSG Trial 8. Breast Cancer Res Treat 2005; 94:S10.
36. Punglia RS, Kuntz KM, Winer EP, Weeks JC, Burstein HJ. Optimizing adjuvant endocrine therapy in postmenopausal women with early-stage breast cancer: a decision analysis. J Clin Oncol 2005; 23(22):5178–5187.
37. Winer EP, Hudis C, Burstein HJ, et al. American Society of Clinical Oncology technology assessment on the use of aromatase inhibitors as adjuvant therapy for postmenopausal women with hormone receptor-positive breast cancer: status report 2004. J Clin Oncol 2005; 23(3):619–629.
38. Fisher B, Dignam J, Bryant J, Wolmark N. Five versus more than five years of tamoxifen for lymph node-negative breast cancer: updated findings from the National Surgical Adjuvant Breast and Bowel Project B-14 randomized trial. J Natl Cancer Inst 2001; 93(9):684–690.
39. Baum M, Budzar AU, Cuzick J, et al. Anastrozole alone or in combination with tamoxifen versus tamoxifen alone for adjuvant treatment of postmenopausal women with early breast cancer: first results of the ATAC randomised trial. Lancet 2002; 359(9324):2131–2139.
40. Whelan TJ, Goss PE, Ingle JN, et al. Assessment of quality of life in MA.17: a randomized, placebo-controlled trial of letrozole after 5 years of tamoxifen in postmenopausal women. J Clin Oncol 2005; 23(28):6931–6940.
41. Felson DT, Cummings SR. Aromatase inhibitors and the syndrome of arthralgias with estrogen deprivation. Arth Rheum 2005; 52(9):2594–2598.
42. Geiger AM, Chen W, Bernstein L. Myocardial infarction risk and tamoxifen therapy for breast cancer. Br J Cancer 2005; 92(9):1614–1620.
43. Kataja V, Hietanen P, Joensuu H, et al. The effects of adjuvant anastraxole, exemestane, tamoxifen, and toremifene on serum lipids in post-menopausal women with breast cancer—a randomised study. Breast Cancer Res Treat 2002; 76:S156.
44. Elisaf MS, Bairaktari ET, Nicolaides C, et al. Effect of letrozole on the lipid profile in postmenopausal women with breast cancer. Eur J Cancer 2001; 37(12):1510–1513.
45. Wojtacki J, Lesniewski-Kmak K, Piotrowska M, Rolka-Stempniewicz G, Kubik M, Wroblewska M. Effect of anastrozole on serum levels of apolipoprotein A-I and B in patients with early breast cancer: additional data on lack of atherogenic properties. Breast Cancer Res Treat 2004; 88:S238.
46. Wasan KM, Goss PE, Pritchard PH, et al. The influence of letrozole on serum lipid concentrations in postmenopausal women with primary breast cancer who have completed 5 years of adjuvant tamoxifen (NCIC CTG MA.17L). Ann Oncol 2005; 16(5):707–715.
47. Nordenskjold B, Rosell J, Rutqvist LE, et al. Coronary heart disease mortality after 5 years of adjuvant tamoxifen therapy: results from a randomized trial. J Natl Cancer Inst 2005; 97(21):1609–1610.
48. Eiermann W, Paepke S, Appfelstaedt J, et al. Preoperative treatment of postmenopausal breast cancer patients with letrozole: a randomized double-blind multicenter study. Ann Oncol 2001; 12(11):1527–1532.
49. Ellis MJ, Coop A, Singh B, et al. Letrozole is more effective neoadjuvant endocrine therapy than tamoxifen for ErbB-1 and/or ErbB-2-positive, estrogen receptor-positive primary breast cancer: evidence from a phase III randomized trial. J Clin Oncol 2001; 19(18):3808–3816.
50. Smith IE, Dowsett M, Ebbs SR, et al. Neoadjuvant treatment of postmenopausal breast cancer with anastrozole, tamoxifen, or both in combination: the Immediate Preoperative Anastrozole, Tamoxifen, or Combined with Tamoxifen (IMPACT) multicenter double-blind randomized trial. J Clin Oncol 2005; 23(22):5108–5116.
51. Ellis MJ. Neoadjuvant endocrine therapy for breast cancer: more questions than answers. J Clin Oncol 2005; 23(22):4842–4844.
52. van't Veer LJ, Dai H, van de Vijver MJ, et al. Gene expression profiling predicts clinical outcome of breast cancer. Nature 2002; 415(6871):530–536.

53. Sorlie T, Tibshirani R, Parker J, et al. Repeated observation of breast tumor subtypes in independent gene expression data sets. Proc Natl Acad Sci USA 2003; 100(14):8418–8423.

54. Ravdin PM, Green S, Dorr TM, et al. Prognostic significance of progesterone receptor levels in estrogen receptor-positive patients with metastatic breast cancer treated with tamoxifen: results of a prospective Southwest Oncology Group study. J Clin Oncol 1992; 10(8):1284–1291.

55. Elledge RM, Green S, Pugh R, et al. Estrogen receptor (ER) and progesterone receptor (PgR), by ligand-binding assay compared with ER, PgR and pS2, by immuno- histochemistry in predicting response to tamoxifen in metastatic breast cancer: a Southwest Oncology Group Study. Int J Cancer 2000; 89(2):111–117.

56. Bardou VJ, Arpino G, Elledge RM, Osborne CK, Clark GM. Progesterone receptor status significantly improves outcome prediction over estrogen receptor status alone for adjuvant endocrine therapy in two large breast cancer databases. J Clin Oncol 2003; 21(10):1973–1979.

57. Konecny G, Pauletti G, Pegram M, et al. Quantitative association between HER-2/neu and steroid hormone receptors in hormone receptor-positive primary breast cancer. J Natl Cancer Inst 2003; 95(2):142–153.

58. Cui X, Zhang P, Deng W, et al. Insulin-like growth factor-I inhibits progesterone receptor expression in breast cancer cells via the phosphatidylinositol 3-kinase/Akt/mammalian target of rapamycin pathway: progesterone receptor as a potential indicator of growth factor activity in breast cancer. Mol Endocrinol 2003; 17(4):575–588.

59. Tovey S, Dunne B, Witton CJ, Forsyth A, Cooke TG, Bartlett JM. Can molecular markers predict when to implement treatment with aromatase inhibitors in invasive breast cancer? Clin Cancer Res 2005; 11(13):4835–4842.

60. Osborne CK, Shou J, Massarweh S, Schiff R. Crosstalk between estrogen receptor and growth factor receptor pathways as a cause for endocrine therapy resistance in breast cancer. Clin Cancer Res 2005; 11(Pt 2):865s–870s.

61. Shou J, Massarweh S, Osborne CK, et al. Mechanisms of tamoxifen resistance: increased estrogen receptor-HER2/neu cross-talk in ER/HER2-positive breast cancer. J Natl Cancer Inst 2004; 96(12):926–935.

62. Dowsett M, Cuzick J, Wale C, Howell T, Houghton J, Baum M. Retrospective analysis of time to recurrence in the ATAC trial according to hormone receptor status: an hypothesis-generating study. J Clin Oncol 2005; 23(30):7512–7517.

63. Viale G, Regan M, Dell'Orto P, et al. Central review of ER, PgR and HER-2 in BIG 1-98 evaluating letrozole vs. tamoxifen as adjuvant endocrine therapy for postmenopausal women with receptor-positive breast cancer. Breast Cancer Res Treat 2005; 94:S13–S14.

64. Coombes RC, Hall E, Gibson LJ, et al. A randomized trial of exemestane after two to three years of tamoxifen therapy in postmenopausal women with primary breast cancer. N Engl J Med 2004; 350(11):1081–1092.

65. Goss PE, Ingle JN, Tu D. NCIC CTG MA17: disease free survival according to estrogen receptor and progesterone receptor status of the primary tumor. Breast Cancer Res Treat 2005; 94(suppl 1):S98.

66. Itoh T, Karlsberg K, Kijima I, et al. Letrozole-, anastrozole-, and tamoxifen-responsive genes in MCF-7aro cells: a microarray approach. Mol Cancer Res 2005; 3(4):203–218.

67. Loi S, Piccart M, Halbe-Kains B, et al. Prediction of early distant relapses on tamoxifen in early-stage breast cancer (BC): a potential tool for adjuvant aromatase inhibitor (AI) tailoring. J Clin Oncol 2005. ASCO Annual Meeting Proceedings. Part I of II (June 1 Supplement), 2005; 23(165):509.

68. Miller WR, Krause A, Evans DB, et al. Phenotypes for endocrine resistance can be identified by RNA microarray of sequential biopsies and are more variable than those predicting for tumour response. Breast Cancer Res Treat 2005; 94:S17.

69. Knox SK, Ingle JN, Suman VJ, et al. Cytochrome P450 2D6 status predicts breast cancer relapse in women receiving adjuvant tamoxifen (Tam). J Clin Oncol 2006; 24(18S):504.

70. Garber JE, Halabi S, Kaplan E, et al. Factor V Leiden (FVL) mutations and thromboembolic events (TE) in women with breast cancer on adjuvant tamoxifen. J Clin Oncol 2005. ASCO Annual Meeting Proceedings. Part I of II (June 1 Supplement), 2005; 23(165):508.

71. Losordo DW, Isner JM. Estrogen and angiogenesis: a review. Arterioscler Thromb Vasc Biol 2001; 21(1):6–12.
72. Manders P, Beex LV, Tjan-Heijnen VC, Span PN, Sweep CG. Vascular endothelial growth factor is associated with the efficacy of endocrine therapy in patients with advanced breast carcinoma. Cancer 2003; 98(10):2125–2132.
73. Ryden L, Jirstrom K, Bendahl PO, et al. Tumor-specific expression of vascular endothelial growth factor receptor 2 but not vascular endothelial growth factor or human epidermal growth factor receptor 2 is associated with impaired response to adjuvant tamoxifen in premenopausal breast cancer. J Clin Oncol 2005; 23(21):4695–4704.
74. Traina TA, Dickler MN, Caravelli JF, et al. A phase II trial of letrozole in combination with bevacizumab, an anti-VEGF antibody, in patients with hormone receptor-positive metastatic breast cancer. Breast Cancer Res Treat 2005; 94:S93.

15 Fulvestrant: A Novel Hormonal Agent

Rebecca A. Miksad

Division of Hematology–Oncology, Beth Israel Deaconess Medical Center and Harvard Medical School, Boston, Massachusetts, U.S.A.

Steven E. Come

Breast Cancer Program, Beth Israel Deaconess Medical Center and Harvard Medical School, Boston, Massachusetts, U.S.A.

INTRODUCTION

Endocrine therapy plays a crucial role in the systemic treatment of hormone receptor-positive breast cancer. The selective estrogen receptor (ER) modulator tamoxifen is widely used as a treatment for ER positive breast cancer and for risk reduction. However, tamoxifen possesses both antagonistic and agonist effects on the ER (1,2). Fulvestrant, a pure ER antagonist, was initially developed to overcome the agonist-based limitations of tamoxifen and to treat tamoxifen-resistant tumors. Further, fulvestrant may modulate the interaction between the ER and growth factor signaling pathways by downregulating ER expression. This action may be important in developing an optimal strategy for using endocrine therapy—in sequence, in combination, or paired with other biologically targeted agents. This chapter reviews the pharmacological properties of fulvestrant, evaluates the preclinical and clinical data, and describes the role of fulvestrant today in the context of other available hormonal and biologic therapies.

THE UNIQUE MECHANISMS OF ACTION OF FULVESTRANT

As a steroidal analog of 17β-estradiol, fulvestrant has a chemical structure that is similar to that of estradiol, but distinct from tamoxifen and other nonsteroidal hormonal agents. Both tamoxifen and fulvestrant competitively inhibit the binding of estradiol to the ER. In contrast to tamoxifen, fulvestrant has no agonist effect and downregulates the expression of the ER.

With estradiol as the comparator, fulvestrant's ER binding affinity (0.89) is much greater than tamoxifen's (0.025) (3,4). The conformational changes induced in the ER receptor by fulvestrant are distinct from those induced by estradiol or by tamoxifen. The ER–fulvestrant complex decreases dimerization of the ER (5–7), reduces nuclear uptake of the drug–receptor complex (8), and, through its relatively unstable complex, accelerates degradation of the ER (8,9).

Fulvestrant disables both the AF1 and AF2, which are functional regions that recruit the co-activator and co-repressor proteins required for expression of targeted genes to the ER transcription complex (10). When tumors are exposed to fulvestrant, transcription of ER-regulated genes is abrogated (4,11). In contrast, estradiol activates both AF1 and AF2 (12), and tamoxifen blocks AF2 but activates AF1 (11,13).

The decrease in progesterone receptor (PgR) levels in cells treated with fulvestrant provides evidence for fulvestrant's lack of an estrogen-agonist effect (4,14,15). Tamoxifen increases PgR levels (14). In a phase I trial ($n = 30$), a single injection of fulvestrant 250 mg given 14 days prior to estrogen administration did not produce estrogenic changes in the endometrium and also inhibited normal estrogen-stimulation effects (16).

PRECLINICAL EFFICACY STUDIES

In nude mice, fulvestrant doubles the median time to progression (TTP) of MCF-7 tumor cells compared with tamoxifen (200 vs. 104 days) (11). Tamoxifen-resistant, ER positive tumors from the MCF-7 human breast cancer cell line are inhibited by fulvestrant in both tissue culture and nude mice xenografts (4,17–19).

FORMULATION AND PHARMACOKINETIC ISSUES

Oral fulvestrant has low bioavailability (20) and has a low aqueous solubility (21). Therefore, fulvestrant was developed as a long-acting intramuscular (IM) injection given in a castor-oil-based vehicle (21). Pharmacokinetic substudies in phase III trials demonstrate that plasma fulvestrant concentrations remain in a narrow range and above the predicted biologic threshold for at least 28 days after depot IM injection (21–23).

The original fulvestrant phase III trial in the United States of 250 mg fulvestrant utilized two 2.5 mL injections (one in each buttock), instead of the single 5 mL injection used in the concurrent European-based study (24,25). These two dosing options (2×2.5 mL and 1×5 mL) yield similar plasma concentrations, areas under the curve, and predicted steady-state plasma concentrations (21,22). The parenteral formulation of fulvestrant potentially increases patient compliance in comparison with oral therapy and may improve access to treatment for patients who lack prescription medication coverage.

NEOADJUVANT BIOLOGIC DATA

In a partially blind, randomized, multi-center study, postmenopausal women with breast cancer ($n = 200$) scheduled for curative-intent surgery were pretreated with fulvestrant (50, 125, or 250 mg IM once), tamoxifen (20 mg per os (PO) daily), or matching tamoxifen placebo for 14 to 21 days prior to surgery. In comparison of fulvestrant with placebo, ER, PgR, and Ki67LI (Ki67 proliferation associated antigen labeling index, a measure of cell proliferation) were significantly decreased in the surgical specimen when compared with the diagnostic biopsy (14). Compared with tamoxifen, fulvestrant produced greater reductions in ER at all doses but was statistically significant only for the 250 mg dose. Tamoxifen decreased Ki67LI to a similar degree as fulvestrant and increased PgR (14). The reduction in the cell turnover index (a composite measure of apoptosis and proliferation) was significantly greater in surgically removed tumors pretreated with fulvestrant instead of tamoxifen (26).

CLINICAL EVIDENCE

Early Clinical Data

Phase II data of fulvestrant demonstrated a 36% partial response (PR) rate and a 31% stable disease (SD) rate for postmenopausal women with tamoxifen-resistant advanced breast cancer (ABC) (27). In this open-label, dose escalation study ($n = 19$), 15 patients received 250 mg of fulvestrant for the entire treatment period. The median duration of response (DOR) was 25 months (23,27). Responses were seen regardless of whether tamoxifen was utilized as adjuvant therapy or as treatment for ABC.

Clinical Trials in the Second-Line (Post-Tamoxifen) Setting

The clinical efficacy of fulvestrant as a second-line agent was established by two phase III trials (Trials 0020 and 0021) (24,25). Trial 0020 was an open-label trial that recruited patients in Europe, Australia, and South Africa (25). Trial 0021 was a double-blind, double-placebo trial conducted in North America (24). Although the two trials differed in geography and in blinding status, they were designed to run concurrently and to be analyzed with individual as well as pooled data.

By the time fulvestrant was ready for phase III testing, the third generation aromatase inhibitors (AIs) were regarded as the standard second-line treatment for tamoxifen-resistant breast cancer in postmenopausal women (28–34). Therefore, anastrozole was the comparative agent.

Both trials were large, multi-center, parallel group trials of postmenopausal women, with locally advanced or metastatic breast cancer, who failed prior endocrine therapy (adjuvant or first-line for advanced disease). All patients had either documented prior response to endocrine therapy or positive ER and/or PgR. The trials were powered to show superiority of fulvestrant over anastrozole, and patients were followed until death (24,25).

Patients were initially randomized to fulvestrant (either 250 or 125 mg IM) or to anastrozole 1 mg PO (24,25). In a planned preliminary interim analysis, fulvestrant 125 mg did not demonstrate clinical activity and recruitment to this arm was stopped (24,25). The final protocol for both trials compared fulvestrant 250 mg (1 × 5 mL or 2 × 2.5 mL monthly IM injections) with anastrozole 1 mg PO daily given until disease progression or withdrawal. The primary endpoint was TTP. Secondary endpoints included objective response (OR), clinical benefit (CB) (complete responders + partial responders + those with SD ≥24 weeks), and DOR.

Trial 0020

In the European trial ($n = 451$, median follow-up = 14.4 months), there was no difference in TTP for fulvestrant and anastrozole [HR, 0.98; 95.14% confidence interval (CI), 0.80–1.21; $P = 0.84$] (25). The median TTP was 5.5 months for fulvestrant and 5.1 months for anastrozole, with a similar CB in both arms (44.6% and 45.0%, respectively).

The data suggested an advantage for fulvestrant for some secondary endpoints. Fulvestrant had a numerically superior OR, compared with anastrozole: OR = 20.7% and 15.7%, respectively (odds ratio, 1.38; 95.14% CI, 0.84–2.29; $P = 0.20$) (25). In addition, the DOR was significantly greater for fulvestrant than for anastrozole (ratio of average response durations, 1.27; 95% CI, 1.05–1.55; $P = 0.01$). For responders, the median DOR was 15 months for fulvestrant ($n = 48$) and 14.5 months for anastrozole ($n = 39$) (25).

Trial 0021
The results of the North American trial ($n = 400$, median follow-up $= 16.8$ months) were similar to those of Trial 0020 (24). There was no difference in the TTP between fulvestrant and anastrozole (HR, 0.92; 95.14% CI, 0.74–1.14; $P = 0.43$) (24). The median TTP was 5.4 months for fulvestrant and 3.4 months for anastrozole, with a CB of 42.2% and 36.1%, respectively.

In contrast to the European trial, the OR rate did not show a numerical advantage for fulvestrant (OR $= 17.5$% in both arms). However, the DOR was significantly greater for fulvestrant than for anastrozole [ratio of average DOR, 1.35 (95% CI, 1.10–1.67; $P < 0.01$)] (24). For responders, the median DOR was 19.0 months for fulvestrant ($n = 36$) and 10.8 months for anastrozole ($n = 34$) (24). The difference in the DOR for responders was larger than that observed in Trial 0020.

Updated Combined Analysis of Trials 0020 and 0021
The updated combined analysis of Trials 0020 and 0021 ($n = 821$) was prospectively planned and the results were comparable with those from the individual trials (24,25,35,36). The prior treatment exposure for patients in both trials was similar, with the majority of women in each arm receiving prior tamoxifen (>96%) and prior chemotherapy (>52%) (36). The treatment groups were generally well matched in terms of other patient characteristics (36). At an extended median follow-up of 15.1 months, there was no difference for combined TTP, OR, or CB (36).

At a median follow-up of 27.0 months (range 0–66.9 months), there was no difference between fulvestrant and anastrozole for the combined median overall survival: 27.4 and 27.7 months, respectively (HR, 0.98; 95% CI, 0.84–1.15; $P = 0.809$) (35). Because the upper CI was <1.25, fulvestrant was described as noninferior to anastrozle for overall survival (35). On the basis of this phase III data, fulvestrant 250 mg IM injection gained approval by the United States Food and Drug Administration in April 2002 (37) and received marketing approval for the European Union in March 2004 (10). Fulvestrant is presently indicated for the treatment of hormone receptor-positive metastatic breast cancer in postmenopausal women with disease progression following anti-estrogen therapy (37). The monthly dose may be given as a single 5 mL IM injection or as two 2.5 mL injections into each buttock (37).

Clinical Data in the First-Line (Endocrine Naïve) Setting
Second-line fulvestrant is as effective as anastrozole, and first-line anastrozole possesses benefits over tamoxifen for postmenopausal women (24,25,38–40). Therefore, researchers hypothesized that first-line fulvestrant may also have benefits over tamoxifen.

Trial 0025 was a multi-center, double-blind, double-placebo randomized trial ($n = 587$) that compared monthly fulvestrant 250 mg IM with daily tamoxifen 20 mg PO as first-line therapy for postmenopausal women with ABC (40). Although patients known to be ER and PgR negative were excluded, confirmed receptor positivity was not required. Patients had not received prior endocrine or cytotoxic chemotherapy for ABC and had not received adjuvant endocrine therapy within the prior 12 months. Only 22% of patients in the fulvestrant arm and 24.8% of patients in the tamoxifen arm had received adjuvant tamoxifen (40). The primary endpoint was TTP.

At a median follow-up of 14.5 months, no significant difference was noted between TTP for fulvestrant and tamoxifen: 6.8 and 8.3 months, respectively

(95% CI 0.98–1.44; $P = 0.088$) (40). Although there was no difference in OR, secondary endpoint analysis favored tamoxifen: the CB was 54.3% for fulvestrant and 62% for tamoxifen ($P = 0.026$) (40).

A prospectively planned subset analysis of the women with known ER and/or PgR positive tumors (78.9% and 77.4% of women in the fulvestrant and tamoxifen arms, respectively) did not demonstrate a difference for TTP, OR, or CB (40). An unplanned exploratory analysis of TTP in patients with both ER and PgR positive tumors ($n = 245$) suggested a possible benefit of fulvestrant over tamoxifen (HR = 0.85, with 95% CI, 0.63–1.15; $P = 0.31$) (40). Trial 0025 did not demonstrate superiority of fulvestrant over tamoxifen, and, consequently, AIs remain favored as first-line endocrine therapy for postmenopausal women with ABC.

SAFETY ISSUES
Injection Site Events

Although there were initial concerns in the United States about a single 5 mL IM injection, these concerns were not confirmed in clinical trials. In the European phase III study (Trial 0020), injection site events occurred with 1.1% of all monthly injections (25). Most events were mild (transient injection site pain, inflammation, hemorrhage, and hypersensitivity reaction), and only one patient withdrew because of an event (25). In the North American phase III study (Trial 0021), a set of two 2.5 mL IM injections was administered each month. Injection site reactions occurred in 4.6% of the monthly injection sets (24). Placebo injections reaction rates were similar (24).

Adverse Events

Fulvestrant is well tolerated overall and its side effect profile is similar to other endocrine therapies for breast cancer. At a 27-month follow-up, combined analysis of most predefined adverse events (AEs) in Trials 0020 and 0021 did not demonstrate significant differences between fulvestrant and anastrozole: gastrointestinal disturbances (48.7% vs. 45.4%, respectively), hot flashes (21.7% vs. 22.2%), thrombo-embolic disease (3.5% vs. 4.5%), urinary tract infection (8.7% vs. 5.9%), vaginitis (2.6% vs. 1.9%), and weight gain (1.4% vs. 2.1%) (35). The only event found to be significantly different between the two arms was joint disorders. Joint disorders occurred less often in patients receiving fulvestrant (8.3%) than in those receiving anastrozole (12.8%) ($P = 0.0234$) (35).

A similar proportion of patients on the fulvestrant and anastrozole arms reported AEs (46.1% and 40.4%, respectively), although withdrawal due to a drug-related AEs was low (0.9% and 1.2%, respectively) (36). AE analysis directly comparing fulvestrant and tamoxifen showed no difference between these two agents. There was no difference in quality of life between treatment arms for Trials 0020, 0021, or 0025 (24,25,40).

The three reported phase III fulvestrant trials did not prospectively define bone density, hyperlipidemia, or cardiac events as adverse events for statistical analysis (36,40). Trial 0025 reported hyperlipidemia in 1% of patients in the fulvestrant arm and in 10% of patients in the tamoxifen arm. Bone fracture and cardiac events were not reported as occurring in ≥2% of patients in Trials 0020, 0021, or 0025. Given that these adverse events are now of concern for AIs, further clinical evidence is needed for fulvestrant.

OPTIMAL DOSING

The results for first-line fulvestrant in postmenopausal women with ABC were unexpected. The observation that the Trial 0025 Kaplan–Meier curves for TTP separate early raised questions about fulvestrant's pharmacokinetics. The greatest separation between the curves occurred at three months, suggesting a relatively high rate of early progression.

Clinical data for fulvestrant provided evidence for serum drug accumulation and a dose-dependent relationship with serum concentration (23,41). Pharmacokinetic profiling from a combined subset analysis of Trials 0020 and 0021 ($n = 219$) showed that the plasma steady state for fulvestrant 250 mg monthly IM injection is achieved after six doses (six months) (21). The majority of drug accumulation occurs after three doses (21). In comparison, the steady-state plasma concentration for tamoxifen is reached in 4 weeks (42) and for an AI in ~8 to 10 days (43).

A prolonged interval prior to attainment of a plasma steady state may correlate with a delay in achieving the maximal downregulation of ER. Decreased expression of the ER (as well as decreased PgR H-scores and Ki67LI) has a dose-dependent relationship with a single dose of fulvestrant 50, 125, or 250 mg given to untreated postmenopausal women (14). Biopsies obtained four to six weeks and six months after the initiation of monthly fulvestrant 250 mg IM showed a trend for increased ER downregulation over time (44). Decreased ER expression was sustained for at least six months in responders (44). In contrast, ER expression was detectable in all tumors at disease progression and in all women who never responded to fulvestrant (44). These data suggest a relationship between ER suppression and fulvestrant's CB.

Fulvestrant Loading Dose

A loading dose regimen may achieve the plasma steady state sooner and, perhaps, earlier treatment responses. Several ongoing phase III trials (discussed below) utilize loading dose regimens: patients receive a total of 1000 mg IM fulvestrant during the first month of treatment and 250 mg per month thereafter (500 mg on day 0, 250 mg on day 14 and day 28, and then 250 mg every 28 days) (10).

Higher Dose Fulvestrant

Higher doses of fulvestrant may enhance the efficacy of fulvestrant without adding significant toxicities. Given the formulation of fulvestrant, administration of more than two 5 mL injections (500 mg) at a single time point appears impractical. Several ongoing trials will evaluate the tolerability, safety, and efficacy of fulvestrant 500 mg IM. The Comparison of "Faslodex^TM" Recurrent or Metastatic breast cancer (CONFIRM) trial is a phase III, randomized, double-blind, dose comparison, parallel assignment, industry-sponsored efficacy trial that compares monthly 500 mg IM fulvestrant with monthly 250 mg IM fulvestrant for postmenopausal women with ABC who have failed one prior endocrine therapy (45).

Neoadjuvant trials provide the benefit of convenient collection of tissue for biomarker assessment. In postmenopausal women, the Neoadjuvant Endocrine Therapy for Women with Estrogen Sensitive Tumors (NEWEST) trial will compare 500 versus 250 mg IM fulvestrant given for four months prior to surgery (10). Other fulvestrant dosing regimes alone and in combination with an AI are under investigation.

Loading Dose Combined with Higher Dose Fulvestrant

Further benefit may be obtained by combining loading dose and high dose fulvestrant. In a nonrandomized, phase II trial, postmenopausal women with hormone receptor-positive ABC are given 500 mg IM fulvestrant on day 1, day 14, and then every 28 days (46). Response and pharmacokinetic parameters are measured (46). Eligibility criteria include no endocrine therapy in the metastatic setting and relapse at least 12 months after adjuvant endocrine therapy (46).

These loading dose and high dose fulvestrant trials may establish a more advantageous dosing strategy for fulvestrant.

FULVESTRANT AFTER AROMATASE INHIBITORS
Preclinical Data

The mechanisms by which tumors become resistant to AIs are not fully characterized, but differ, at least in part, from those involved in tamoxifen resistance because AIs lack the agonist effect associated with tamoxifen. Both estrogen hypersensitivity and crosstalk between growth factor pathways may contribute to endocrine resistance. In current practice patterns, AIs are often used in the first-line setting for adjuvant treatment or for advanced ABC in postmenopausal women. Therefore, fulvestrant is often used after an AL, a scenario without phase III clinical trial data available.

Two laboratory model systems describe the effect of fulvestrant on tumors deprived of estrogen or treated with an AI. In the long-term estrogen-deprived (LTED) model, MCF-7 cells are grown in steroid-deplete medium (47). LTED cells develop "adaptive hypersensitivity" and grow in response to low estrogen levels both in vivo and in vitro (47). This hypersensitivity is associated with upregulation of ERα (47,48), enhancement of nongenomic, plasma membrane-mediated pathways (47), and synergy of downstream interactions (47). Several proteins have been implicated: mitogen-activated protein kinase (MAPK) (47–50), phosphoinosital 3 kinase (PI3-K) (47,48), v-erb-b2 erythroblastic leukemia viral oncogene homolog 2 (ErbB2), human epidermal growth factor receptor 2 (HER2) (48,49), v-akt murine thymona viral oncogene homolog 1 (AKT) (49,51), and mammalian target of rapamycin (mTOR) (47).

Fulvestrant inhibits the growth of LTED cells, indicating possible efficacy and suggesting that this benefit may be related to its ability to negate ER signaling in the setting of AI-induced estrogen depletion (52). These laboratory data may support the continuation of AI therapy in order to maintain ligand suppression when fulvestrant is added for progressive disease (52).

The bell-shaped estrogen growth response curve is markedly shifted toward the left for LTED cells. Exogenous estradiol produces a 60% reduction in cell growth in LTED cells through increased apoptosis (53). This result raises the possibility that higher levels of estradiol induced by AI withdrawal or obtained by exogenous estradiol administration may shift the estrogen response growth curve back toward the right. This change may permit the emergence of an estrogen-sensitive clone responsive to fulvestrant.

In the long-term letrozole-treated (LTLT) model, MCF-7 cells are transfected with aromatase (MCF-7Ca) and are then treated with letrozole (50). LTLT cells also initially adapt to estrogen deprivation with upregulation of ER signaling, leading to activation of transcription and cell-proliferation kinase proteins (50). Fulvestrant inhibits tumor growth in mice bearing MCF-7Ca, prior to prolonged letrozole exposure (54). However, after exposure to letrozole for 56 weeks, ERs were downregulated and fulvestrant was unable to reverse resistance in LTLT cells (55). These LTLT data mirror the relatively low clinical OR rate for fulvestrant after an AI.

In the LTLT model, the combination of fulvestrant and letrozole treatment before the development of AI resistance provides superior results to single-agent letrozole treatment or sequential therapy with tamoxifen or higher dose letrozole (56). MCF-7Ca xenograft tumors regressed by 45% over the 29-week treatment period for those mice treated with combination therapy (56). This additive effect suggests that some transcription may occur via the ER during single-agent fulvestrant treatment (50). Fulvestrant may counteract AI-induced estradiol hypersensitivity and crosstalk by inhibiting the binding of remaining ligand for the ER, by downregulating the ER, and by minimizing crosstalk with growth factor pathways.

Clinical Evidence
Fulvestrant After an Aromatase Inhibitor
The fulvestrant compassionate use program (CUP) provided the first prospective data regarding the benefit of fulvestrant in postmenopausal women previously exposed to an AI. Evaluation of a multi-center CUP ($n = 339$) showed that monthly 250 mg IM fulvestrant given after multiple prior endocrine therapies (93% previously exposed to an AI) produced a CB of 38.4% (57). The OR rate was 11.8%, with no women obtaining a complete response (57).

A North Central Cancer Treatment Group (NCCTG) phase II trial evaluated fulvestrant in postmenopausal women with measurable hormone-positive ABC who had progressed on a third-generation AI and had not received more than one hormonal agent or cytotoxic chemotherapy ($n = 77$) (58). The median number of cycles administered was two (1 to ≥ 10). No complete responses were observed and only 14.3% of women obtained a PR (58). The CB was 35%, with a median TTP of three months and a median survival of 20.2 months (58). The subset of women who had only been treated with an AI in the past fared better than those previously exposed to both an AI and to tamoxifen (PR = 28.6% and 8.9%, respectively, and CB = 52.4% and 28.6%, respectively) (58). The Swiss Group for Clinical Cancer Research reported a phase II multi-center trial ($n = 67$), in which 250 mg IM fulvestrant was given monthly to postmenopausal women ($n = 67$) with ABC after progression on an AI. A CB of 28.4% (CR = 0% and PR = 1%) was observed (59).

With the majority of the CB being SD, these data demonstrate a low clinical response to fulvestrant after an AI. In an effort to improve this response, a small phase II trial will assess the OR, safety, and tolerability of administering up to 12 weeks of estradiol after AI failure and prior to fulvestrant treatment (46).

Fulvestrant After Aromatase Inhibitor vs. Fulvestrant Combined with an Aromatase Inhibitor vs. Additional Aromatase Inhibitor
To specifically address question raised by preclinical data, two phase III trials are enrolling patients in order to assess sequencing and combination issues for fulvestrant after AI failure. In the Evaluation of "Faslodex^{TM}" versus Exemestane Clinical Trial (EFECT), postmenopausal women with hormone-positive ABC that recurs or progresses on a nonsteriodal AI are randomized to exemestane monotherapy or to fulvestrant with a loading dose (500 mg IM on day 1, 250 mg IM on days 14 and 28, and 250 mg IM/month thereafter) (10). Exemestane is used as the comparator

agent because phase II data suggest that after progression on a nonsteroidal AI, exemestane produces a CB of 24.3% (CR = 1.2% and PR = 5.4%) and a median DOR of 37 weeks (60).

The Study of "Faslodex^{TM}" versus Exemestane with/without "Arimidex" (SOFEA) trial utilizes the same entry criteria and the same fulvestrant loading dose regimen but adds a third treatment arm (10). Women may also be randomized to treatment with combination therapy with fulvestrant and an AI (10).

Combination Fulvestrant and Aromatase Inhibitor Before the Development of Aromatase Inhibitor Resistance

In light of the preclinical data demonstrating superiority of combination fulvestrant and AI before the development of AI resistance, two trials have been developed. The Southwest Oncology Group (SWOG) S0226 trial is randomizing postmenopausal women with hormone receptor-positive ABC who progressed on adjuvant tamoxifen therapy to fulvestrant plus anastrozole or anastrozole alone. Importantly, crossover from the anastrozole alone arm to the combination arm is allowed. The "Faslodex^{TM}" and "Arimidex" in Combination Trial (FACT) is similar to the SWOG trial, but it allows prior adjuvant treatment with tamoxifen or a nonsteroidal AI and there is no crossover (10).

FULVESTRANT RESISTANCE
Endocrine Therapy Following Fulvestrant
Preclinical Data

Fulvestrant-resistant MCF-7 cells lose ERα expression and upregulate epidermal growth factor receptor (EGFR) expression, leading to changes in gene expression patterns (61,62). The increase in EGFR may allow cells to develop estradiol-independent signaling pathways. However, the re-emergence of ER expression after progression on fulvestrant also supports a trial of subsequent endocrine therapies (44).

Clinical Evidence

Retrospective assessment suggests that women may respond to endocrine therapy after failure on fulvestrant. Investigators of Trials 0020 and 0021 were asked to report, for each patient deriving a CB from fulvestrant, the response to subsequent therapy (63). Follow-up data were available on 66 (35%) patients (63). Fifty-four patients (82%) were treated with endocrine therapy (mainly AIs) after progression and 25 again derived a CB (PR = 4 and SD = 21) (63). Although this study was a nonrandomized, retrospective analysis, the results suggest incomplete cross-resistance between fulvestrant and other endocrine therapies.

NOVEL AGENTS IN COMBINATION WITH FULVESTRANT
Crosstalk as a Target
Preclinical Data

ER activation can be achieved through epidermal growth factor (EGF) and the MAPK-signaling pathways (48,61,64,65). Fulvestrant-resistant cells lose ERα expression (61), demonstrate a decline in ER-mediated transcription (62), and appear to have an increased dependence on the EGF/MAPK pathways (61,62). Fulvestrant resistance can be reversed with the addition of the EGFR tyrosine kinase inhibitor gefitinib (62). Combination treatment with gefitinib and fulvestrant decreased proliferation in MCF-7 cells (66).

Crosstalk between ER and HER2 offers a potential target for combination therapy. Although both single-agent fulvestrant and single-agent trastuzumab inhibit the growth of tamoxifen resistant, HER2 overexpressing cells, the combination is superior (67). Other targeted agents with preclinical evidence of benefit in combination with fulvestrant include lapatinib, a dual kinase inhibitor that disrupts both EGFR and HER2 (68), and tipifarnib, which inhibits farnesyl transferase, an enzyme involved downstream of EGFR and HER2 (10).

Clinical Evidence

Several targeted agents are being combined with fulvestrant in clinical trials. A phase II, open-label Eastern Cooperative Oncology Group (ECOG 4101) trial will assess gefinitib in combination with 250 mg fulvestrant versus gefinitib in combination with anastrozole in hormone-positive postmenopausal women with ABC (10). Trial treatment may be first- or second-line. A separate phase II trial will evaluate the efficacy of trastuzumab alone, high dose fulvestrant alone, and the combination of the two agents in HER2 positive, hormone-positive postmenopausal women with ABC (10).

The combination of lapatinib and loading dose fulvestrant will be assessed in a phase III, placebo-controlled trial by the Cancer and Leukemia Group B (CALGB 40302) (10). The comparator will be fulvestrant alone and eligibility criteria include postmenopausal status, hormone-positive tumors, HER2- or EGFR-positive ABC, and prior exposure to an AI (10). An additional phase II trial will investigate the utility of combining fulvestrant and tipifarnib in the second-line setting after failure of a prior endocrine treatment for postmenopausal, hormone receptor-positive women with ABC (10).

PREMENOPAUSAL WOMEN

There are little preclinical and clinical data on the utility of fulvestrant in premenopausal women, and fulvestrant does not have an indication for this group. A phase II, second-line trial is investigating the 500 mg IM dose of fulvestrant in premenopausal women with hormone receptor-positive ABC who have not been exposed to endocrine therapy. Up to three courses of chemotherapy for metastatic disease are allowed (69). A phase II neoadjuvant study comparing 750 mg IM fulvestrant (single dose) versus 20 mg tamoxifen daily for two weeks prior to surgery will assess tumor marker changes in premenopausal women (10).

SUMMARY

Fulvestrant has been established by two phase III trials to be at least as effective as anastrozole for second-line endocrine treatment in postmenopausal women with ABC. However, fulvestrant has not been shown to be superior in the first-line setting. High dose or loading dose fulvestrant may improve fulvestrant's performance in both first and second line settings, without compromising its tolerability. Ongoing trials will address these questions.

Fulvestrant's unique mode of action as a pure anti-estrogen make it an ideal candidate for combination therapy with AIs as well as with agents that inhibit the growth factor signaling pathways. The optimal sequencing position for fulvestrant in a multi-agent endocrine therapy strategy has not been established. Ongoing and future trials should help to clarify these issues.

REFERENCES

1. Gottardis MM, Jordan VC. Development of tamoxifen-stimulated growth of MCF-7 tumors in athymic mice after long-term antiestrogen administration. Cancer Res 1988; 48:5183–5187.
2. Johnston SR, Haynes BP, Smith IE, et al. Acquired tamoxifen resistance in human breast cancer and reduced intra-tumoral drug concentration. Lancet 1993; 342:1521–1522.
3. Wakeling AE, Bowler J. Steroidal pure antioestrogens. J Endocrinol 1987; 112:R7–R10.
4. Wakeling AE, Dukes M, Bowler J. A potent specific pure antiestrogen with clinical potential. Cancer Res 1991; 51:3867–3873.
5. Parker MG. Action of "pure" antiestrogens in inhibiting estrogen receptor action. Breast Cancer Res Treat 1993; 26:131–137.
6. Pink JJ, Jordan VC. Models of estrogen receptor regulation by estrogens and antiestrogens in breast cancer cell lines. Cancer Res 1996; 56:2321–2330.
7. Fawell SE, Lees JA, White R, Parker MG. Characterization and colocalization of steroid binding and dimerization activities in the mouse estrogen receptor. Cell 1990; 60: 953–962.
8. Dauvois S, White R, Parker MG. The antiestrogen ICI 182780 disrupts estrogen receptor nucleocytoplasmic shuttling. J Cell Sci 1993; 106(Pt 4):1377–1388.
9. Nicholson RI, Gee JM, Manning DL, Wakeling AE, Montano MM, Katzenellenbogen BS. Responses to pure antiestrogens (ICI 164384, ICI 182780) in estrogen-sensitive and -resistant experimental and clinical breast cancer. Ann N Y Acad Sci 1995; 761:148–163.
10. Howell A. Fulvestrant ("Faslodex"): current and future role in breast cancer management. Crit Rev Oncol Hematol 2006; 57:265–273.
11. Osborne CK, Coronado-Heinsohn EB, Hilsenbeck SG, et al. Comparison of the effects of a pure steroidal antiestrogen with those of tamoxifen in a model of human breast cancer. J Natl Cancer Inst 1995; 87:746–750.
12. Kumar V, Green S, Stack G, Berry M, Jin JR, Chambon P. Functional domains of the human estrogen receptor. Cell 1987; 51:941–951.
13. Tzukerman MT, Esty A, Santiso-Mere D, et al. Human estrogen receptor transactivational capacity is determined by both cellular and promoter context and mediated by two functionally distinct intramolecular regions. Mol Endocrinol 1994; 8:21–30.
14. Robertson JF, Nicholson RI, Bundred NJ, et al. Comparison of the short-term biological effects of 7alpha-[9-(4,4,5,5,5-pentafluoropentylsulfinyl)-nonyl]estra-1,3,5, (10)-triene-3,17beta-diol (Faslodex) versus tamoxifen in postmenopausal women with primary breast cancer. Cancer Res 2001; 61:6739–6746.
15. Wakeling AE. Similarities and distinctions in the mode of action of different classes of antioestrogens. Endocr Relat Cancer 2000; 7:17–28.
16. Addo S, Yates RA, Laight A. A phase I trial to assess the pharmacology of the new oestrogen receptor antagonist fulvestrant on the endometrium in healthy postmenopausal volunteers. Br J Cancer 2002; 87:1354–1359.
17. Lykkesfeldt AE, Madsen MW, Briand P. Altered expression of estrogen-regulated genes in a tamoxifen-resistant and ICI 164,384 and ICI 182,780 sensitive human breast cancer cell line, MCF-7/TAMR-1. Cancer Res 1994; 54:1587–1595.
18. Osborne CK, Jarman M, McCague R, Coronado EB, Hilsenbeck SG, Wakeling AE. The importance of tamoxifen metabolism in tamoxifen-stimulated breast tumor growth. Cancer Chemother Pharmacol 1994; 34:89–95.
19. Hu XF, Veroni M, De Luise M, et al. Circumvention of tamoxifen resistance by the pure anti-estrogen ICI 182,780. Int J Cancer 1993; 55:873–876.
20. Harrison M, Laight A, Clarke DA, Giles P, Yates RA. Pharmacokinetics and metabolism of fulvestrant after oral, intravenous and intramuscular administration in healthy volunteers [abstr 311]. Proc Am Soc Clin Oncol 2003; 22:78.

21. Robertson JF, Erikstein B, Osborne KC, et al. Pharmacokinetic profile of intramuscular fulvestrant in advanced breast cancer. Clin Pharmacokinet 2004; 43:529–538.
22. Robertson JF, Harrison MP. Equivalent single-dose pharmacokinetics of two different dosing methods of prolonged-release fulvestrant ("Faslodex") in postmenopausal women with advanced breast cancer. Cancer Chemother Pharmacol 2003; 52:346–348.
23. Howell A, DeFriend DJ, Robertson JF, et al. Pharmacokinetics, pharmacological and anti-tumour effects of the specific anti-oestrogen ICI 182780 in women with advanced breast cancer. Br J Cancer 1996; 74:300–308.
24. Osborne CK, Pippen J, Jones SE, et al. Double-blind, randomized trial comparing the efficacy and tolerability of fulvestrant versus anastrozole in postmenopausal women with advanced breast cancer progressing on prior endocrine therapy: results of a North American trial. J Clin Oncol 2002; 20:3386–3395.
25. Howell A, Robertson JF, Quaresma Albano J, et al. Fulvestrant, formerly ICI 182,780, is as effective as anastrozole in postmenopausal women with advanced breast cancer progressing after prior endocrine treatment. J Clin Oncol 2002; 20:3396–3403.
26. Bundred NJ, Anderson E, Nicholson RI, Dowsett M, Dixon M, Robertson JF. Fulvestrant, an estrogen receptor downregulator, reduces cell turnover index more effectively than tamoxifen. Anticancer Res 2002; 22:2317–2319.
27. Howell A, DeFriend D, Robertson J, Blamey R, Walton P. Response to a specific antioestrogen (ICI 182780) in tamoxifen-resistant breast cancer. Lancet 1995; 345:29–30.
28. Jonat W, Howell A, Blomqvist C, et al. A randomised trial comparing two doses of the new selective aromatase inhibitor anastrozole (Arimidex) with megestrol acetate in postmenopausal patients with advanced breast cancer. Eur J Cancer 1996; 32A:404–412.
29. Buzdar AU, Jones SE, Vogel CL, Wolter J, Plourde P, Webster A. A phase III trial comparing anastrozole (1 and 10 milligrams), a potent and selective aromatase inhibitor, with megestrol acetate in postmenopausal women with advanced breast carcinoma. Arimidex Study Group. Cancer 1997; 79:730–739.
30. Buzdar AU, Jonat W, Howell A, et al. Anastrozole versus megestrol acetate in the treatment of postmenopausal women with advanced breast carcinoma: results of a survival update based on a combined analysis of data from two mature phase III trials. Arimidex Study Group. Cancer 1998; 83:1142–1152.
31. Robertson JF, Howell A, Buzdar A, von Euler M, Lee D. Static disease on anastrozole provides similar benefit as objective response in patients with advanced breast cancer. Breast Cancer Res Treat 1999; 58:157–162.
32. Dombernowsky P, Smith I, Falkson G, et al. Letrozole, a new oral aromatase inhibitor for advanced breast cancer: double-blind randomized trial showing a dose effect and improved efficacy and tolerability compared with megestrol acetate. J Clin Oncol 1998; 16:453–461.
33. Buzdar A, Douma J, Davidson N, et al. Phase III, multicenter, double-blind, randomized study of letrozole, an aromatase inhibitor, for advanced breast cancer versus megestrol acetate. J Clin Oncol 2001; 19:3357–3366.
34. Kaufmann M, Bajetta E, Dirix LY, et al. Exemestane is superior to megestrol acetate after tamoxifen failure in postmenopausal women with advanced breast cancer: results of a phase III randomized double-blind trial. The Exemestane Study Group. J Clin Oncol 2000; 18:1399–1411.
35. Howell A, Pippen J, Elledge RM, et al. Fulvestrant versus anastrozole for the treatment of advanced breast carcinoma: a prospectively planned combined survival analysis of two multicenter trials. Cancer 2005; 104:236–239.
36. Robertson JF, Osborne CK, Howell A, et al. Fulvestrant versus anastrozole for the treatment of advanced breast carcinoma in postmenopausal women: a prospective combined analysis of two multicenter trials. Cancer 2003; 98:229–238.
37. Bross PF, Baird A, Chen G, et al. Fulvestrant in postmenopausal women with advanced breast cancer. Clin Cancer Res 2003; 9:4309–4317.
38. Bonneterre J, Buzdar A, Nabholtz JM, et al. Anastrozole is superior to tamoxifen as first-line therapy in hormone receptor positive advanced breast carcinoma. Cancer 2001; 92:2247–2258.

39. Nabholtz JM, Buzdar A, Pollak M, et al. Anastrozole is superior to tamoxifen as first-line therapy for advanced breast cancer in postmenopausal women: results of a North American multicenter randomized trial. Arimidex Study Group. J Clin Oncol 2000; 18: 3758–3767.

40. Howell A, Robertson JF, Abram P, et al. Comparison of fulvestrant versus tamoxifen for the treatment of advanced breast cancer in postmenopausal women previously untreated with endocrine therapy: a multinational, double-blind, randomized trial. J Clin Oncol 2004; 22:1605–1613.

41. DeFriend DJ, Howell A, Nicholson RI, et al. Investigation of a new pure antiestrogen (ICI 182780) in women with primary breast cancer. Cancer Res 1994; 54:408–414.

42. AstraZeneca. Nolvadex (Tamoxifen citrate). Medication Guide, approved by the US Food and Drug Administration. Wilmington, DE 19850: AstraZeneca Pharmaceuticals LP, 2003 (revised March 2005).

43. Smith IE, Dowsett M. Aromatase inhibitors in breast cancer. N Engl J Med 2003; 348:2431–2442.

44. Gutteridge E, Robertson JFR, Cheung KL, Pinder S, Wakeling A. Effects of fulvestrant on estrogen receptor levels during long-term treatment of patients with advanced breast cancer final results [abstr 4086]. 27th Annual San Antonio Breast Cancer Symposium, San Antonio, Dec 10, 2004.

45. ClinicalTrials.gov. A Comparison of the Efficacy and Tolerability of Fulvestrant (FASLODEX™) 500mg With Fulvestrant (FASLODEX™) 250mg in Postmenopausal Women With Oestrogen Receptor Positive Advanced Breast Cancer Progressing or Relapsing After Previous Endocrine Therapy. Vol. 2006, U.S. National Institute of Health, 2006.

46. Come SE, Borges VF. Role of fulvestrant in sequential hormonal therapy for advanced, hormone receptor-positive breast cancer in postmenopausal women. Clin Breast Cancer 2005; 6(suppl 1):S15–S22.

47. Santen RJ, Song RX, Zhang Z, et al. Long-term estradiol deprivation in breast cancer cells up-regulates growth factor signaling and enhances estrogen sensitivity. Endocr Relat Cancer 2005; 12(suppl 1):S61–S73.

48. Martin LA, Farmer I, Johnston SR, Ali S, Marshall C, Dowsett M. Enhanced estrogen receptor (ER) alpha, ERBB2, and MAPK signal transduction pathways operate during the adaptation of MCF-7 cells to long term estrogen deprivation. J Biol Chem 2003; 278:30458–30468.

49. Gutierrez MC, Detre S, Johnston S, et al. Molecular changes in tamoxifen-resistant breast cancer: relationship between estrogen receptor, HER-2, and p38 mitogen-activated protein kinase. J Clin Oncol 2005; 23:2469–2476.

50. Brodie A, Jelovac D, Sabnis G, Long B, Macedo L, Goloubeva O. Model systems: mechanisms involved in the loss of sensitivity to letrozole. J Steroid Biochem Mol Biol 2005; 95:41–48.

51. Yue W, Wang JP, Conaway MR, Li Y, Santen RJ. Adaptive hypersensitivity following long-term estrogen deprivation: involvement of multiple signal pathways. J Steroid Biochem Mol Biol 2003; 86:265–274.

52. Martin LA, Pancholi S, Chan CM, et al. The anti-oestrogen ICI 182,780, but not tamoxifen, inhibits the growth of MCF-7 breast cancer cells refractory to long-term oestrogen deprivation through down-regulation of oestrogen receptor and IGF signalling. Endocr Relat Cancer 2005; 12:1017–1036.

53. Song RX, Mor G, Naftolin F, et al. Effect of long-term estrogen deprivation on apoptotic responses of breast cancer cells to 17beta-estradiol. J Natl Cancer Inst 2001; 93:1714–1723.

54. Lu Q, Liu Y, Long BJ, Grigoryev D, Gimbel M, Brodie A. The effect of combining aromatase inhibitors with antiestrogens on tumor growth in a nude mouse model for breast cancer. Breast Cancer Res Treat 1999; 57:183–192.

55. Jelovac D, Sabnis G, Long BJ, Macedo L, Goloubeva OG, Brodie AM. Activation of mitogen-activated protein kinase in xenografts and cells during prolonged treatment with aromatase inhibitor letrozole. Cancer Res 2005; 65:5380–5389.

56. Jelovac D, Macedo L, Goloubeva OG, Handratta V, Brodie AMH. Additive antitumor effect of aromatase inhibitor letrozole and antiestrogen fulvestrant in a postmenopausal breast cancer model. Cancer Res 2005; 65:5439–5444.

57. Steger GG, Gips M, Simon SD, et al. Fulvestrant ("Faslodex"): clinical experience from the Compassionate Use Programme. Cancer Treat Rev 2005; 31(suppl 2):S10–S16.
58. Ingle JN, Suman VJ, Rowland KM, et al. Fulvestrant in women with advanced breast cancer after progression on prior aromatase inhibitor therapy: North Central Cancer Treatment Group Trial N0032. J Clin Oncol 2006; 24:1052–1056.
59. Perey L, Paridaens R, Nolé F, et al. Fulvestrant ("Faslodex") as hormonal treatment in postmenopausal patients with advanced breast cancer (ABC) progressing after treatment with tamoxifen and aromatase inhibitors: update of a phase II SAKK trial. [abstr 6048]. Breast Cancer Res Treat 2004; 88:S236.
60. Lonning PE, Bajetta E, Murray R, et al. Activity of exemestane in metastatic breast cancer after failure of nonsteroidal aromatase inhibitors: a phase II trial. J Clin Oncol 2000; 18:2234–2244.
61. Sommer A, Hoffmann J, Lichtner RB, Schneider MR, Parczyk K. Studies on the development of resistance to the pure antiestrogen Faslodex in three human breast cancer cell lines. J Steroid Biochem Mol Biol 2003; 85:33–47.
62. McClelland RA, Barrow D, Madden TA, et al. Enhanced epidermal growth factor receptor signaling in MCF7 breast cancer cells after long-term culture in the presence of the pure antiestrogen ICI 182,780 (Faslodex). Endocrinology 2001; 142:2776–2788.
63. Vergote I, Robertson JF, Kleeberg U, Burton G, Osborne CK, Mauriac L. Postmenopausal women who progress on fulvestrant ("Faslodex") remain sensitive to further endocrine therapy. Breast Cancer Res Treat 2003; 79:207–211.
64. Levin ER. Bidirectional signaling between the estrogen receptor and the epidermal growth factor receptor. Mol Endocrinol 2003; 17:309–317.
65. Pietras RJ. Interactions between estrogen and growth factor receptors in human breast cancers and the tumor-associated vasculature. Breast J 2003; 9:361–373.
66. Gee JM, Harper ME, Hutcheson IR, et al. The antiepidermal growth factor receptor agent gefitinib (ZD1839/Iressa) improves antihormone response and prevents development of resistance in breast cancer in vitro. Endocrinology 2003; 144:5105–5117.
67. Kunisue H, Kurebayashi J, Otsuki T, et al. Anti-HER2 antibody enhances the growth inhibitory effect of anti-oestrogen on breast cancer cells expressing both oestrogen receptors and HER2. Br J Cancer 2000; 82:46–51.
68. Johnston SR. Clinical efforts to combine endocrine agents with targeted therapies against epidermal growth factor receptor/human epidermal growth factor receptor 2 and mammalian target of rapamycin in breast cancer. Clin Cancer Res 2006; 12:1061s–1068s.
69. ClinicalTrials.gov. Fulvestrant in premonpausal women with hormone receptor-positive breast cancer. Vol. 2006, U.S. National Institute of Health, 2006.

16 HER2-Positive Breast Cancer: Current Treatment Strategies

Edith A. Perez and Mansoina Baweja
Mayo Clinic, Jacksonville, Florida, U.S.A.

INTRODUCTION

Human epidermal growth factor receptor 2 (HER2) has been found to be an important prognostic and predictive marker of treatment response in women with breast cancer in the adjuvant setting and advanced disease. The *HER2* gene is amplified and the HER2 protein is overexpressed in ~20% to 25% of breast cancers with resulting poor prognosis and shortened overall survival (OS) (1). The *HER2* gene, also known as HER2/neu or c-erbB2, is located on chromosome 17q and belongs to the human epithelial receptor (HER) family of genes. It encodes a 185 kDa transmembrane tyrosine kinase growth factor receptor, which mediates signaling for cell proliferation and survival (2).

HER2 gene amplification and resultant protein overexpression are associated with a more aggressive clinical course. Although normal cells have about 24,000 HER2 proteins and only two copies of the *HER2* gene, overexpressed tissue may demonstrate as many as 2,400,000 protein molecules or 50 to 100 copies of the gene, which precipitate ligand-independent activation of the HER2 kinase (3).

Several murine monoclonal antibodies against the extracellular domain of the HER2 protein have been found to inhibit proliferation of cells overexpressing HER2 (4). However, to minimize immunogenicity, the antigen-binding region of one of the more effective antibodies was fused to the framework region of the human IgG leading to trastuzumab. Trastuzumab® (Herceptin, Genentech Inc., South San Francisco, California, U.S.A.) is a humanized monoclonal antibody that binds to the HER2. It was approved in 1998 by the U.S. Food and Drug Administration (FDA) for the treatment of HER2-positive metastatic breast cancer (MBC) in the first-line setting in combination with paclitaxel, or as monotherapy for patients who had received at least one prior chemotherapy regimen for HER2-positive MBC. Trastuzumab is now predominantly used in combination with chemotherapy in the first-line setting of metastatic disease due to its clear advantage in improving clinical outcome. Recent data related to the impact of adding this agent to chemotherapy as adjuvant therapy for HER2-positive breast cancer have altered the standard of treatment for these patients. Studies in combination with hormonal therapy and other biological agents are ongoing.

METHODOLOGIES FOR HUMAN EPIDERMAL GROWTH FACTOR RECEPTOR 2 TESTING

Guidelines established by American Society of Clinical Oncology (ASCO) (5) and the College of American Pathologists strongly suggest that HER2 status be checked in all newly diagnosed patients with invasive breast cancer. One of the most critical aspects of selecting patients for this targeted therapy is the methodology used to detect HER2 overexpression in tumor tissue. In order to clinically evaluate trastuzumab as therapy for HER2-positive breast cancer, it was necessary to simultaneously develop and validate testing methods that could confirm HER2 amplification or overexpression in the primary tumor. Immunohistochemical (IHC) analysis and fluorescence in situ hybridization (FISH) are the two most widely used methods used to evaluate HER2 status in breast cancer tissue.

Initially, IHC testing was used to select patients for trastuzumab therapy. IHC is performed on formalin-fixed, paraffin-embedded tissue and occasionally on frozen samples and measures cell surface HER2 protein as a surrogate for *HER2* gene amplification. Specimens are scored as 0, 1+, 2+, or 3+ on the basis of the extent and location of cellular staining, with 3+ indicating the strongest possible result. In the initial clinical trials of trastuzumab, patients whose tumors scored 2+ or 3+ for HER2 overexpression by IHC were enrolled. IHC is fast, widely available, relatively inexpensive, and uses light microscopy. However, the result can vary between laboratories depending on the antibodies used and the technique also uses subjective judgment criteria. Therefore, to obtain consistent, reproducible results with fewest false-positive or false-negative results, it is essential to choose a laboratory with extensive experience. The IHC tests typically used are HercepTest® (DAKO, Carpinteria, California, U.S.A.) and Pathway™ (Ventana, Tucson, Arizona, U.S.A.).

FISH directly tests for gene copies in tumor cell. Fluorescent DNA probes are used to visualize formalin-fixed, paraffin-embedded tissue with fluorescence microscope. Cells with *HER2/neu* gene over amplification demonstrate as many as 50 to 100 copies of the gene and this results in the overexpression of the p185$^{HER2/neu}$ at both the mRNA and the protein levels. FISH requires extra time when compared with IHC, but is nonradioactive and needs very little tissue. Additionally, it needs special equipment and may not be available at all hospitals, is also more expensive than IHC, and there may be limited community experience. Currently, there are two FISH-based assays for the assessment of *HER2* gene amplification: PathVysion® (Vysis, Downers Grove, Illinois, U.S.A.) and INFORM® (Ventana, Tucson, Arizona, U.S.A.).

Chromogenic in situ hybridization (CISH) is a new method to detect HER2 overexpression. Although it makes use of the in situ hybridization technology of FISH, it also takes advantage of the chromogenic signal detection of IHC that can be detected with the ordinary light microscope. CISH is potentially able to detect *HER2/neu* gene amplification and to minimize, if not eliminate, the false-positive fraction with the IHC procedure. It also costs one-quarter as much as FISH. CISH is emerging as a practical, cost-effective, and valid alternative to FISH in testing for gene alteration, especially in centers primarily working with IHC.

Both false-negative and false-positive HER2 testing results can have significant clinical impact: patients may be denied the potential benefits of treatment with trastuzumab on the basis of a false-negative HER2 result, whereas patients may be exposed to the potential side effects and cost of trastuzumab without the possibility of clinical benefit on the basis of a false-positive HER2 result. Therefore, the accurate assessment of the *HER2* gene amplification or protein overexpression is critical in patient management.

ISSUES WITH HUMAN EPIDERMAL GROWTH FACTOR RECEPTOR 2 TESTING

Discordance Between Immunohistochemical Analysis and Fluorescence In Situ Hybridization

Retrospective analyses of major trials using HER2 targeted therapy find that either IHC 3+ or a positive FISH is equally predictive of benefit for trastuzumab. A fairly general recommendation is that 2+ IHC should be confirmed by FISH, and most recently that FISH results are corroborated with IHC, although there are no data to document benefit of trastuzumab in the subset of patients with positive FISH but negative protein overexpression (7).

Concordance Between Local and Central Laboratories

Data published by Perez et al. showed that in the North Central Cancer Treatment Group (NCCTG) N9831 trial, when local and central evaluation used the same methodology, the level of concordance was 80.6% for HercepTest IHC and 87% for FISH. Concordance between local testing by non-HercepTest IHC and central testing by IHC or FISH was 73.9%. Among the discordant cases examined at the reference laboratory, there was 94.5% agreement for IHC (0, 1+, and 2+) and 95.1% agreement for FISH regarding nonamplified samples. Paik et al. had reported high level of discordance between local and central IHC testing. But when IHC is performed in experienced laboratories (those performing more than 100 tests per month), the concordance rate of local versus central IHC increased to 98% (8). These data indicate discordance between local and central testing for both IHC and FISH but a high degree of agreement between the central and reference laboratories regarding the discordant cases and support the importance of using high-volume, experienced laboratories for HER2 testing to improve the process of selecting patients likely to benefit from trastuzumab therapy (8a).

The predictability of different testing methods has been evaluated in various studies, including an analysis conducted by the FDA utilizing the data from the original and pivotal H0648 g trial, which evaluated chemotherapy versus chemotherapy and trastuzumab in patients with HER2-positive breast cancer (at that time defined as 2+ or 3+ via the clinical trial assay).

Sponsor analysis of the H0648 g trial in data presented to the FDA shows that IHC 3+ benefited irrespectively of FISH status (i.e., both FISH+ and FISH− derived benefit with trastuzumab). However, 2+ did not derive benefit, again irrespective of FISH status. Similarly, FISH+ patients (regardless of IHC scores) derived greater clinical benefit from the addition of trastuzumab to chemotherapy than did patients with FISH− tumors.

TRASTUZUMAB IN METASTATIC BREAST CANCER

Monotherapy

Single-agent trastuzumab was tested in phase I clinical trials since 1992. Subsequent phase II trials in patients pretreated with chemotherapy or without prior chemotherapy showed response rates of 12% to 26% and median time to progression from 3 to 5.1 months (9–12).

Trastuzumab is usually administered as a loading dose of 4 mg/kg intravenously (IV), followed by a 2 mg/kg maintenance dose at weekly intervals (9). However, the half-life of trastuzumab appears to be longer than previously thought, 25 versus five to six days. Early reports suggest that every three-week administration (loading dose of 8 mg/kg IV followed by 6 mg/kg every 21 days) is active, tolerable, and increases patient convenience. However, as expected, mean trough trastuzumab concentrations were lower and peak levels were higher with three-weekly trastuzumab compared with weekly treatments (12,13). As it may take several weeks to achieve steady state levels with the every week regimen, it is advisable to start with the weekly approach—especially in patients with symptomatic breast cancer. Regulatory approval of the every three weeks regimen has not been granted in the United States.

Combination with Cytotoxic Agents

Preclinical studies suggest additive or synergistic interactions between trastuzumab and multiple cytotoxic agents. These data provide the rationale for exploring combination therapy. Pegram et al. (14) found laboratory evidence of synergy for the combination of trastuzumab with carboplatin, cyclophosphamide, docetaxel, and vinorelbine and additive effect for trastuzumab with doxorubicin, epirubicin, and paclitaxel. Although preclinical data are interesting, it is most important to follow the data from clinical trials.

Two important phase III trials have evaluated the addition of trastuzumab to chemotherapy in women with HER2 overexpressing MBC.

In a pivotal clinical trial reported by Slamon et al., patients received chemotherapy with either doxorubicin and cyclophosphamide (AC) or single-agent paclitaxel with or without trastuzumab. The combination of chemotherapy and trastuzumab resulted in significantly higher overall response rates with a longer median time to disease progression and OS time than with chemotherapy alone (15). An improvement in median OS from 20.3 to 25.1 months ($P = 0.046$) was seen in the trastuzumab arm. About two-thirds of the patients in the chemotherapy-alone arm crossed over to receive trastuzumab at disease progression.

Another phase III trial evaluated single-agent docetaxel with or without trastuzumab, as first-line therapy for MBC also showed an improvement in median OS from 22.7 to 31.2 months ($P = 0.0325$) (16). Patients who went on to receive trastuzumab at progression had a worse survival, compared with those who received the combination initially.

A quality of life (QOL) study designed to compare the effects of chemotherapy with chemotherapy plus trastuzumab reported a significant improvement in fatigue and improved global QOL in patients treated with the combination (17).

An increasing number of phase II studies and a phase III study support incorporation of carboplatin as a standard agent in the management of patients eligible to receive first-line chemotherapy for MBC. The rationale for combining carboplatin with a taxane is based on their single-agent activities in MBC, their complementary mechanisms of action, and their activity in other malignancies. In addition to a possible synergistic interaction, in vitro data suggest that trastuzumab may also reverse primary platinum resistance by modulating HER2/neu activity (18). In addition, when used in combination, paclitaxel appears to have a platelet-sparing action that reduces the thrombocytopenia seen with carboplatin alone (19).

The NCCTG protocol 98-32-52 by Perez et al. (20) was a randomized phase II trial that tested carboplatin/docetaxel/trastuzumab as first-line chemotherapy in patients overexpressing HER2 with MBC. Patients received either every three-week therapy consisting of paclitaxel 200 mg/m^2, carboplatin AUC 6, and trastuzumab administered every 21 days for eight cycles, or weekly therapy consisting of paclitaxel 80 mg/m^2 and carboplatin AUC 2 for three of four weeks, with weekly trastuzumab administered every four weeks for six cycles. Trastuzumab was continued until disease progression or toxicity. The objective response rate (ORR) with the three-week therapy versus the weekly therapy was 65% (90% CI; 51–77%) and 81% (90% CI; 70–90%), with a median time to disease progression of 9.9 versus 13.8 months and median OS of 2.1 versus 3.2 years. Toxicities occurred significantly less frequently with weekly versus three-week therapy.

A phase III randomized trial tested the addition of carboplatin to paclitaxel and trastuzumab. The trial enrolled 188 patients and showed an improvement in response rate (RR) from 36% to 52% and time to tumor progression time to tumor progression (TTP) from 6.9 to 14.6 months with a trend in the OS in favor of the triplet of 42.1 versus 30.6 months ($P = 0.11$) (21). However, in the absence of a statistically significant survival benefit and without a comparison arm that automatically crossed over the nonplatinum group to platinum-containing therapy, it is difficult to assess the best combination.

TRASTUZUMAB BEYOND DISEASE PROGRESSION

Although treatment beyond progression represents a new paradigm in oncologic therapy, the novel and targeted action of trastuzumab and its synergy with a number of standard chemotherapy agents may support this approach. Only retrospective and uncontrolled data on RR and TTP are available for this strategy so far.

To obtain additional data on the safety of trastuzumab in combination with chemotherapy, patients in the pivotal H0648 g trial were given the opportunity to receive trastuzumab in a companion treatment-extension trial (H0659 g) at the time of disease progression. The patients originally assigned to chemotherapy alone crossed over to receive trastuzumab in the extension trial. A clinical benefit rate (complete response (CR) + partial response (PR) + stable disease) of 32% was seen in the arm that was trastuzumab naïve and a benefit of 22% was seen in the second arm, which consisted of patients who had been receiving trastuzumab in the initial trial. The median duration of treatment was 30 weeks (range 0–185 weeks) in the first group and 26 weeks (range 0–184 weeks) in the second group (22).

Additional ongoing trials that are comparing chemotherapy alone (vinorelbine in one study and capecitabine in another) or chemotherapy with trastuzumab in patients whose disease is progressing on taxane plus trastuzumab should give us more information about the independent contribution of trastuzumab.

Data with a novel anti HER2 agent, lapatinib, were reported in 2006. The data were based on a well conducted randomized phase III study comparing capecitabine alone vs. capecitabine in combination with lapatinib in more than 300 patients previously treated with anthracyclines, taxane, and trastuzumab. The reports demonstrated clinical and statistically significant improvements in response rate and progressive-free survival for patients receiving the lapatinib. Formal peer-reviewed publication of these data is forthcoming, but the results of the trial are expected to yield regulatory approval of lapatinib in the setting of disease progression to trastuzumab in the near future.

ADJUVANT TRASTUZUMAB

Recent clinical trials and consensus meetings have established that adjuvant therapy improves survival in women with invasive breast cancer. But there is not yet agreement on the optimal treatment for this patient population. Combination therapy with an anthracycline and cyclophosphamide (AC) is widely used. Taxanes can enhance the efficacy of AC. Clinical trials such as the BCIRG 001, CALGB 9344, PACS-01, National Surgical Adjuvant Breast and Bowel Project (NSABP) B-28, and others have demonstrated that the addition of docetaxel or paclitaxel to AC improves disease-free survival (DFS) in women with Stage II–III breast cancer.

Findings presented at ASCO 2005 indicated a clear, if not striking, benefit for trastuzumab in the adjuvant setting. The key trial findings presented were from a joint analysis of the (NSABP) B-31 trial with the NCCTG N9831 trial, additional data from NCCTG N9831, and the HERceptin Adjuvant (HERA) trial.

National Surgical Adjuvant Breast and Bowel Project B-31 and North Central Cancer Treatment Group N9831

The NSABP B-31 study randomized patients into two treatment groups (23). The chemotherapy group received four cycles of standard AC followed by four cycles of paclitaxel at 175 mg/m^2 q three weeks. The trastuzumab group received the same chemotherapy regimen, but also received weekly trastuzumab for 52 weeks, starting with the first paclitaxel dose. Trastuzumab was given at an initial loading dose of 4 mg/kg the first week and 2 mg/kg for the remaining 51 weeks. The protocol was later amended to allow the use of either weekly paclitaxel at 80 mg/m^2 for 12 doses or q three-week paclitaxel at 175 mg/m^2 as per the choice of the treating physician. Patients in the NCCTG N9831 trial received AC followed by weekly paclitaxel, but it also included a third group of patients who received trastuzumab after the completion of all chemotherapy, so the effects of giving trastuzumab sequentially versus concurrently could be assessed. However, outcome of this sequential group was not included in the joint interim analysis.

The combined interim analysis included 3351 patients: 1736 from NSABP B-31, who had been followed for a median of 2.4 years, and 1615 from N-9831, who had been followed up for a median of 1.5 years. Three-year DFS was 87% in the trastuzumab group versus 75% in the chemotherapy-alone group, for a hazard ratio (HR) of 0.48. There was also a significantly longer time to first distant recurrence among patients on trastuzumab versus those on chemotherapy alone. Three-year rate of distant recurrence was 90% versus 81%; HR, 0.47 (two-sided $P = 8 \times 10^{-10}$).

There was a clear trend towards improved DFS for patients receiving trastuzumab in concurrent instead of sequential fashion with chemotherapy in NCCTG N9831. The trial indicated a 36% decreased recurrence with concurrent versus sequential treatment ($P = 0.0114$). With regard to OS, the preliminary data indicate longer OS for patients receiving trastuzumab compared with patients receiving chemotherapy alone, with a four-year survival of 91% versus 87%, HR, 0.67, which is statistically significant ($P = 0.015$).

Herceptin Adjuvant Trial

Piccart-Gebhart et al. (24) presented data with a one-year median follow-up for the HERA trial, an international collaborative trial including 5090 HER2-positive patients. The HERA study compared one versus two years of adjuvant trastuzumab versus no trastuzumab. In contrast to the NSABP B-31 and NCCTG N9831 trials, patients in the HERA trial received adjuvant chemotherapy and radiation therapy prior to enrolling in the trial and receiving trastuzumab.

Median follow-up during presentation was one year; thus, no data from the two-year trastuzumab arm were available in 2006. DFS was significantly higher among patients following one year of trastuzumab versus the observation cohort. The estimated two-year DFS was 85.8% versus 77.4% (HR, 0.54; 95% CI, 0.43–0.67; $P < 0.0001$).

BCIRG 006

The BCIRG 006 trial compared a standard treatment arm of four cycles of AC followed by docetaxel for six cycles (AC-T) with two trastuzumab containing regimens after initial surgery. One arm included the above regimen with one year of trastuzumab (AC-TH) and the other was a nonanthracycline regimen of taxotere plus carboplatin plus one year of trastuzumab where trastuzumab was started concomitantly with chemotherapy (TCH). The trial randomized 3222 women, ~30% with node-negative disease. At 23 months of follow-up, there had been 322 events and 84 deaths. The data are not yet mature enough to assess OS. Results presented at the 2005 San Antonio Breast Cancer Symposium (SABCS) showed that the relative reduction in the risk of relapse was 51% (95% CI, 35–63%) and 39% (95% CI, 21–53%) for the AC-TH and TCH arms respectively, compared with the AC-T control arm. There was no statistically significant difference in DFS between AC-TH and TCH. This study is the first to evaluate trastuzumab in combination with a nonanthracycline-containing chemotherapy regimen in the adjuvant setting. The results also showed a 0.95% incidence of cardiotoxicity in the AC-T arm, compared with a 2.34% incidence in the AC-TH arm ($P = 0.016$ vs. AC-TH). In the TCH arm, the incidence of cardiotoxicity was 1.33% ($P = 0.1$ vs. AC-TH). The overall incidence of grade 3/4 hematological adverse events was similar among the three treatment arms, with more neutropenia and leukopenia in the anthracycline-containing arms and more anemia and thrombocytopenia in the TCH arm.

Additionally, results from mapping of HER2 in a subset of patients showed that coamplification of the topoisomerase II alpha gene occurred in ~35% of HER2-positive patients and may confer a therapeutic benefit with respect to anthracycline-based/trastuzumab combination regimens. Moreover, HER2-positive tumors that were not coamplified for topoisomerase II alpha, ~65%, did not appear to derive this same benefit, and further research is needed to determine whether they may be candidates for nonanthracycline-containing, trastuzumab-based adjuvant regimens (25). More data and follow-up are required to corroborate these findings.

FinHer Trial

The FinHer trial was published in 2006. This multicenter randomized trial investigated the safety and efficacy of trastuzumab given for only nine weeks concomitantly with chemotherapy in early breast cancer. A total of 1010 women from 17 centers with axillary node positive breast cancer or tumor more than 2.0 cm that was progesterone receptor negative were accrued for a median follow-up of 38 months. Women were randomly assigned to receive either 3 three-weekly cycles of docetaxel (100 mg/m^2) or eight-weekly cycles of vinorelbine (25 mg/m^2) as adjuvant therapy. Single-agent docetaxel/vinorelbine was followed in both arms by 3 three-weekly cycles of cyclophosphamide, epirubicin, and 5-fluorouracil (F_{600} E_{60} C_{600}). Patients whose tumor showed HER2 amplification by chromogen in situ hybridization had a second randomization to receive nine weekly cycles of trastuzumab (2 mg/kg after loading 4 mg/kg) concomitantly with either docetaxel or vinorelbine, or to no trastuzumab.

Distant and locoregional recurrence was less frequent among patients treated with docetaxel/cyclophosphamide; epirubicin; 5-fluorouracil (CEF) than among those treated with vinorelbine/FEC (39/502 vs. 68/507, HR 0.58). Adjuvant nine-week trastuzumab was effective in preventing breast cancer recurrence (11/115 vs. 26/116, HR 0.46). Three-year distant DFS was 93% for patients who had received trastuzumab when compared with 76% for those that did not ($P = 0.0078$, HR 0.43). Most importantly, trastuzumab was well tolerated and the left ventricular ejection fractions (LVEFs) were maintained during the three-year follow-up (26). Although the data appear very intriguing, further study is required.

Overall, these trials demonstrate that the use of trastuzumab can be extended to the management of patients with early breast cancer with a significant impact on progression-free and OS. The duration of time for which trastuzumab should be given is still unclear. Right now we know that one year of therapy is effective, but we do not know whether less than one year or more than two years will be more or less effective.

NEOADJUVANT TRASTUZUMAB

At present, neoadjuvant chemotherapy is a part of standard multimodality management of inflammatory and locally advanced breast cancer. It is also appropriate in patients with operable disease who desire tumor "down-staging" to facilitate breast conservation or a better cosmetic outcome. Neoadjuvant trastuzumab-containing regimens have shown encouraging activity in phase II trials in the treatment of HER2-positive early breast cancer with an acceptable safety profile and pathological CR rates ranging from 18% to 35% (27–32).

A small phase III trial conducted at MD Anderson Cancer Center provides preliminary evidence that the addition of trastuzumab to chemotherapy significantly increases treatment effectiveness over chemotherapy alone in patients with HER2-positive breast cancer (33). Forty-two patients were randomized to four cycles of paclitaxel followed by four cycles of FEC-75 with or without concomitant weekly trastuzumab (2 mg/kg) for 24 weeks. This was followed by definitive surgery. The pathological CR rates in the breast in the chemotherapy and the chemotherapy/trastuzumab arms were 26.3% and 65.2%. This high pathological CR may be explained by the duration of this study, six months versus around three months in most other studies.

CARDIAC DYSFUNCTION

An unexpected adverse event observed during the pivotal trials of trastuzumab was cardiac dysfunction. It was found that treatment with trastuzumab may result in the development of clinically manageable left ventricular systolic dysfunction and occasionally advanced congestive heart failure (CHF). The incidence and severity were greatest in patients receiving trastuzumab in combination with an anthracycline and cyclophosphamide (7). The monitoring of left ventricular function in all patients before and during trastuzumab treatment is now recommended.

Retrospective Analysis

Reports of trastuzumab-related cardiotoxicity during the pivotal clinical trials of this agent prompted a retrospective analysis of all data collected from seven phase II and III clinical trials for trastuzumab (34). The analysis was performed by an independent Cardiac Review and Evaluation Committee. The severity of these events was categorized using the New York Heart Association functional classification system. Patients treated with trastuzumab were found to be at an increased risk for cardiac dysfunction. The incidence was greatest in patients receiving concomitant trastuzumab and AC (27%). The risk was substantially lower in patients receiving paclitaxel and trastuzumab (13%) or trastuzumab alone (3–7%); however, most of these patients had received prior anthracycline therapy. Cardiac dysfunction was noted in 8% of patients receiving AC and 1% receiving paclitaxel alone. Most trastuzumab-treated patients developing cardiac dysfunction were symptomatic (75%) and most patients improved with standard treatment for CHF (79%). The use of anthracyclines after stopping therapy with trastuzumab may also carry a higher risk of cardiac toxicity. Pharmacokinetic data suggest that the half-life of trastuzumab is significantly longer than previously calculated (25 vs. 5–6 days) and that trastuzumab may persist in the circulation for up to 18 weeks after discontinuing treatment (35).

Discontinuation of trastuzumab is generally recommended when clinically significant CHF occurs. However, most patients who developed CHF during the pivotal trials responded to appropriate medical therapy, which often included discontinuation of trastuzumab. Tripathy et al. recently reported more detailed information regarding cardiac dysfunction from the pivotal trial of chemotherapy plus trastuzumab, including data on those patients who continued to receive trastuzumab after the development of CHF. CHF improved in 75% of the patients with treatment for a median of 25 weeks. Moreover, 33 patients continued to receive trastuzumab after the development of cardiac dysfunction, 21 (64%) of whom had no further decrease in cardiac function (36).

Recent Data

Updated results for trastuzumab in the adjuvant setting were presented at the 2005 SABCS and included data on 2999 of the enrolled 3505 patients in N9831. Adjuvant trastuzumab after anthracycline-based chemotherapy leads to an approximate three-year cumulative incidence rate of 2.5% to 3.5% significant clinical cardiac events. A higher proportion of patients experienced ≥15% decrease in the LVEF at any time point in the trastuzumab containing arms when compared with the nontrastuzumab containing arm (arm A: 6.7%, arm B: 14.2%, and arm C: 17.3%). There was a trend towards a higher cardiac toxicity with increasing age. A total of 77.8% of patients received more than nine months of trastuzumab and 72.7% completed trastuzumab therapy. Approximately 15% of patients randomized to concurrent trastuzumab and paclitaxel regimen (arm C), who had a satisfactory post-AC cardiac evaluation, had to discontinue trastuzumab due to symptomatic or asymptomatic cardiac adverse events. There appeared to be no correlation between radiation therapy and the risk of cardiac toxicity (37).

The decision to treat patients with trastuzumab involves an analysis of its potential risks and benefits.

HUMAN EPIDERMAL GROWTH FACTOR RECEPTOR 2 AND RESPONSE TO ENDOCRINE THERAPY

Preclinical studies suggest physiologic "cross-talk" between the HER2 and the ER signal transduction pathways. Some clinical trials have suggested relative resistance to adjuvant endocrine therapy but conflicting data have been reported (38–40).

Although the data are conflicting, the clinical evidence does not support the hypothesis that HER2/neu amplification and/or overexpression results in a hormone-independent phenotype in women with ER-positive breast cancer. An expert panel convened by the ASCO recommended that HER2 expression should not be used to make decisions regarding hormone therapy in either the adjuvant or the metastatic disease setting (41). At this time, the selection of endocrine therapy should be based upon established markers such as ER and PR. Larger, more definitive studies are underway to determine whether HER2 status should be used to select either selected estrogen receptor modulator (SERM) or aromatase inhibitor therapy.

The recent report by Kaufman et al.[a] in the fall of 2006 documented the low response rate of the aromatase inhibitor anastrozole (7%) or in combination with trastuzumab (21%) in patients with ER-positive and HER2-positive metastatic breast cancer. Further follow-up of this trial is indicated.

HUMAN EPIDERMAL GROWTH FACTOR RECEPTOR 2 AND RESPONSE TO CHEMOTHERAPY

Women whose tumors overexpress HER2 appear to be relatively resistant to alkylating agent-based adjuvant therapy and might derive greater benefit from anthracycline-based adjuvant therapy (42). Although the available data are far from conclusive, it is reasonable to assess HER2 status on all primary breast tumors at the time of diagnosis. Anthracycline-based therapy may be better in women with HER2-positive breast cancers in the adjuvant setting, unless such therapy is contraindicated, or in women who received prior anthracycline therapy for a previous breast cancer (43).

It has also been hypothesized that HER2 is to be viewed as a marker for the real anthracycline target, topoisomerase II α (TOP2A). The *TOP2A* gene is located next to the *HER2* gene on chromosome 17q12–q21. In vitro studies have shown that amplification of TOP2A leads to overexpression of the topoisomerase II α and increased sensitivity to anthracyclines (44). In a retrospective analysis of topoisomerase II α amplifications and deletions as a predictive marker for epirubicin sensitivity in the Danish Breast Cancer Group trial 89D, Knoop et al. (45) found TOP2A amplifications and possibly deletions to be a predictive marker for the effect of

---

[a]Kaufman B, et al. Trastuzumab plus anastrozole prolongs progression-free survival in post-menopausal women with HER2-positive, hormone-dependent metastatic breast cancer (MBC) presented at the 2006 Congress of the European Society for Medical Oncology October 2006.

adjuvant epirubicin containing therapy in primary breast cancer. However, these data need to be confirmed by a confirmative study or meta-analysis.

In women with metastatic disease, there is no conclusive evidence to suggest that women whose tumors overexpress HER2 are more likely to derive greater benefit from therapy with anthracycline-containing or taxane-containing regimens (46).

CONCLUSION

In MBC, the aims of treatment are symptom control and prolongation of survival. Although the debate concerning combination therapy versus sequential single agent continues, targeted biologics, such as trastuzumab, provide a compelling argument for the use of these agents in combination with traditional chemotherapeutics. Trastuzumab combined with chemotherapy offers the possibility of achieving these goals at the price of acceptable toxicity. Its targeted nature has relevant implications in the selection of patients to be treated with this agent.

Also, the integration of trastuzumab in the adjuvant setting has begun to show promise. Trastuzumab combined with chemotherapy results in increased disease-free survival and overall survival when compared with chemotherapy alone. Although methods to assess HER2 status may vary, the test in question must be validated by regular internal and external quality control. Much research needs to be done to determine the appropriate duration of administration to afford maximum benefit and to avoid unnecessary toxicity and expense. Cardiotoxicity mandates accurate evaluation of risk factors and measurement of cardiac function before and during treatment. Mechanisms of trastuzumab resistance, either primary or acquired during treatment, need to be determined in order to further exploit its efficacy with other forms of targeted therapy.

As we enter an era where HER2-positive breast cancer is treated as a distinct entity, the question quickly arises as to whether HER2-positive disease in the presence of trastuzumab behaves the same as HER2-negative disease in the absence of trastuzumab. To date, there are few data on this matter but emerging information suggests that trastuzumab (and potentially lapatinib) radically changes the natural history of HER2-positive MBC. Although women with HER2-positive tumors have historically been thought of as having worse prognosis, the advent of trastuzumab means that they appear to do better in response to chemotherapy than do patients with HER2-negative tumors, exhibiting higher rates of response and improved OS.

Anti-HER therapy has brought significant changes for the treatment of HER2-positive breast cancer patients. Investigating the mechanisms of response will help provide insight into cancer biology. Ongoing clinical trials and translational research are sure to provide illuminating information into further application of this exciting therapeutic approach.

REFERENCES

1. Slamon DJ, Clark GM, Wong SG, Levin WJ, Ullrich A, McGuire WL. Human breast cancer: correlation of relapse and survival with amplification of the HER-2/neu onco-gene. Science 1987; 235(4785):177–182.

2. Seidman AD, Fornier MN, Esteva FJ, et al. Weekly trastuzumab and paclitaxel therapy for metastatic breast cancer with analysis of efficacy by HER2 immunophenotype and gene amplification. J Clin Oncol 2001; 19(10):2587–2595.

3. Pegram M, Slamon D. Biological rationale for HER2/neu (c-erbB2) as a target for monoclonal antibody therapy. Semin Oncol 2000; 27(suppl 9):13–19.

4. Shepard HM, Lewis GD, Sarup JC, et al. Monoclonal antibody therapy of human cancer: taking the HER2 protooncogene to the clinic. J Clin Immunol 1991; 11(3):117–127.

5. Bast RC Jr, Ravdin P, Hayes DF, et al. 2000 update of recommendations for the use of tumor markers in breast and colorectal cancer: clinical practice guidelines of the American Society of Clinical Oncology. J Clin Oncol 2001; 19(6):1865–1878.

6. Jacobs TW, Gown AM, Yaziji H, Barnes MJ, Schnitt SJ. Comparison of fluorescence in situ hybridization and immunohistochemistry for the evaluation of HER-2/neu in breast cancer. J Clin Oncol 1999; 17(7):1974–1982.

7. Paik S, Bryant J, Tan-Chiu E, et al. Real-world performance of HER2 testing—National Surgical Adjuvant Breast and Bowel Project experience. J Natl Cancer Inst 2002; 94(11):852–854.

8. Baselga J, Tripathy D, Mendelsohn J, et al. Phase II study of weekly intravenous recombinant humanized anti-p185HER2 monoclonal antibody in patients with HER2/neu-overexpressing metastatic breast cancer. J Clin Oncol 1996; 14(3):737–744.

8a. Ingle JN, Suman VJ, Rowland KM, et al. Fulvestrant in women with advanced breast cancer and progression on prior aromatase inhibitor therapy: North Central Cancer Treatment Group trial N0032. J Clin Oncol 2006; 24(7):1052–1056.

9. Cobleigh MA, Vogel CL, Tripathy D, et al. Multinational study of the efficacy and safety of humanized anti-HER2 monoclonal antibody in women who have HER2-overexpressing metastatic breast cancer that has progressed after chemotherapy for metastatic disease. J Clin Oncol 1999; 17(9):2639–2648.

10. Vogel CL, Cobleigh MA, Tripathy D, et al. Efficacy and safety of trastuzumab as a single agent in first-line treatment of HER2-overexpressing metastatic breast cancer. J Clin Oncol 2002; 20(3):719–726.

11. Baselga J, Carbonell X, Castaneda-Soto NJ, et al. Phase II study of efficacy, safety, and pharmacokinetics of trastuzumab monotherapy administered on a 3-weekly schedule. J Clin Oncol 2005; 23(10):2162–2171.

12. Leyland-Jones B, Gelmon K, Ayoub JP, et al. Pharmacokinetics, safety, and efficacy of trastuzumab administered every three weeks in combination with paclitaxel. J Clin Oncol 2003; 21(21):3965–3971.

13. Pegram MD, Konecny GE, O'Callaghan C, et al. Rational combinations of trastuzumab with chemotherapeutic drugs used in the treatment of breast cancer. J Natl Cancer Inst 2004; 96(10):739–749.

14. Slamon DJ, Leyland-Jones B, Shak S, et al. Use of chemotherapy plus a monoclonal antibody against HER2 for metastatic breast cancer that overexpresses HER2. N Engl J Med 2001; 344(11):783–792.

15. Marty M, Cognetti F, Maraninchi D, et al. Randomized phase II trial of the efficacy and safety of trastuzumab combined with docetaxel in patients with human epidermal growth factor receptor 2-positive metastatic breast cancer administered as first-line treatment: the M77001 study group. J Clin Oncol 2005; 23(19):4265–4274.

16. Osoba D, Slamon DJ, Burchmore M, et al. Effects on quality of life of combined trastuzumab and chemotherapy in women with metastatic breast cancer. J Clin Oncol 2002; 20(14):3106–3113.

17. Perez EA, Hillman DW, Stella PJ, et al. A phase II study of paclitaxel plus carboplatin as first-line chemotherapy for women with metastatic breast carcinoma. Cancer 2000; 88(1):124–131.

18. Pertusini E, Ratajczak J, Majka M, et al. Investigating the platelet-sparing mechanism of paclitaxel/carboplatin combination chemotherapy. Blood 2001; 97(3):638–644.

19. Perez EA, Rowland KM, Suman VJ. N98-32-52: efficacy and tolerability of two schedules of paclitaxel, carboplatin and trastuzumab in women with HER2 positive metastatic breast cancer: an NCCTG randomized phase II trial [abstr 216]. Breast cancer Res Treat 2003; 82:S47.

20. Perez EA, Suman VJ, Rowland KM, et al. Two concurrent phase II trials of paclitaxel, carboplatin and trastuzumab (weekly or every 3 week schedule) as first line therapy in women with HER2 positive metastatic breast cancer: NCCTG study 98-32-52. Clin Breast Cancer 2005; 6(5):425–432.
21. Tripathy D, Slamon DJ, Cobleigh M, et al. Safety of treatment of metastatic breast cancer with trastuzumab beyond disease progression. J Clin Oncol 2004; 2(6): 1063–1070.
22. Romond EH, Perez EA, Bryant J, et al. Trastuzumab plus adjuvant chemotherapy for operable HER2-positive breast cancer. N Engl J Med 2005; 353(16):1673–1684.
23. Piccart-Gebhart MJ, Procter M, Leyland-Jones B, et al. Trastuzumab after adjuvant chemotherapy in HER2-positive breast cancer. N Engl J Med 2005; 353(16):1659–1672.
24. Smith I. Trastuzumab following adjuvant chemotherapy in HER2-positive early breast cancer (HERA Trial): disease-free and overall survival after 2 year median follow-up. Presented at: American Society of Clinical Oncology Annual Meeting Scientific Special Session; June 3, 2006; Atlanta, Georgia.
25. Slamon D, Eiermann W, Robert N, et al.; BCIRG 006 study. Program and abstracts of the 28th Annual San Antonio Breast Cancer Symposium, San Antonio, Texas, 2005 [abstr 1].
26. Joensuu H, Kellokumpu-Lehtinen P, Bono P, et al. Adjuvant docetaxel or vinorelbine with or without trastuzumab for breast cancer. N Engl J Med 2006; 354(8):809–820.
27. Burstein HJ, Harris LN, Gelman R, Lester SC. Preoperative therapy with trastuzumab and paclitaxel followed by sequential adjuvant doxorubicin/cyclophosphamide for HER2 overexpressing stage II or III breast cancer: a pilot study. J Clin Oncol 2003; 21(1):46–53.
28. Harris LN, Burstein HJ, Gelman R, et al. Preoperative trastuzumab and vinorelbine is highly active, well-tolerated regimen for HER2 3+/FISH+ stage II/III breast cancer [abstr 86]. Proc Am Soc Clin Oncol 2003; 22 (abstract no. 86).
29. Hurley J, Philomena D, Reis I, et al. Docetaxel, cisplatin, and trastuzumab as primary systemic therapy for human epidermal growth factor receptor 2-positive locally advanced breast cancer. J Clin Oncol 2006; 24(12):1831–1838.
30. Van Pelt AF, Mohsin S, Elledge RM, et al. Neoadjuvant trastuzumab and docetaxel in breast cancer: preliminary results. Clin Breast Cancer 2003; 4:348–353.
31. Limentani SA, Brufsky AM, Erban JK, et al. Dose-dense neoadjuvant treatment of women with breast cancer utilizing docetaxel, vinorelbine and trastuzumab with growth factor support. Breast Cancer Res Treat 2003; 82:S55.
32. Carey LA, Dees EC, Sawyer L, et al. Response to trastuzumab given with paclitaxel immediately following 4AC as initial therapy for primary breast cancer. Proceedings of the 24th San Antonio Breast Cancer Symposium, 2002.
33. Buzdar AU, Ibrahim NK, Francis D, et al. Significantly higher pathologic complete remission rate after neoadjuvant therapy with trastuzumab, paclitaxel, and epirubicin chemotherapy: results of a randomized trial in human epidermal growth factor receptor 2-positive operable breast cancer. J Clin Oncol 2005; 23(16):3676–3685.
34. Seidman A, Hudis C, Pierri MK, et al. Cardiac dysfunction in the trastuzumab clinical trials experience. J Clin Oncol 2002; 20(5):1215–1221.
35. Tripathy D, Seidman A, Keefe D, et al. Effect of cardiac dysfunction on treatment outcomes in women receiving trastuzumab for HER2-overexpressing metastatic breast cancer. Clin Breast Cancer 2004; 5(4):293–298.
36. Perez EA, Suman VJ, Davidson NE, et al. Exploratory analysis from NCCTG N9831: do clinical and laboratory characteristics predict cardiac toxicity of trastuzumab when administered as a component of adjuvant therapy? (Abstract # 2038) Breast Cancer Res Treat 2005; 94(suppl 1):S96.
37. Bianco AR, De Laurentiis M, Carlomagno C, et al. 20 years update of the Naples GUN Trial of adjuvant breast cancer therapy: evidence of interaction between c-erbB-2 expression and tamoxifen efficacy [abstr]. Proc Am Soc Clin Oncol 1998; 17:97a.
38. Ellis MJ, Coop A, Singh B, et al. Letrozole is more effective neoadjuvant endocrine therapy than tamoxifen for ErbB-1- and/or ErbB-2-positive, estrogen receptor-positive primary breast cancer: evidence from a phase III randomized trial. J Clin Oncol 2001; 19:3808.

39. Pritchard KI, Levine MN, Tu D. neu/erbB-2 overexpression and response to hormonal therapy in premenopausal women in the adjuvant breast cancer setting: will it play in Peoria? Part II. J Clin Oncol 2003; 21:399.
40. Bast RC Jr, Ravdin P, Hayes DF, et al. 2000 Update of recommendations for the use of tumor markers in breast and colorectal cancer: clinical practice guidelines of the American Society of Clinical Oncology. J Clin Oncol 2001; 19:1865.
41. Allred DC, Clark G, Tandon A, et al. HER-2/neu in node-negative breast cancer: prognostic significance of overexpression influenced by the presence of in situ carcinoma. J Clin Oncol 1992; 10:599.
42. Paik S, Bryant J, Park C, et al. erbB-2 and response to doxorubicin in patients with axillary lymph node-positive, hormone receptor-negative breast cancer. J Natl Cancer Inst 1998; 90:1361.
43. Jarvinen TA, Tanner M, Rantanen V, et al. Amplification and deletion of topoisomerase I alpha associate with ErbB-2 amplification and affect sensitivity to topoisomerase II inhibitor doxorubicin in breast cancer. Am J Pathol 2000; 156(3):839–847.
44. Knoop AS, Knudsen H, Balslev E, et al. Retrospective analysis of topoisomerase IIa amplifications and deletions as predictive markers in primary breast cancer patients randomly assigned to cyclophosphamide, methotrexate, and fluorouracil or cyclophosphamide, epirubicin, and fluorouracil: Danish Breast Cancer Cooperative Group. J Clin Oncol 2005; 23(30):7483–7490.
45. Sjostrom J, Collan J, von Boguslawski K, et al. C-erbB-2 expression does not predict response to docetaxel or sequential methotrexate and 5-fluorouracil in advanced breast cancer. Eur J Cancer 2002; 38:535.

Is There a Role for ErbB Dual Kinase Inhibition?

Carmel S. Verrier and Kimberly Blackwell

Departments of Medicine and Radiation Oncology, Duke University Medical Center, Durham, North Carolina, U.S.A.

BIOLOGY OF ErbB RECEPTORS

The ErbB family of receptors belong to the type I superfamily of receptor tyrosine kinases. To date, four members of this family have been identified: epidermal growth factor receptor (EGFR) or ErbB1/HER1, ErbB2/Neu/HER2, ErbB3/HER3, and ErbB4/HER4. They are expressed in a variety of tissues including epithelial, mesenchymal, and neural origin, where they exert effects on development, cellular proliferation, and differentiation (1). Structurally, all ErbB receptors share in common an extracellular domain, a membrane-spanning domain, and an intracellular domain that encompasses the tyrosine kinase activity. Through a complex network of downstream cascades, their dysregulation confers poorer prognosis in breast and other solid tumors that overexpress them (2–6).

Activation of ErbB receptors occurs via specific ligand binding. An extended family of ligands that include epidermal growth factor (EGF), TGF-alpha, amphiregulin, betacellulin, epiregulin, epigen, heparin-binding EGF, and the neuregulins selectively bind to EGFR, ErbB3, and ErbB4 (Table 1). Thus far, no ligand has been identified for ErbB2. Its dimerization domain is constitutively exposed making it a preferred heterodimerization partner with the other ErbB receptors (7). With ligand binding, ErbB receptors form either homo- or heterodimers resulting in autophosphorylation of specific tyrosine residues within the conserved catalytic kinase domains of ErbB receptors. These phosphorylated tyrosine residues serve as docking sites for Src-homology 2 and phosphotyrosine binding-domain containing proteins that link activated ErbB receptors to downstream cell proliferation via mitogen-activated protein kinase (MAPK) and survival via phosphatidyl-inositol-3-phosphate (PI3K/Akt) pathways (8). Activation of the latter can then modulate cell growth and survival by affecting apoptosis, migration, growth, adhesion, differentiation, and angiogenesis (Fig. 1).

Through analysis of genetically modified mice, the ErbB receptors have also been shown to play a crucial role in development. Loss of ErbB1 leads to embryonic or perinatal lethality in mice with abnormalities apparent in multiple organs including brain, skin, lung, and gastrointestinal tract (9–11). ErbB2 null mice, on the other hand, die at midgestation due to heart malformation (12), a feature that is also displayed by ErbB4 knockout mice (13). In the case of ErbB3, the null mice have defective heart valves and lack Schwann cells (14,15). In the adult organism, studies elucidating the roles of these receptors are limited given the lethality associated with their deletions. In the mammary gland, at least, given the specific patterns of expression of all four ErbB receptors in that tissue (16,17), it is inferred that their function is vital to the normal development of that organ. Indeed, mutations in the ErbB1 kinase

TABLE 1   ErbB Family and Their Small Molecule Inhibitors

Target receptor	Ligand(s)	Inhibitor	Phase of clinical development in breast cancer
ErbB1	EGFR	AG1478/PD158780/EKB569	I
	TGF-alpha	Gefitinib/Erlotinib	II
	Amphiregulin	CI1033(Canertinib)	II
	Epiregulin	Lapatinib(GW572016)	III
	Betacellulin		
	HB-EGF		
ErbB2	–	AG1478/PD158780/EKB569	I
		Lapatinib(GW572016)	III
ErbB3	Epiregulin		
	Neuregulin1/2		
ErbB4	Neuregulin 1/2		II
	CI1033(Canertinib)		
	Neuregulin 3/4		I
	PD158780		
	Epiregulin		
	Betacellulin		
	HB-EGF		

Abbreviations: EGFR, epidermal growth factor receptor; HB-EGF, heparin-binding EGF; TGF, transforming growth factor.

domain or dominant-negative ErbB1 in the mammary gland show defective ductal formation (18–20). For ErbB2 and ErbB4, data accumulated thus far seem to support a role for them in lobuloalveolar differentiation and lactation (21,22).

The notion of ErbB receptors serving as target for anti-cancer therapy is one that is over 20-years-old (23). The reason for such proposal is supported by

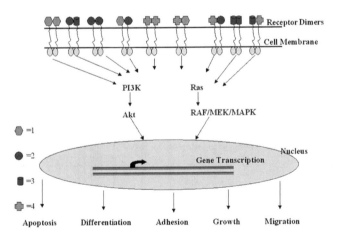

FIGURE 1   Ligand binding to ErbB family receptors induce the formation of either homo- or heterodimers resulting in autophosphorylation of specific tyrosine residues within the conserved catalytic kinase domains of ErbB receptors. Multiple cytoplasmic signaling pathways, including the Ras/Raf mitogen-activated protein kinase pathway and the phosphoinositol 3′-kinase/AKT pathway, transduce signals into the nucleus leading to various biological effects. *Abbreviations*: MAPK, mitogen-activated protein kinase; MEK, map-erk kinase.

(*i*) the finding of EGFR overexpression in many human tumors; (*ii*) poor outcome in some malignancies when EGFR displays increased expression; (*iii*) increased receptor content associated with increased ligand production by the tumor cells (24–26). An extensive body of literature links ErbB2 as a key mediator of tumor cell growth and survival predicting a poor clinical outcome in 25% to 30% of patients that either overexpress it or display gene amplification (5). Recent data also suggest that ErbB1 expression is linked to activation of ErbB2 in human breast cancers (27). Consequently, treatment strategies to inhibit ErbB receptors have focused on developing monoclonal antibodies that interfere with signaling or serve as carriers of prodrugs or toxins, tyrosine kinase inhibitors (TKIs) that abrogate downstream signaling effects, competitive receptor antagonists, antisense oligonucleotides, and vaccines. Of these approaches, monoclonal antibodies and TKIs are in the most advanced stage of clinical development.

PRECLINICAL AND CLINICAL STUDIES LEADING TO DUAL ErbB RECEPTOR BLOCKADE

The anti-tumor activity of monoclonal antibodies (MoAbs) is probably multifactorial in nature. MoAbs in part exert their effects on ErbB receptors by binding to the extracellular domain preventing its proteolytic cleavage and thereby promoting down-modulation of the receptors (28). In addition, MoAbs are able to inhibit angiogenesis through downregulation of vascular endothelial growth factor (VEGF) and cause an immune-mediated cell cytotoxicity via Fc receptors on tumor cells (28). Unfortunately, resistance to the only currently approved ErbB2-targeted MoAb, trastuzumab, has been well demonstrated prompting a greater need to evaluate other targets for treatment, including small molecule TKIs.

No specific ErbB1 TKIs are approved to date in the treatment of breast cancer though significant activity in various cancer cell lines has been demonstrated (1). In a number of breast cancer cell lines, gefitinib has shown inhibitory effect that is additive when combined with taxanes and anthracyclines (29,30). Moreover, gefitinib appears to have synergy when combined with trastuzumab (31), and reverses hormone therapy resistance (32) in animal models of established breast cancer. In a phase II trial of gefitinib in heavily pretreated patients with metastatic breast cancer (MBC), minimal clinical activity was seen (33). Other phase II trials of gefitinib in ductal carcinoma in situ (DCIS), advanced and tamoxifen-resistant breast cancer (34,35), as well as erlotinib in locally advanced or MBC (36) have also been done, but to date, none has shown substantial single agent activity in the studied cohorts. This suggests that targeting of a single ErbB receptor in the absence of other anti-cancer or targeted therapy might not be sufficient to hamper ErbB-receptor mediated cell growth/survival. In addition, single pathway blockade might lead to accelerated resistance as compared to when ErbB blockade is combined with either traditional chemotherapy or other targeted agents. By widening the number of ErbB receptor inhibition, more dimer types can be prevented from activating downstream signaling pathways for an overall result of more effective anti-tumor activity (1).

AGENTS TARGETING MULTIPLE ErbB RECEPTORS

In various tumor cell lines, including breast cancer lines, that express either ErbB1 or ErbB2, dual ErbB1/ErbB2 inhibitors have demonstrated anti-tumor activity and are shown to induce apoptosis in the tumor cells (37,38). To date, in breast cancer, several agents that target multiple members of the ErbB family are being studied. These combined agents include dual inhibitors of both ErbB1 and ErbB2, such as AG1478 and EKB569 (both in phase I trials). Multiple receptor inhibitors are also being studied and include PD158780, an inhibitor of ErbB1, ErbB2, and ErbB4. CI-1033 (canertinib) is an irreversible nonselective EGFR inhibitor and produces rapid inhibition of all members of the EGFR family (39). At low nanomolar range, canertinib inhibits EGFR kinase activity and displays anti-tumor activity in ErbB1- and ErbB2-dependent preclinical models (40). Though canertinib is nonselective against ErbB receptors and also has activity against ErbB3 and ErbB4, these effects on the ErbB receptor TKIs appear highly specific against ErbB family members as no effect is seen with this drug on other tyrosine kinases (41). When tested against a variety of breast carcinomas in vitro and in vivo tumor xenograft models, canertinib has anti-tumor activity (42). Currently, phase II trials with canertinib in MBC are still ongoing.

LAPATINIB IN PRECLINICAL STUDIES

The dual small molecule TKI in the most advanced phase of development is the orally available agent, lapatinib (GW572016). It is a reversible potent inhibitor of ErbB1 and ErbB2 receptor tyrosine kinase phosphorylation in intact cells and ErbB-driven tumor growth in tissue culture and animal models (37,43). In preclinical models, lapatinib's possible efficacy against cancer cells was encouraged by the findings of synergistic cell growth inhibition when both ErbB1 and ErbB2 receptor TKIs were targeted. Specifically, treatment of the ErbB2 overexpressed, EGFR-coexpressing breast cancer cell lines SKBR-3 and BT-474 with gefitinib and the ErbB2 MoAb, trastuzumab, resulted in synergistic cell growth inhibition (30). This fueled further testing of lapatinib efficacy against breast cancer cell lines whose ErbB1/2 status are well characterized. Indeed, cells with the highest ErbB1/2 activation are most sensitive to lapatinib and apoptosis is triggered in ErbB2-overexpressing breast cancer cell lines like BT-474 (37,43). Interestingly, when lapatinib is combined with anti-ErbB2 antibodies, an enhanced apoptotic effect is seen in response to the combination of drugs (44). This effect appears to be mediated via inhibition of survivin, a protein that appears to protect tumors from programmed cell death following activation of apoptotic pathways (45,46).

An increasing body of literature indicate that both ErbB1 and ErbB2 are involved in cellular and tissue responses to radiation and that overexpression/dysregulation of either one of these receptors is linked to developing radio resistance (47). Growth alteration as well as increased radiosensitization of the cells were therefore tested in the presence of lapatinib (43,48). Potent inhibition of growth was seen in either ErbB1 or ErbB2 expressing cell lines. Radiosensitizing effects were most prominent for ErbB1-expressing cell lines as ErbB2-expressing lines were extremely sensitive to lapatinib even without radiation therapy (48). Interestingly, these effects appear to be modulated by inhibition of the Ras-MAPK and the PI3K-Akt pathways as one cell line resistant to lapatinib failed to demonstrate inhibition of these two downstream pathways (48).

LAPATINIB IN CLINICAL STUDIES

In phase I dose escalation studies, lapatinib administered up to 1800 mg/day on a once-daily schedule was well tolerated and the most frequent side effects included rash, nausea, diarrhea, fatigue, and anorexia. In a randomized, multicenter, phase IB study of lapatinib in patients with EGFR- and/or HER2-overexpressing advanced solid tumors, four patients achieved a partial response from the 30 patients with pretreated MBC (49). Biological response assessment in those that achieved a PR showed significant decline in phosphorylated EGFR and HER2 as well as in phosphorylated downstream signal transducers, namely Akt and Erk. These changes correlated with increased tumor cell apoptosis as assessed by TUNEL analysis.

Two open-labeled phase II studies in heavily pretreated patients with ErbB2-expressing previously treated MBC (EGF20002, EGF20008), demonstrated single agent activity with lapatinib. In EGF20002, patients had to have progressed on a trastuzumab-containing regimen in the first- or second-line setting. At the time of a planned interim analysis of EGF20002, a clinical benefit rate was demonstrated in 17 of 78 patients (22%) in the studied cohort. Using a classification tree for exploratory analysis of predictive markers to response to lapatinib in EGF20002, the presence of the extracellular domain of ErbB2, shorter duration of prior trastuzumab therapy (less than six months), and the absence of estrogen receptor and/or progesterone receptor all accounted for a higher response to therapy. Interestingly, a decrease in the serum level of shed ErbB2 extracellular domain also predicted response to therapy (50). EGF20008, led by Dr. Burstein and colleagues, examined the activity of lapatinib in both ErbB2-overexpressing and nonoverexpressing ErbB2 MBC patients that had progressed on therapies containing anthracyclines, taxanes, and capecitabine. An interim analysis of that trial demonstrated a response or stable disease at 16 weeks in 18/140 (13%) ErbB2-positive patients who had received anthracycline, taxanes, and capecitabine (50). Interestingly, no objective responses have been observed in 89 patients with normal ErbB2 status.

ONGOING STUDIES WITH LAPATINIB
First Line and Refractory Metastatic Breast Cancer

Combination chemotherapy with trastuzumab is now standard of care for first line treatment of women with ErbB2-overexpressing breast cancer (51). With the potential benefits of small molecules being examined, there are a number of ongoing trials that will evaluate for potential increased efficacy, response to treatment when lapatinib is used alone, added to chemotherapy or hormonal therapy. As first line, EGF20009 is comparing two schedules of lapatinib alone in patients that have not had any prior therapy for their MBC and whose tumors were all ErbB2 FISH amplified. In that trial, lapatinib as a single agent demonstrated confirmed PRs in 5 of 13 patients (38%), and stable disease greater than eight weeks in six of 13 patients (46%) (52). This trial was recently updated by George Sledge at the San Antonio Breast Cancer Symposium (SABCS) in December of 2005. An interim analysis of the first 40 patients randomized to either 500 mg twice daily versus 1500 mg daily of lapatinib was conducted. No unexpected toxicity was seen. Confirmed PRs was apparent in 12 patients (30%) by investigator review and 14 patients (35%) by independent review. Stable disease lasting at least eight weeks was seen in 13 patients (32.5%) by investigator review and 14 patients (35%) by independent review (SABCS, Abstract 1071). This activity level is still encouraging and represents similar activity to the original single agent trastuzumab studies reported in previously untreated ErbB2-overexpressing MBC (53).

As first-line therapy for MBC, combining lapatinib with hormonal therapy is being evaluated as well. The estrogen receptor (ER) signals not only through genomic pathways that involve ER binding to specific estrogen response elements, it can also act via nongenomic mechanisms. This nongenomic ER action occurs when membrane-associated receptor activates downstream signaling cascades that are in common with ErbB signaling. This interplay between these two receptor systems is also supported by the finding of an inverse relationship between ER expression and expression of ErbB1, ErbB2, and/or ErbB3 as assessed by immunohistochemistry (54). Indeed, overexpression of ErbB2 has been found to decrease responsiveness to hormonal therapy in patients with breast cancer (55) and estrogen depletion can increase the expression of ErbB1 in breast cancer cell lines (56). Given these observations, when tested in preclinical models, lapatinib restored the sensitivity of breast cancer cells to tamoxifen, and inhibited the growth of tamoxifen-resistant, ErbB2-overexpressing MCF-7 xenografts (57). In another study, treatment of MCF-7/ErbB2 xenografts with single agent gefitinib, trastuzumab, or pertuzumab significantly impaired tamoxifen-stimulated tumor growth (58). These findings support a beneficial role in combining lapatinib with hormonal treatment in breast cancer. Ongoing studies utilizing this approach include EGF30008 and CALGB40302. EGF30008 is a phase III trial that will compare letrozole/lapatinib to letrozole alone in patients with hormone receptor-positive MBC. Of note, this trial does not require ErbB2 overexpression. CALGB40302 will examine fulvestrant/lapatinib versus fulvestrant alone in MBC that has progressed through therapy with an aromatase inhibitor. This trial does require that the patient's tumor have some level of ErbB1 or ErbB2 overexpression.

Additional first line treatment trials include the phase III trial EGF104383, in which paclitaxel/trastuzumab/lapatinib will be compared to paclitaxel/trastuzumab in patients with ErbB2-overexpressing tumors. Finally, as first line therapy, a large, international phase III trial (EGF104535) is assessing lapatinib/paclitaxel with paclitaxel alone in previously untreated advanced or MBC with ErbB2-overexpressing tumors. This last study will offer valuable information about the activity of small molecule inhibitors in combination with chemotherapy and will offer a standard upon which to compare the older studies involving trastuzumab and paclitaxel.

In refractory disease, a phase II trial, EGF10161 is comparing lapatinib/docetaxel/trastuzumab with docetaxel/trastuzumab in ErbB2-amplified MBC. A large phase III trial, EGF100151, is looking at lapatinib/capecitabine with capecitabine alone in patients with previously treated MBC.

Early Stage Breast Cancer

Given the high amounts of activity seen with lapatinib, the next step will be to incorporate its use in the treatment of early-stage breast cancer (ESBC). Although little data is available with regards to its long-term use, minimal to no cardiac and other toxicities have been seen with its use in MBC. Two large studies are being planned in the adjuvant therapy setting of ErbB2 overexpressing breast cancer. Both studies will incorporate standard anthracycline-taxane based chemotherapy in combination with either trastuzumab alone, lapatinib alone, or the combination of trastuzumab and lapatinib. Enrollment to both studies is scheduled to begin sometime in late 2006.

CONCLUSIONS

The ErbB family of receptor tyrosine kinases has quickly become one of the most important signaling pathways found in human breast cancer. Its dysregulation leads to a more aggressive cancer phenotype and its inhibition can act as a highly effective therapeutic strategy. Trastuzumab has set the standard by which new approaches to inhibiting this pathway will be compared. To date, there are a number of small molecule tyrosine kinase inhibitors with documented activity in ErbB2-overexpressing breast cancer that are being tested for improved efficacy in the treatment of breast cancer. The small molecule inhibitor with the most clinical data is a dual ErbB1/2 inhibitor, lapatinib with which multiple clinical trials are still ongoing. As more knowledge is gained regarding the anti-cancer activity and safety of multiple ErbB family member inhibitors, these drugs will be incorporated into therapies for both ESBC and MBC. Hopefully, these multiple targeted pathway approaches will result in more effective, convenient, and safe treatment for breast cancer patients worldwide.

REFERENCES

1. Hynes NE, Lane HA. ERBB receptors and cancer: the complexity of targeted inhibitors. Nat Rev Cancer 2005; 5:341–354.
2. Klijn JG, Berns PM, Schmitz PI, Foekens JA. The clinical significance of epidermal growth factor receptor (EGF-R) in human breast cancer: a review on 5232 patients. Endocr Rev 1992; 13:3–17.
3. Klijn JG, Look MP, Portengen H, Alexieva-Figusch J, van Putten WL, Foekens JA. The prognostic value of epidermal growth factor receptor (EGF-R) in primary breast cancer: results of a 10 year follow-up study. Breast Cancer Res Treat 1994; 29:73–83.
4. Paik S, Hazan R, Fisher ER, et al. Pathologic findings from the National Surgical Adjuvant Breast and Bowel Project: prognostic significance of erbB-2 protein overexpression in primary breast cancer. J Clin Oncol 1990; 8:103–112.
5. Slamon DJ, Clark GM, Wong SG, Levin WJ, Ullrich A, McGuire WL. Human breast cancer: correlation of relapse and survival with amplification of the HER-2/neu oncogene. Science 1987; 235:177–182.
6. Holbro T, Civenni G, Hynes NE. The ErbB receptors and their role in cancer progression. Exp Cell Res 2003; 284:99–110.
7. Garrett TP, McKern NM, Lou M, et al. The crystal structure of a truncated ErbB2 ectodomain reveals an active conformation, poised to interact with other ErBB receptors. Mol Cell 2003; 11:495–505.
8. Yarden YS, Sliwkowski MX. Untangling the ErbB signaling network. Nat Rev Mol Cell Biol 2001; 2:127–137.
9. Miettinen PJ, Berger JE, Meneses J, et al. Epithelial immaturity and multiorgan failure in mice lacking epidermal growth factor receptor. Nature 1995; 376:337–341.
10. Sibilia M, Steinbach JP, Stingl L, Aguzzi A, Wagner EF. A strain-independent postnatal neurodegeneration in mice lacking the EGF receptor. EMBO J 1998; 17:719–731.
11. Sibilia M, Wagner EF. Strain-dependent epithelial defects in mice lacking the EGF receptor. Science 1995; 269:234–238.
12. Lee KF, Simon H, Chen H, Bates B, Hung MC, Hauser C. Requirement for neuregulin receptor erbB2 in neural and cardiac development. Nature 1995; 378:394–398.
13. Gassmann M, Casagranda F, Orioli D, et al. Aberrant neural and cardiac development in mice lacking the ErbB4 neuregulin receptor. Nature 1995; 378:390–394.
14. Erickson SL, O'Shea KS, Ghaboosi N, et al. ErbB3 is required for normal cerebellar and cardiac development: a comparison with ErbB2-and heregulin-deficient mice. Development 1997; 124:4999–5011.
15. Riethmacher D, Sonnenberg-Riethmacher E, Brinkmann V, Yamaai T, Lewin GR, Birchmeier C. Severe neuropathies in mice with targeted mutations in the ErbB3 receptor. Nature 1997; 389:725–730.

16. Darcy KM, Zangani D, Wohlhueter AL, et al. Changes in ErbB2 (her-2/neu), ErbB3, and ErbB4 during growth, differentiation, and apoptosis of normal rat mammary epithelial cells. J Histochem Cytochem 2000; 48:63–80.
17. Schroeder JA, Lee DC. Dynamic expression and activation of ERBB receptors in the developing mouse mammary gland. Cell Growth Differ 1998; 9:451–464.
18. Fowler KJ, Walker F, Alexander W, et al. A mutation in the epidermal growth factor receptor in waved-2 mice has a profound effect on receptor biochemistry that results in impaired lactation. Proc Natl Acad Sci USA 1995; 92:1465–1469.
19. Wiesen JF, Young P, Werb Z, Cunha GR. Signaling through the stromal epidermal growth factor receptor is necessary for mammary ductal development. Development 1999; 126:335–344.
20. Xie W, Paterson AJ, Chin E, Nabell LM, Kudlow JE. Targeted expression of a dominant negative epidermal growth factor receptor in the mammary gland of trans-genic mice inhibits pubertal mammary duct development. Mol Endocrinol 1997; 11:1766–1781.
21. Jones FE, Stern DF. Expression of dominant-negative ErbB2 in the mammary gland of transgenic mice reveals a role in lobuloalveolar development and lactation. Oncogene 1999; 18:3481–3490.
22. Jones FE, Welte T, Fu XY, Stern DF. ErbB4 signaling in the mammary gland is required for lobuloalveolar development and Stat5 activation during lactation. J Cell Biol 1999; 147:77–88.
23. Kawamoto T, Sato JD, Le A, Polikoff J, Sato GH, Mendelsohn J. Growth stimulation of A431 cells by epidermal growth factor: identification of high-affinity receptors for epidermal growth factor by an anti-receptor monoclonal antibody. Proc Natl Acad Sci USA 1983; 80:1337–1341.
24. Mendelsohn J. Targeting the epidermal growth factor receptor for cancer therapy. J Clin Oncol 2002; 20:1S–13S.
25. Moscatello DK, Holgado-Madruga M, Godwin AK, et al. Frequent expression of a mutant epidermal growth factor receptor in multiple human tumors. Cancer Res 1995; 55:5536–5539.
26. Salomon DS, Brandt R, Ciardiello F, Normanno N. Epidermal growth factor-related peptides and their receptors in human malignancies. Crit Rev Oncol-Hematol 1995; 19:183–232.
27. DiGiovanna MS, Stern DF, Edgerton, SM, Whalen SG, Moore D, Thor AD. Relationship of epidermal growth factor receptor expression to ErbB-2 signaling activity and prognosis in breast cancer patients. J Clin Oncol 2005; 23:1152–1160.
28. Rabindran SK. Antitumor activity of HER-2 inhibitors. Cancer Lett 2005; 227:9–23.
29. Ciardiello F, Caputo R, Borriello, G. ZD1839 (Iressa), an EGFR-selective tyrosine kinase inhibitor, enhances taxane activity in bcl-2 overexpressing, multidrug-resistant MCF-7 ADR human breast cancer cells. Int J Cancer 2002; 98:463–369.
30. Moulder SY, Yakes FM, Muthuswamy, SK. Epidermal growth factor receptor (HER1) tyrosine kinase inhibitor ZD1839 (Iressa) inhibits HER2/neu-overexpressing breast cancer cells in vitro and in vivo. Cancer Res 2001; 61:8887–8895.
31. Normanno N, Campiglio M, DeLuca, A. Cooperative inhibitory effect of ZD1839 (Iressa) in combination with trastuzumab (Herceptin) on human breast cancer cell growth. Ann Oncol 2002; 13:65–72.
32. McClelland RA, Barrow D, Madden TA. Enhanced epidermal growth factor receptor signaling in MCF7 breast cancer cells after long-term culture in the presence of the pure antiestrogen ICI 182,780 (Faslodex). Endocrinology 2001; 142:2776–2788.
33. Albain K, Elledge R, Gradishar, WJ, et al. Open-label, phase II, multicenter trial of ZD1839 (Iressa) in patients with advanced breast cancer. Breast Cancer Res Treat 2002; 76:S33 (abstract 20).
34. Baselga J, Albanell J, Ruiz, A. Phase II and tumor pharmacodynamic study of gefitinib (ZD1839) in patients with advanced breast cancer [abstract 24]. Proc Am Soc Clin Oncol 2003; 22:7.
35. Robertson JF, Gutteridge E, Cheung KL. Gefitinib (ZD1839) is active in acquired tamoxifen-resistant oestrogen receptor positive and ER-negative breast cancer: results from a phase II study [abstract 23]. Proc Am Soc Clin Oncol 2003; 22:7.

36. Winer EC, Dickler M. Phase II multicenter study to evaluate the efficacy and safety of Tarceva (erlotinib) in women with previously treated locally advanced or metastatic breast cancer [abstract 445]. Breast Cancer Res Treat 2002; 76(suppl 1):S115.
37. Rusnak DW, Lackey K, Affleck K, et al. The effects of the novel, reversible epidermal growth factor receptor/ErbB-2 tyrosine kinase inhibitor, GW2016, on the growth of human normal and tumor-derived cell lines in vitro and in vivo. Mol Cancer Ther 2001; 1:85–94.
38. Traxler P, Allegrini PR, Brandt R, et al. AEE788: a dual family epidermal growth factor receptor/ErbB2 and vascular endothelial growth factor receptor tyrosine kinase inhibitor with antitumor and antiangiogenic activity. Cancer Res 2004; 64: 4931–4941.
39. Ranson M. Epidermal growth factor receptor tyrosine kinase inhibitors. Br J Cancer 2004; 90:2250–2255.
40. Slichenmyer WJ, Elliott WL, Fry DW. CI-1033, a pan-erbB tyrosine kinase inhibitor. Semin Oncol 2001; 28:80–85.
41. Thomas SM, Grandis JR. Pharmacokinetic and pharmacodynamic properties of EGFR inhibitors under clinical investigation. Cancer Treat Rev 2004; 30:255–268.
42. Allen LF, Lenehan PF, Eiseman IA, Elliott WL, Fry DW. Potential benefits of the irreversible pan-erbB inhibitor, CI-1033, in the treatment of breast cancer. Semin Oncol 2002; 29:11–21.
43. Xia W, Mullin RJ, Keith BR, et al. Anti-tumor activity of GW572016: a dual tyrosine kinase inhibitor blocks EGF activation of EGFR/erbB2 and downstream Erk1/2 and AKT pathways. Oncogene 2002; 21:6255–6263.
44. Xia W, Gerard CM, Liu L, Baudson NM, Ory TL, Spector NL. Combining lapatinib (GW572016), a small molecule inhibitor of ErbB1 and ErbB2 tyrosine kinases, with therapeutic anti-ErbB2 antibodies enhances apoptosis of ErbB2-overexpressing breast cancer cells. Oncogene 2005; 24:6213–6221.
45. Li F, Ackermann EJ, Bennett CF, et al. Pleiotropic cell-division defects and apoptosis induced by interference with survivin function. Nat Cell Biol 1999; 1:461–466.
46. Tamm I, Wang Y, Sausville E, et al. IAP-family protein survivin inhibits caspase activity and apoptosis induced by Fas (CD95), Bax, caspases, and anticancer drugs. Cancer Res 1998; 58:5315–5320.
47. Ethier SP, Lawrence TS. Epidermal growth factor receptor signaling and response of cancer cells to ionizing radiation. J Natl Cancer Inst 2001; 93:890–891.
48. Zhou H, Kim YS, Peletier A, McCall W, Earp HS, Sartor CI. Effects of the EGFR/HER2 kinase inhibitor GW572016 on EGFR- and HER2-overexpressing breast cancer cell line proliferation, radiosensitization, and resistance. Int J Radiat Oncol, Biol, Phys 2004; 58:344–352.
49. Burris H III, Hurwitz H, Dees EC, et al. Phase I safety, pharmacokinetics, and clinical activity study of lapatinib (GW572016), a reversible inhibitor of epidermal growth factor receptor tyrosine kinases in heavily pretreated patients with metastatic carcinomas. J Clin Oncol 2005; 23:2502–2512.
50. Blackwell KL, Burstein M, Pegram M, et al. Determining relevant biomarkers from tissue and serum that may predict response to single agent lapatinib in trastuzumab refractory metastatic breast cancer [abstract 3006]. Proc Am Soc Clin Oncol 2005; 23(suppl):203s.
51. Slamon DJ, Leyland-Jones B, Shak S, et al. Use of chemotherapy plus a monoclonal antibody against HER2 for metastatic breast cancer that overexpresses HER2. N Engl J Med 2001; 344:783–792.
52. Gomez H, Chavez M, Doval D. A phase II randomized trial using the small molecule tyrosine kinase inhibitor lapatinib as a first-line treatment in patients with FISH positive advanced or metastatic breast cancer [abstract 3046]. J Clin Oncol 2005; 23(suppl):203s.
53. Vogel C, Cobleigh M, Tripathy D. Efficacy and safety of trastuzumab as a single agent in first-line treatment of HER2-overexpressing metastatic breast cancer. J Clin Oncol 2002; 20:719–726.
54. Witton CJ, Reeves JR, Going JJ, Cooke TG, Bartlett JM. Expression of the HER1-4 family of receptor tyrosine kinases in breast cancer. J Pathol 2003; 200:290–297.

55. De Placido S, De Laurentiis M, Carlomagno C, et al. Twenty-year results of the Naples GUN randomized trial: predictive factors of adjuvant tamoxifen efficacy in early breast cancer. Clin Cancer Res 2003; 9:1039–1046.
56. Yarden RI, Wilson MA, Chrysogelos SA. Estrogen suppression of EGFR expression in breast cancer cells: a possible mechanism to modulate growth. J Cell Biochem 2001; 81:232–246.
57. Chu I, Blackwell KL, Chen S, et al. The dual ErbB1/ErbB2 inhibitor, lapatinib, cooperates with tamoxifen to inhibit both cell proliferation and estrogen-dependent gene expression in anti-estrogen resistant breast cancer. Cancer Res 2005; 65:18–25.
58. Arpino G, Weiss H, Wakeling A, et al. Complete disappearance of ER+/HER2+ breast cancer xenografts with the combination of gefitinib, trastuzumab, and pertuzumab to block HER2 cross-talk with ER and restore tamoxifen inhibition [abstract 23]. Breast Cancer Res Treat 2004; 88(suppl 1):S15.

18 Anti-Epidermal Growth Factor Receptor Strategies for Advanced Breast Cancer

Susana M. Campos

Department of Breast and Gynecology, Dana-Farber Cancer Institute, Harvard University, Boston, Massachusetts, U.S.A.

INTRODUCTION

Significant progress has been achieved in the treatment of breast cancer with therapeutics focused on DNA replication or cell division. Despite the armamentarium of cytotoxic agents, enthusiasm for these agents has been tempered by their lack of tumor cell selectivity, toxicity profile, and almost uniformly the emergence of resistance.

In recent years, the focus has shifted to an understanding of cellular signaling pathways involved in carcinogenesis and tumor growth in hopes of allowing the development of targeted cancer drugs. The epidermal growth factor receptor (EGFR) has emerged as an attractive target for the design of targeted therapeutics due to several findings implicating their involvement in the development and progression of cancer (1–3). The activation of EGFR signaling pathways is known to increase proliferation, angiogenesis, and decrease apoptosis. Several strategies directed at the EGFR have been investigated in the clinical setting. These include monoclonal antibodies that block ligand binding to receptors and small molecule adenosine triphosphate (ATP) competitive inhibitors of the receptor tyrosine kinase.

This chapter will review the current data on tyrosine kinase inhibitors in the management of advanced breast cancer. Attention will be directed at understanding the molecular mechanisms of these agents balanced with their application to clinical practice.

EPIDERMAL GROWTH FACTOR
Epidermal Growth Factor Ligands

Growth factor receptors such as the EGFR bind one or more growth factor proteins or other molecules that regulate the activity of the receptor. Most ligands of the ErbB family are synthesized as transmembrane precursors that are proteolytically cleaved to release the soluble form of the peptide (4–8). These peptides share a domain of homology that is required for the ErbB family receptor binding and activation. Ligands for the EGFR include the epidermal growth factor (EGF), transforming growth factor-alpha (TGF-alpha), amphiregulin, heparin-binding EGF, epiregulin, heregulin subfamily, and betacellulin (9). EGF and TGF-alpha are believed to be the main endogenous ligands that result in EGFR-mediated stimulation.

EGF ligands are expressed in a variety of tissues and can act on both normal and tumor cells. In vitro and in vivo data have revealed that overproduction of growth factors can result in transformation of various cell types. Tumor cells can secrete growth factors and in an autocrine manner augment EGFR-mediated growth and/or differentiation (10).

Some ligands bind exclusively to one ErbB member, whereas others bind with multiple ErbB members. As such, substantial functional redundancy and specificity within the EGF family exists. In addition, substantial differences in the biological activity of these ligands exist. Although TGF-alpha and EGF bind exclusively to Erb-B1, TGF-alpha is more potent than EGF as an angiogenic factor in vivo (4,11–14).

The Epidermal Growth Factor Receptor

The human EGFR is the result of a gene that encodes a 170 kD membrane-spanning glycoprotein. It is composed of three distinct regions: (*i*) an extracellular region consisting of a glycosylated domain; (*ii*) a transmembrane domain; and (*iii*) an intracellular region containing the catalytic tyrosine kinase domain responsible for the generation and regulation of intracellular signaling (15). The EGFR has several roles, namely, a key mediator in the maintenance of normal cellular function and survival and a regulator of tumor cell survival, apoptosis, angiogenesis, motility, and invasiveness. It is expressed on the cell surface of many normal tissues but is known to be elevated in a variety of human tumors including breast cancer (16,17). Studies have suggested that EGFR is overexpressed in 16% to 48% of human breast cancers and that overexpression and/or mutation of the EGFR receptor is associated with aggressive clinical behavior and a worse prognosis (16,18).

The human EGFR family is composed of four members sharing a common molecular architecture: (*i*) ErbB1; (*ii*) ErbB2; (*iii*) ErbB3; and (*iv*) ErbB4. The ErbB1 (EGFR) was the first ErbB receptor family to be described (19). It plays a pivotal role in the regulation of normal cell growth and differentiation. ErbB1 is expressed on normal cells at levels ranging from 20,000 to 200,000 receptors per cell (12). In contrast, MDA-468 breast cancer cells express up to two million surface receptors per cell (15). High levels of EGFR expression have also been observed in tumors in which the EGFR gene is not amplified (20). The overexpression of the ErbB1 receptor may occur by different means such as the amplification of the growth factor receptor genes (21,22), mutations that increase ErbB1 transcription and mRNA translation (20,23). Its dysregulation confers a proliferative advantage and malignant potential. The receptor transmits growth regulatory signals on binding of EGF ligands, particularly EGF and TGF-alpha, thereby having a significant effect on several essential processes including stromal and vascular invasion (24,25), tumor cell survival and apoptotic pathways, and angiogenesis (14,25,26). In addition, the overexpression of ErbB1 is often accompanied by production of its ligand (27). These events produce an autocrine system that maintains tumor viability. Continued EGF stimulation has been shown to protect against apoptosis triggered by Fas, a cell death receptor (28).

Several variants of the ErbB1 receptor have been associated with human malignancies. The most common variant is a mutation of the ErbB1 receptor known as EGFR vIII that is caused by deletion of exons two to seven (29). This variant is not found in normal tissues but is expressed on the cell membrane of certain tumors including up to 78% of breast carcinomas (30). The mutation results in the deletion of a part of the extracellular domain that renders the receptor incapable of binding ligands. However, this variant possesses a constitutively activated tyrosine kinase that results in ligand-independent transmission (31).

The second member of the ErbB2 family (HER2/neu) shares considerable homology to ErbB1, is believed to be a more potent oncoprotein than other members of the ErbB family, but has no known high-affinity ligands (32–34). Transfection of the *ErbB2* gene into human breast and ovarian tumor cell lines resulted in more aggressive characteristics such as increased DNA synthesis and metastatic potential in nude mice (35). It differs from other family members in that it triggers ligand-independent activation of the tyrosine kinase domain. ErbB2 overexpression or amplification has been demonstrated in 20% to 25% of invasive ductal breast cancer (36) and is correlated with other negative features such as tumor size, lymph node involvement, high nuclear grade, aneuploidy, and lower disease free and overall survival (35–37). Interestingly, ErbB2 overexpression is reported in early forms of breast cancer such as ductal carcinoma in situ suggesting that alteration in ErbB2 represents, but one factor in the malignant phenotype transformation (35–37).

ErbB3 (HER3) and ErbB4 (HER4) are structurally related family members (4–8). ErbB3 is catalytically inactive because of its lack of tyrosine kinase activity. It is activated by tyrosine kinases on other receptors (38). Recent studies have suggested that ErbB3-dependent signaling through ErbB3/ErbB2 heterodimers can contribute to metastasis by enhancing tumor cell invasion and intravasation in vivo (39). The ErbB-4 receptor is overexpressed in 7% to 13% of breast cancers and is often associated with tumors that have a more differentiated phenotype. Isoforms of the ErbB4 have been identified that differ in the composition and structure of their juxtamembrane regions and C-terminal tails. This has been shown to result in differences in the downstream signaling protein recruitment (40). Interestingly, a recent study suggested that the absence of HER4 expression predicts recurrence of ductal carcinoma in situ of the breast (41).

Ligand:Receptor Interactions

Ligand binding leads to receptor aggregation, dimerization, autophosphorylation, and activation of the intrinsic tyrosine kinase of the EGFR. The interaction results in the mediation of a network that transmits extracellular signals to downstream signal transduction pathways such as the mitogen-activated protein kinase (MAPK) and the phosphotidylinositol-3-kinase pathways (PI3K) (15).

Signal diversity is achieved at multiple levels. This occurs as a result of not only the ability of the ErbB receptor family to undergo homodimerization and heterodimerization, but also as the result of differences in the amino acid sequences of the C-terminal domains of the receptors that serve as docking sites for proteins involved in signal transduction (42–45).

In addition to signal diversity, the potency of responses initiated by ligand binding is a result of multiple factors. These include the identity of the ligand, the specific dimer, the concentration of the ligand and receptor, the affinity of the receptor dimerization, the receptor kinase activity, and the rate of receptor internalization.

EPIDERMAL GROWTH FACTOR EXPRESSION: PROGNOSTIC SIGNIFICANCE

Numerous studies (16,18,46–48) have been conducted to determine if EGFR can serve as a prognostic factor. In part, conflicting data has resulted from variability in methods used to assay the EGFR protein and the heterogeneity of clinical studies.

Unlike ErbB2 (HER2), which has a Food and Drug Administration approved testing assay [immunohistochemistry (IHC) or fluorescence in situ hybridization (FISH)], no defined analysis exists for the expression of EGFR. EGFR can be evaluated at the DNA, RNA, and protein level (49–52). Several techniques have included IHC (49), Western blotting (49), or enzyme immunoassay (EIA) (53). EGFR protein levels in serum, from breast cancer patients, have been examined using EIA and have been reported to be elevated in 67.5% of patients (53). Radioimmunohistochemistry (RIHC) has also been used to determine EGFR expression and has yielded an overall higher positive rate of EGFR expression (54). Northern analysis and reverse transcriptase polymerase chain reaction can be utilized to detect levels of the EGFR RNA transcript (55). However, as noted by Rampaul et al. (56), such levels may not reflect the levels of protein produced. Kersting et al. (51) studied the correlation between EGFR gene amplification and protein expression in breast cancer utilizing variable technology. The majority of cases that reported EGFR protein overexpression lacked amplifications.

In addition to the variable data that surrounds EGFR testing, clinical studies have not yielded any comforting data regarding the prognostic and predicative value of this marker. A large meta-analysis by Klijn et al. (16) examined EGFR expression in breast cancer from 1984 to 1992 and reported on over 5000 patients. The authors found univariate significance in five studies. EGFR expression correlated with tumor grade in 10 of 18 studies, tumor size in 2 of 17 studies, nodal status in 5 to 9 of 20 studies and proliferative index in 3 of 9 studies. Associations between relapse-free survival and EGFR expression were dependent on time of follow-up with more significant correlations found for short-term follow-up than for long-term follow-up. Fox et al. (57) examined 370 patients with a median follow-up of 18 months. No correlation was reported with size, stage, or grade. Rampaul et al. (58) examined a cohort of patients with primary breast cancer (median follow-up of 222 months) who did not receive adjuvant treatment. Twenty percent of the cases (56; $n = 255$) were positive for EGFR by IHC. Univariate analysis showed a significant correlation among grade ($P < 0.004$), Nottingham Prognostic Index (NPI) ($P < 0.001$), tumor type ($P < 0.037$), and patient age ($P < 0.006$) and a highly significant inverse correlation was noted between EGFR and estrogen receptor (ER) ($P < 0.001$). Multivariate analysis showed significance for only NPI and grade (58).

As illustrated by the studies described, larger scale studies are warranted to strengthen correlations between EGFR and prognosis, metastatic potential and survival.

THE ErbB RECEPTOR FAMILY: A TARGET FOR THERAPEUTIC DEVELOPMENT

The ErbB family of receptors and ligands serve as targets for the therapeutic development of agents against malignant disease. Numerous investigators are attempting to control the growth of cancer cells using agents that target all levels of signal transduction: the receptor itself, the signal transduction cascade, gene expression and translation.

Since growth factors are an integral component of the EGF-signaling pathways, a logical approach to therapy is to interfere with growth factor receptor-mediated autocrine/paracrine growth stimulation. A variety of approaches have been developed to target the EGFR. These include monoclonal antibodies directed against the receptor, synthetic tyrosine kinase inhibitors that act directly on the cytoplasmic domain of the EGFR, ligand conjugates which bind specifically to the EGFR, immunoconjugates (anti-EGFR antibody conjugated to ricin), and antisense oligonucleotides.

Given the broad scope of this topic, this chapter focuses specifically on small molecule tyrosine kinase inhibitors.

SMALL MOLECULE TYROSINE KINASE INHIBITORS

Tyrosine kinase activity is required for EGFR-mediated tumorigenicity. Overexpression of protein tyrosine kinase receptors correlates with a poor prognosis and a shorter survival time in patients with breast cancer. Recent research has focused on therapies that ablate this function.

Quinazoline compounds represent a class of competitive inhibitors of the ATP-binding site that are orally active, potent, and selective tyrosine kinase inhibitors (59). These small molecule tyrosine kinase inhibitors competitively block the ATP-binding site on the receptor and subsequently prevent signal transduction. These agents also target the highly tumorigenic EGFR mutant vIII that may be inaccessible to monoclonal antibodies.

In breast cancer, several tyrosine kinase inhibitors are being investigated. These include gefitinib (Iressa®; AstraZeneca Pharmaceuticals, Wilmington, Delaware, U.S.A.), erlotinib (Tarceva®; Genentech Inc., South San Francisco, California, U.S.A.), lapatinib (Tykerb®; GlaxoSmithKline, Research Triangle Park, North Carolina, U.S.A.), and CI-1033 (Pfizer, New York, U.S.A.). The principle differences among these tyrosine kinase inhibitors are that gefitinib and erlotinib are specific for the ErbB-1, and are reversible inhibitors; whereas lapatinib is a reversible dual inhibitor that targets ErbB1 and ErbB2. CI-1033 is an irreversible inhibitor that blocks a region of the catalytic site conserved among all ErbB receptors and is referred to as a Pan-Erb inhibitor.

Gefitinib in Breast Cancer

Gefitinib is a low molecular weight, highly selective, and reversible tyrosine kinase inhibitor of the EGFR (60). It is a potent inhibitor of proliferation not only in cells overexpressing EGFR, but also in those that additionally overexpress HER2, possibly mediated by gefitinib reduction of EGFR/HER2 heterodimer phosphorylation (61–63).

In the clinical setting, phase I trials of gefitinib have been generally well tolerated with the majority of events being that of grade 1 and 2 gastrointestinal or skin toxicities (64–67). Anti-tumor activity was demonstrated in a broad range of tumors including the observation of prolonged stable disease in patients with breast cancer.

A phase II study by Albain et al. (68) evaluated the efficacy and safety of gefitinib in patients with metastatic breast cancer who had progressed on previous hormonal and cytotoxic agents. Gefitinib was delivered at 500 mg/day until disease progression or toxicity. The primary objective of the study was to evaluate the clinical benefit rate (defined as complete response plus partial response plus stable disease greater than or equal to six months). Sixty-three patients were enrolled. The median age of the patients was 52 years (range: 34–81). Patient characteristics included 27 (43%) patients with hormone receptor-positive disease and 17 patients (27%) with HER2/neu overexpressing tumors. Seventy-nine percent of patients had involvement of the viscera. The majority of individuals (78%) had received at least two prior cytotoxic treatments and all ErbB2 positive patients (36%) had been previously treated with trastuzumab. The treatment was well tolerated with the exception of diarrhea. The results, however, noted minimal response. One patient had a partial response and five patients had stable disease lasting at least four months in duration. Median overall survival was 144 days (range: 110–242 days). Median progression-free survival was 57 days (range: 16–205+ days). The authors noted that some patients experienced an improvement in symptoms such as bone pain. Five patients (42%) experienced palliation of pain. Similar to previous studies, toxicities consisted of grade 3 diarrhea, nausea, vomiting, and a rash. Skin rash occurred in 44% of patients ($n = 28$), four of which had grade 3 rash. Four patients required a dose reduction of gefitinib to 250 mg/day. The authors noted that several hypotheses could have accounted for the low-response rate observed in this trial, namely, a heavily pretreated patient population with chemotherapy and hormonal therapy, the lack of activating mutations as found in nonsmall cell lung cancer and perhaps an inferior dose of the agent.

Von Minckwitz et al. (69) reported on 46 breast cancer patients treated with gefitinib. Again, the dose utilized was 500 mg/day. After 12 weeks of therapy, one (2.2%) patient had partial response and three (6.5%) patients had stable disease. Forty-two patients experienced progressive disease.

Baselga et al. (70) reported a multicenter phase II trial and pharmacodynamic study of gefitinib in patients with advanced breast cancer. In this study, patients received gefitinib 500 mg/day, apart from day 1 when patients received gefitinib 500 mg/day followed a second dose 12 hours later. Each treatment cycle was 28 days. Patients received treatment until disease progression, unacceptable toxicity, or withdrawal of consent. The primary objective was to assess the objective response rate of this agent in patients with locally advanced or metastatic disease. The pharmacodynamic profile of gefitinib in skin and tumor tissues as well as the safety profile of the drug were secondary objectives. Patients enrolled in this clinical trial were women with histologically confirmed stage IIIb/IV advanced breast cancer that were resistant to one or two prior chemotherapy regimens. The trial aimed at achieving a patient cohort that was at least 50% EGFR-positive. A two-stage design was employed. Several pharmacodynamic markers were assessed. These included EGFR expression, activated/phosphorylated EGFR (pEFGR), the ligand TGF-alpha, the downstream signaling markers including phosphorylated MAPK (pMAPK) and protein kinase B (pAKT), the proliferation markers Ki67 and the cyclin-dependent kinase inhibitor, p27. All markers were evaluated by IHC. Of the 31 evaluable patients who received treatment for a median duration of eight weeks, 12 (38.7%) patients had stable disease including three (9.7%) patients with recurrent breast cancer that had stable disease for six months or greater. The duration of stable disease was 84 to 349 days. No complete or partial responses were noted. Progressive disease occurred in 19 (61.3%) patients with a median time to progression of 55 days (95% CI, 42–88). Median overall survival was 503 days. The most prevalent drug-related adverse effects included diarrhea, skin rash, and asthenia.

Pretreatment tumor samples were available in all patients. EGFR expression was detected in 15 (48%) patients. A significant relationship was established between EGFR expression and the expression of TGF-alpha ($P = 0.007$), p-EGFR

($P < 0.001$), p-MAPK ($P = 0.033$), and Ki67 ($P = 0.036$) utilizing a Spearman's correlation test in pretreatment tumors. Correlative studies including basal expression of EGFR, pEGFR, pMAPK, TGF-alpha, Ki67, and p27 were analyzed in skin biopsies compared with expression on day 28 following gefitinib treatment. Gefitinib inhibited the phosphorylation of EGFR and MAPK, decreased the expression of Ki67, and resulted in an increase in expression of inhibitor p27 in the skin keratinocytes. In tumor samples, treatment with gefitinib inhibited phosphorylation of EGFR and MAPK in tumor biopsies. Gefitinib did not result in inhibition of pAKT and did not decrease proliferation or increase p27 levels. There was discordance in the skin and the tumor samples between Ki67 and p27. Of note, in EGFR-positive tumors, treatment with gefitinib increased the apoptotic index. In addition, the authors did not appreciate any significant difference in EGFR expression between patients with stable disease versus those with progressive disease.

Robertson et al. (71) also evaluated the activity of gefitinib in breast cancer patients. The authors noted that gefitinib was active in breast cancer patients with tamoxifen-resistant breast cancer. A disease control rate of 66.6% was observed in a small cohort of ER+ tamoxifen-resistant breast cancer patients. Toxicities were similar to previous studies with skin rash, diarrhea and nausea, and vomiting being the most prevalent adverse event.

Erlotinib

Erlotinib (Tarceva®; OSI-774) is another orally active quinazoline that reversibly inhibits EGFR tyrosine kinase function (72,73). In preclinical studies, erlotinib demonstrated impressive anti-tumor activity both in vitro and in vivo. It was well tolerated at doses ranging from 10 to 200 mg/kg/day and had a favorable pharmacokinetic profile. Several phase I trials (74–77) have been conducted in patients with varying solid tumors. The most common toxicities of erlotinib were similar to other EGFR inhibitors and were noted to be skin rashes, diarrhea, nausea, and headache. The recommended phase II dose based on previous phase I studies was established at 150 mg/day.

Winer et al. (78) reported the efficacy of single agent erlotinib in patients with locally advanced or metastatic breast cancer. Erlotinib was delivered at a dose of 150 mg/day. Two cohorts of patients were studied. Patients in cohort I had progressed after multiple prior therapies containing an anthracycline, a taxane and capecitabine. Patients in cohort II had disease progression on or after at least one prior regimen. Forty-seven patients were accrued to cohort I, and 22 patients were accrued to cohort II. Patients in both cohorts were extensively pretreated. The mean number of prior regimens in cohort I was eight and six in cohort II. Forty percent of patients received prior trastuzumab. In cohort I, one patient achieved a partial response of 23 weeks duration for an objective response of 2%. Two additional patients had stable disease for greater than 12 weeks. In cohort II, one patient had stable disease of greater than eight weeks duration. The most common grade-3 toxicity was diarrhea, asthenia, acneiform, rash, nausea, and vomiting. Unfortunately, erlotinib did not reveal stellar activity in this study in patients with advanced breast cancer.

In studies with EGFR tyrosine kinase inhibitors, skin has been proposed as a surrogate tissue of EGFR expression (79,80). Tan et al. (81) studied the effects of daily-administered erlotinib and correlated it to changes in the EGFR phosphoryl-ation and downstream signaling in patients with metastatic breast cancer. Eighteen patients were treated with erlotinib at 150 mg/day. Ki67, EGFR, pEGFR, pMAPK, and pAKT were studied in skin, buccal mucosa, and tumor biopsies. The biological endpoints were measured at baseline and after one month of treatment. The authors reported that Ki67 in keratinocytes of the epidermis significantly decreased after treatment ($P = 0.0005$). No significant change in proliferation markers was detected in tumor samples. One tumor was EGFR-positive, whereas the remaining speci-mens were EGFR-negative. In the EGFR-positive tumor, pEGFR, pMAPK, and pAKT were reduced after treatment with erlotinib. Interestingly, pEGFR was increased in EGFR-negative tumors.

CI-1033

Unlike the previous tyrosine kinase inhibitors, CI-1033 is a small molecule tyrosine kinase inhibitor that is a potent inhibitor of all catalytically active members of the ErbB family. In addition to inhibiting signaling of all members of the EGFR family, CI-1033 also inhibits the known mutant ErbB receptor known as EGFR vIII (82). A distinction between CI-1033 and erlotinib and gefitinib is that CI-1033 irreversibly inhibits signaling through ErbB receptors by covalently modifying a cysteine residue in the ATP-binding site. CI-1033 prevents the phosphorylation of binding sites for SH2 containing proteins and as such blocks all signal transduction through the EGFR family including the Ras/MAPK pathway and the PI-3 kinase/AKT pathway (83,84). The irreversible property of this agent allows a prolonged suppression of the receptor kinase activity (85).

Preclinical data suggested that CI-1033 had potential in the treatment of breast cancer. In human breast carcinomas grown as xenografts in nude mice, CI-1033 produced complete stasis at 40 mg/kg in the University of Illinois Surgical Oncol-ogy BCA-1 breast tumor and caused tumor regression during treatment in the MDA-MB-468 model (82).

Several clinical phase I studies have been performed to determine the dose-limiting toxicity, maximum tolerated dose, and pharmacokinetics of this pan-erb inhibitor. In one study (86), 53 patients with a variety of solid tumors were treated with CI-1033 for seven consecutive days every three weeks at doses ranging from 50 to 750 mg/day. In this cohort of individuals, there were two patients with metastatic breast cancer that were treated with 130 and 750 mg dose level. The most common adverse events were mild to moderate (grade 1 and 2) and included diarrhea (45%), rash (43%), nausea (42%), mucositis (28%), and vomiting (25%). Additional findings included thrombocytopenia (grade 1–4) in 15 patients (28%) across multiple dose levels and a grade 3 reversible hypersen-sitivity like reaction in one patient at a dose of 560 mg .The maximum tolerated dose of CI-1033 that was administered on this schedule was 750 mg/day at which two grade 3 gastrointestinal dose-limiting toxicities were observed. Clinical activity was observed in this phase I trial and included one partial response (in a patient with squamous cell skin cancer) and stable disease of greater than 12 weeks duration in 18 out of 53 patients (34%). One of the patients with metastatic breast cancer who had received five prior chemotherapy regimens including biological therapy remained on study for 25 weeks without disease progression. Correlative studies using pre- and post-treatment tumors noted ErbB-1 phosphorylation inhibition after seven days of treatment. Interestingly, continued suppression of receptor phosphorylation was observed following the seven-day drug-free period. Other investigators have explored alternative dosing schedules. Nemunaitis et al. (87) examined the tolerability and pharmacokinetics of oral CI-1033 on a two week on one week off schedule. This phase I multicenter trial was conducted in patients with various solid tumors and employed a dose escalation of CI-1033 starting at 300 mg/day. Thirty-two patients were studied. The dose-limiting toxicity mirrored other studies and included diarrhea, rash, and anorexia. Six patients had stable disease. The authors concluded that CI-1033 was suitable for phase II testing at 450 mg/day when administered for 14 days in a 21-day cycle.

Recently completed, yet not reported, is the investigation of CI-1033 in patients with metastatic breast cancer. This phase II study's primary objective was to determine whether CI-1033 had anti-tumor activity in patients previously treated with advanced breast cancer. The primary endpoint was 1-year progression free survival. Secondary endpoints included overall response rate, disease control rates, and duration of response, survival, and changes in subject-reported outcomes. This phase II open label randomized multicenter trial had three cohorts of patients with metastatic breast cancer who expressed at least one member of the ErbB family of receptors and who had progressed following treatment with not more than two cytotoxic chemotherapy regimens. Patients were stratified by hormone receptor status and disease-free interval. Patients were randomized to oral CI-1033 at 50 or 150 mg/day for 21 continuous days in a 21-day cycle or oral CI-1033 at 450 mg for 14 consecutive days followed by seven days of no treatment. The study has reached accrual and publication of the data is pending.

Lapatinib

Lapatinib, like CI-1033, targets more than one EGFR. It is a novel tyrosine kinase inhibitor that targets signaling through ErbB1 and ErbB2 homodimers and heterodimers (15,88). It binds reversibly to the cytoplasmic ATP-binding site of the kinase, thereby preventing receptor autophosphorylation. In addition, it can block the activation of mutated or truncated forms of the receptors. In preclinical studies Xia et al. (89) reported that lapatinib (GW572016) reduced tyrosine phosphorylation of EGFR and ErbB2 and inhibited activation of ERK 1/2 and AKT. A 23-fold increase in apoptosis was noted in ErbB2 overexpressing cells. In addition others have observed that simultaneous inhibition of the EGFR and ErbB2 receptor kinase resulted in synergistic cell growth inhibition (90).

Multiple phase I studies have addressed the safety and tolerability of lapatinib. Versola et al. (91) reported the results of EGF10003, a phase I study of lapatinib in patients with various malignancies. The lapatinib regimen consisted of daily administration of this agent at doses ranging between 175 and 1800 mg/day or 500 to 900 twice a day. No grade 4 toxicities were observed. Most toxicities were grade 1 or 2 with two cases of grade 3 diarrhea observed at the 900 mg twice a day dose. One patient had a complete response, whereas 22 patients had stable disease (data available on 43 patients). Burris et al. (92) recently published the results of a phase I study (EGF10004) in patients with metastatic solid tumors. The median number of prior treatments in this cohort of patients was six. Sixty-seven patients with metastatic solid tumors were treated. Lapatinib was administered at doses ranging from 500 to 1600 mg/day. Five grade 3 toxicities were observed and included gastrointestinal effects and rash. The most common adverse effect was diarrhea (42%) and rash (31%). No significant drug-related reduction in LVEF was noted. One patient experienced an asymptomatic decline in ejection fraction from 37% at baseline to 20%. This was related to underlying disease rather than to the lapatinib. Likewise, no pulmonary toxicity (interstitial pneumonitis) was reported. Fifty-nine out of 67 patients were evaluable. Four patients with breast cancer (trastuzumab-resistant metastatic breast cancer; all HER2 positive, and three of four EGFR-positive) experienced a partial response whereas an additional 24 patients had stable disease, 10 of which had prolonged stable disease. The patients who achieved partial responses had a high expression of activated phosphorylated ErbB2 that was inhibited by lapatinib therapy. The median duration of treatment for patients with a partial response (PR) was 5.5 months (range: 3–8 months).

Evidence of lapatinib activity in solid tumors prompted the initiation of phase II and III trials to examine the benefit of lapatinib in patients with advanced breast cancer. Two nonrandomized, open label, multicenter phase II clinical trials (93,94) are assessing the role of lapatinib in patients who are refractory to trastuzumab and conventional chemotherapy. Efficacy results on the first 81 patients [combined from two studies (93,94)] refractory to trastuzumab noted a 9% response rate. EGF20008 (94) examined the role of lapatinib in women with stage III or IV breast cancer who had also progressed on traditional chemotherapeutic agents with or without trastuzumab. Patients received lapatinib at 1500 mg/day until disease progression or until the presentation of unacceptable toxicity. Patients with ErbB-2 overexpressing tumors had to have been treated with prior anthracyclines, taxanes, capecitabine, and trastuzumab. Patients with ErbB-2 negative tumors had to have been treated with similar agents in cohort I with the exception of trastuzumab. An interim analysis of 40 patients with trastuzumab-refractory disease showed that three (7.5%) patients achieved a partial response and that two (5%) patients had stable disease.

A phase II trial, EGF20009 (95), investigated lapatinib's role as a single agent in women with ErbB-2 overexpressing tumors that had not received prior treatment. Patients were randomized to lapatinib at 1500 mg/day for 12 weeks versus lapatinib at 500 mg twice a day for 12 weeks. Initial findings noted that 38% of the first 13 patients had a partial response to lapatinib monotherapy. An additional six patients had stable disease lasting greater than or equal to eight weeks.

In all of these trials, the adverse effect profile of lapatinib was similar to those observed for other EGFR inhibitors. Gastrointestinal as well as skin events predominated.

One exciting area of research is the potential role of lapatinib in the management of patients with refractory central nervous system (CNS) disease. The EGFR inhibitor, gefitinib, has demonstrated efficacy against brain metastases in patients with lung cancer. A phase II (96) study in 41 patients reported a partial response of 10% and a clinical benefit rate of 27% suggesting that perhaps tyrosine kinase inhibitors could cross the blood–brain barrier. Recently reported by Lin et al. (97) were the results of a phase II trial of lapatinib for brain metastases in patients with HER2 + breast cancer. Eligible patients had HER2/neu + breast cancer with new or progressive brain metastases. Patients received lapatinib at a dose of 750 mg twice a day. All patients enrolled in the study had developed progressive disease on trastuzumab. Two patients achieved a partial response as defined by response evaluation criteria in solid tumors (RECIST) and remained on study for several months. Five patients achieved stable disease lasting greater than 16 weeks. Median time to treatment failure was 3.2 months. The authors concluded that lapatinib was well tolerated in this patient population and that there was evidence that this agent penetrated the central nervous system.

DIFFERENTIAL RESPONSE OF BREAST CARCINOMA TO EPIDERMAL GROWTH FACTOR RECEPTOR INHIBITORS

Until recently, the molecular mechanisms underlying the sensitivity of tyrosine kinase inhibitors remained unknown. Paradoxical associations between EGFR expression and response to treatment lead to further confusion regarding determinants of response to therapy. Recently demonstrated in nonsmall cell lung cancer was the observation that specific mutations in the EGFR tyrosine kinase domain predicted for response to treatment with agents that block EGFR receptors. Two separate study groups (98,99) reported the discovery and the identification of missense and deletion mutations that cause the EGFR to have a much higher affinity for gefitinib and hence lead to an increased responsiveness to the tyrosine kinase inhibitor. Recently reported were the results of Lee et al. (100) who investigated the presence of somatic mutations of ErbB2 kinase domain in gastric, colorectal, and breast carcinomas. The authors concluded that in addition to lung adenocarcinomas, ErbB2 kinase domain mutations occur in breast cancers in addition to other cancers.

EPIDERMAL GROWTH FACTOR RECEPTOR INHIBITORS: OVERCOMING ENDOCRINE RESISTANCE

It has been suggested that EGFR signaling and endocrine resistance may be interrelated. Newby et al. (101), Nicholson et al. (102–106), Knowlden et al. (107), and Martin et al. (108), in independent studies have revealed that EGFR overexpression is associated with endocrine insensitivity. In preclinical studies, McClelland et al. (109) showed that in resistant MCF-7 breast cancer cells developed by prolonged exposure to the tamoxifen or fulvestrant, there was an increase in the expression of EGFR and HER2/neu mRNA and protein. Western blotting revealed increased phosphorylation of the receptors compared to the hormone responsive cell line. Increased basal levels of downstream targets were also noted.

Several studies have tried to ascertain whether targeting the EGFR may overcome or postpone endocrine resistance. Agrawal et al. (110) have in several preclinical studies examined this potential. Based on the results of these preclinical studies, Agrawal et al. embarked on several clinical cancer trials to address the role of EFGR-TKIs in a specific cohort of patients, namely those with endocrine-resistant breast cancer. Clinical trial 57 (1839/0057) studied patients with locally advanced/metastatic disease with either ER+ tamoxifen resistant or ER− carcinomas. Gefitinib was delivered at 500 mg/day. Of the 27 evaluable patients, clinical benefit [PR = 1; stable disease (SD) = 5] was appreciated in the ER+ tamoxifen resistant arm. In the ER− cohort, only 2 out of 18 patients had a response (11%; PR = 1; SD = 1). Median time to progression was longer in the ER+ tamoxifen-resistant group. Correlative studies in trial 57 included tissue biopsies in patients with palpable disease. The authors reported that patients who obtained a clinical response with gefitinib expressed lower pretreatment levels of EGFR than patients with progressive disease. Other correlative studies done in a subset of patients revealed: (*i*) a change in Ki67 marker in patients achieving clinical benefit, and (*ii*) a decreased phosphorylated EGFR during treatment in some patients. Interestingly, patients with progressive disease exhibited increased activity of the signaling molecule AKT, a molecule that Jones et al. (111) have linked with insulin growth factor signaling and gefitinib resistance.

Preclinical studies have observed that acquired resistance to tamoxifen is associated with increased EGFR signaling through the ERK1/2 MAPK pathway. In contrast, cells that were responsive to hormonal manipulation exhibited minimal signaling through the EGFR/MAPK signaling routes. Gee et al. (112) blocked signaling through the ERK1/2 MAPK with the combination of tamoxifen and gefitinib. Based on these findings, Trial 225 was initiated to assess whether combination therapy could improve the inhibitory effect of hormonal manipulation or could possibly delay hormone resistance. Trial 225, a randomized phase II trial of 274 women with ER+ metastatic breast cancer stratifies patients into two groups: (*i*) those with newly diagnosed disease or those who completed adjuvant tamoxifen at least one year prior; or (*ii*) patients with recurrent disease during or after adjuvant aromatase inhibitor (AI) or failing first line treatment with AI. Patients will be then randomized to one of the two arms including tamoxifen and gefitinib or tamoxifen plus placebo. Time to progression is the primary endpoint. Correlative studies planned include IHC examination of downstream players of the ErbB family.

In yet another study, Trial 1839/0004 will explore the role of gefitinib in patients with metastatic breast cancer who have shown resistance to fulvestrant. Two additional phase II trials are examining the combination of gefitinib and fulvestrant in advanced disease. One trial will examine the clinical utility of combination therapy of gefitinib and fulvestrant, while an Eastern Cooperative Oncology Group (ECOG) trial will compare gefitinib and fulvestrant with anastrozole and fulvestrant.

EPIDERMAL GROWTH FACTOR RECEPTOR TYROSINE KINASE INHIBITORS: COMBINATION THERAPY

Given the redundant nature of pathways, numerous studies have now focused on attempting to control the growth of cells utilizing agents that target all levels of signal transduction, namely, the ligand, the receptor, and downstream pathways.

One approach to regulate the proliferation of cancer cells is the blockade of receptor-mediated autocrine/paracrine growth stimulation by the addition of monoclonal antibodies and or tyrosine kinase inhibitors. Numerous clinical trials have established the usefulness of trastuzumab both as a single agent (113,114) and in combination (115–117) with various cytotoxic agents. Recent clinical studies utilizing tyrosine kinase inhibitors have yielded marginal responses in patients with breast cancer (Table 1).

Provocative translational research has provided a signal that combination targeted therapy may be a mechanism to improve responses and circumvent resistance (118,119). Normanno (120) and Moulder (121) recently described the synergistic activity of gefitinib and trastuzumab. They showed that the combination of both of these agents markedly enhanced apoptosis when compared with the results of

TABLE 1 Tyrosine Kinase Inhibitors

Agent	Reference	N	Cancer type	Regimen	Results
Gefitinib	(68)	63	Breast	500 mg/d	PR = 1, SD = 2
	(69)	46	Breast	500 mg/d	PR = 1, SD = 3
	(70)	34	Breast	500 mg/d	MR = 1, SD = 3
	(71)	33	Breast	500 mg/d; loading dose day 1: 1000 mg	PR = 2, SD = 6
Erlotinib	(78)	Cohort 1:47	Breast	150 mg/d	Cohort 1: PR = 1, SD = 6
		Cohort 2:22			Cohort 2: PR = 1, SD = 2
CI-1033	(86)	53	Solid tumors	50–750 mg/d; dose-escalation	PR = 1, SD = 1
	(87)	32	Solid tumors	300–450 mg/d; dose-escalation	SD = 6
Lapatinib	(91)	64	Solid tumors	175–1800 mg/d or 500–900 mg BID	CR = 1, SD = 2
	(92)	67	Solid tumors	500–1600 mg QD	PR = 4, SD = 24
	(128)	27	Breast	750–1500 mg QD + trastuzumab	CR = 1, PR = 5, SD = 10
	(94)	40	Breast	1500 mg/d	PR = 3, SD = 2
	(95)	13	Breast	1500 mg/d or 500 mg BID	PR = 5, SD = 6

Abbreviations: CR, complete response; MR, minor response; PR, partial response; SD, stable disease.

either agent alone. Arpino et al. (122) reported the additional benefit gained when yet another biological agent, in this case pertuzumab, a monoclonal antibody that inhibits the heterodimerization of HER/neu with other HER family members, was combined with trastuzumab, gefitinib, and tamoxifen. In mice, a 71% clinical response was noted. Time to progression was prolonged also with multi-targeted therapy.

Despite provocative preclinical research, a clinical study did not validate the data appreciated in earlier studies. The combined blockade of the ErbB receptor and HER2/neu with gefitinib and trastuzumab, respectively, resulted in a median time to progression of 2.9 months (95% CI: 2.5–4) in chemotherapy naïve patients (121). The poor results of the trial were, in part, attributed to a small sample size and perhaps the induction of HER3 phosphorylation.

Britten et al. (123) recently reported the results of a clinical phase I trial of trastuzumab and erlotinib. In preclinical studies (124), it had been reported that clinically relevant concentrations of trastuzumab and erlotinib demonstrated synergistic activity in several human breast cancer cell lines. In this phase I trial, 16 patients (14 patients were evaluable) received erlotinib at the following doses: 50, 100, and 150 mg. Two previously untreated patients enrolled at the 150 mg dose achieved a confirmed partial response. One patient who had been previously treated with trastuzumab had stable disease that lasted greater than 17 months. A phase II trial of women with previously untreated HER2+ metastatic breast cancer is planned.

Likewise, other ongoing combination trials include the combination of lapatinib in combination with other widely used agents including cytotoxic chemotherapy (125,126), hormonal (127), and trastuzumab (128). The randomized phase II trial EGF30001, will determine the safety and the efficacy of paclitaxel in combination with lapatinib compared to lapatinib alone as first line treatment in patients with advanced or metastatic breast cancer that do not overexpress ErbB2. Patients cannot have received prior treatment for advanced or metastatic breast cancer. The primary endpoint of this trial is time to progression with secondary endpoints being time to response, duration of response, six-month progression-free survival, and overall survival. Trial EGF30008 is a randomized phase III trial utilizing letrozole plus or minus lapatinib in patients with estrogen and or progesterone receptor-positive advanced or metastatic breast cancer. The rationale for this trial centers on previous preclinical studies that suggests crosstalk between the ErbB and estrogen pathways. The primary endpoint of this trial is time to progression.

Storniolo et al. (128) initiated a phase I study to investigate the safety and efficacy of lapatinib and trastuzumab in patients with HER2-overexpressing metastatic breast cancer. Patients received trastuzumab plus escalating doses of lapatinib (750–1500 mg/day). No symptomatic declines in LVEF were noted. One patient had a compete response and five patients achieved a partial response.

Recently reported were the results of EGF100151 (129), a randomized phase III trial of capecitabine plus or minus lapatinib in women with refractory advanced breast cancer. In this phase III trial, the combination of lapatinib and capecitabine had a median time to progression of 36.9 weeks compared to 19.7 weeks for mono-therapy ($P = 0.00016$). Patients eligible for trial were those with HER2+ disease who had been treated with anthracyclines, taxanes, and trastuzumab. The response rate in the intent-to-treat population was 22% in lapatinib and capecitabine group and 14% in the capecitabine group.

CONCLUSIONS

EGFR has emerged as an attractive target for the design of targeted therapeutics. Recent studies employing monoclonal antibodies have revealed improvements in time to progression as well as overall survival. Studies with tyrosine kinase inhibitors have been less revealing but remain in their infancy of development and have provided the basis for continued research.

Despite these advances there are multiple goals for the future. These include a better understanding of the redundant pathways that exist in cell signaling, creative targeting of horizontal and vertical signaling pathways, identification of other predictive markers to better identify a targeted subpopulation of patients that will respond, and an understanding of the underlying mechanisms of resistance. Achieving these goals will be of paramount importance in the study of targeted therapy in breast cancer.

REFERENCES

1. Mendelsohn J, Baselga J. The EFG receptor family as targets for cancer therapy. Oncogene 2000; 19:6550–6565.
2. El-Rayes B, LoRusso T. Targeting the epidermal growth factor receptor. Br J Cancer 2004; 91:418–424.
3. Nahta R, Esteva FJ. Her 2 targeted therapy: lessons learned and future directions. Clin Cancer Res 2003; 9:5078–5084.

4. Schlessinger J. Cell signaling by receptor tyrosine kinases. Cell 2000; 103:211–225.
5. Simon MA. Receptor tyrosine kinases specific outcomes from general signals. Cell 2000; 103:13–15.
6. Daly RJ. Take your partners please: signal diversification by the erbB family of receptor tyrosine kinases. Growth Factors 1999; 16:255–263.
7. Riese DJ II, Stern DF. Specificity within the EGF/ErbB receptor family. Signaling network. Bioessays 1998; 20:41–48.
8. Olayioye MA, Neve RM, Lane HA, et al. The ErbB signaling network receptor hetero-dimerization in development and cancer. EMBO J 2000; 19:3154–3167.
9. Salomon DS, Brandt R, Ciardiello F, et al. Epidermal growth factor related peptides and their receptors in human malignancies. Crit Rev Oncol Hematol 1995; 19:183–232.
10. Sporn MB, Roberts AB. Autocrine secretion-10 years later. Ann Intern Med 1992; 117:408–414.
11. Tzahar E, Pinkas-Kramarski R, Moyer JD, et al. Bivalence of EGF-like ligands drives the ErbB signaling network. EMBO J 1997; 16:4938–4950.
12. Cohen S, Carpenter G. Human epidermal growth factor: isolation and chemical and biological properties. Proc Natl Acad Sci USA 1975; 72:1317–1321.
13. Derynck R. Transforming growth factor alpha. Cell 1988; 54:593–595.
14. Schreiber AB, Winkler ME, Derynck R. Transforming growth factor-alpha: a more potent angiogenic mediator than epidermal growth factor. Science 1986; 232:1250–1253.
15. Ennis BW, Lippman ME, Dickson RB. The EGF receptor system as a target for antitumor therapy. Cancer Invest 1991; 9:553–562.
16. Klijn JG, Berns PM, Schmitz PI, et al. The clinical significance of epidermal growth factor receptor (EGF-R) in human breast cancer: a review of 5232 patients. Endocr Rev 1992; 13:3–17.
17. Bucci B, D'Agnano I, Botti C, et al. EGF-R expression in ductal breast cancer: Proliferation and prognostic implications. Anticancer Res 1997; 17:769–774.
18. Klijn JG, Look MP, Portengan H, et al. The prognostic value of epidermal growth factor receptor (EGF-R) in primary breast cancer: results of a 10-year follow-up study. Breast Cancer Res Treat 1994; 29:73–83.
19. Ullrich A, Coussens L, Hayflick JS, et al. Human epidermal growth factor receptor CDNA sequence and aberrant expression of the amplified gene in A431 epidermoid carcinoma cells. Nature 1984; 309:418–425.
20. Petrides PE, Bock S, Bovens J, et al. Modulation of pro-epidermal growth factor, pro-transforming growth factor alpha and epidermal growth factor gene expression in human renal carcinomas. Cancer Res 1990; 50:3934–3939.
21. Collins VP. Gene amplification in human gliomas. Glia 1995; 15:289–296.
22. Reissman PT, Koga H, Figlin RA, et al. Amplification and overexpression of the cyclin D1 and epidermal growth factor receptor genes in non small cell lung cancer. Lung Cancer Study Group. J Cancer Res Clin Oncol 1999; 125:61–70.
23. Stumm G, Eberwein S, Rostock-Wolf S, et al. Concomitant expression of the EGFR and erbB2 genes in renal cell carcinoma (RCC) is correlated with dedifferentiation and metastasis. Int J Cancer 1996; 69:17–22.
24. Hazan RB, Norton L. The epidermal growth factor receptor modulates the interaction of E-cadherin with the actin cytoskeleton. J Biol Chem 1998; 273:9078–9084.
25. Shibata T, Kawano T, Nagayasu H, et al. Enhancing effects of epidermal growth factor on human squamous cell carcinoma motility and matrix degradation but not growth. Tumour Biol 1996; 17:168–175.
26. de Jong JS, van Diest PJ, van der Valk P, Baak, JP. Expression of growth factors, growth inhibiting factors, and their receptors in invasive breast cancer. II: correlations with proliferation and angiogenesis. J Path 1998; 184:53–57.
27. Morishige K, Kurachi H, Amemiya K, et al. Evidence for the involvement of transforming growth factor alpha and epidermal growth factor receptor autocrine growth mechanism in primary human ovarian cancers in vitro. Cancer Res 1991; 51:5322–5328.

28. Gibson S, Tu S, Oyer R, et al. Epidermal growth factor protects epithelial cells against Fas induced apoptosis: requirement for Akt activation. J Biol Chem 1999; 274:17612–17618.
29. Moscatello DK, Holgado-Madruga M, Emlet DR, et al. Constitutive activation of phosphatidylinositol 3 kinase by a naturally occurring mutant epidermal growth factor receptor. J Biol Chem 1998; 273:200–206.
30. Moscatello DK, Holgado-Madruga M, Godwin AK, et al. Frequent expression of a mutant epidermal growth factor receptor in multiple human tumors. Cancer Res 1995; 55:5536–5539.
31. Chu CT, Everiss KD, Wikstrand CJ, et al. Receptor dimerization is not a factor in signaling activity of a transforming variant epidermal growth factor receptor (EGFR VIII). Biochem J 1997; 324:855–886.
32. Semba K, Kamata N, Toyoshima K, Yamamoto T. A v-erb B related protooncogene, cerbB-2, is distinct from c-erb B/epidermal growth factor receptor gene and is amplified in a human salivary gland adenocarcinoma. Proc Natl Acad Sci USA 1985; 82:6497–6501.
33. Peles E, Bacus SS, Koski RA, et al. Isolation of the neu/HER-2 stimulatory ligand: a 44 kd glycoprotein that induces differentiation of mammary tumor cells. Cell 1992; 69:205–216.
34. Atalay G, Cardoso F, Awada A, Piccart MJ. Novel therapeutic strategies targeting the epidermal growth factor receptor (EGFR) family and its downstream effectors in breast cancer. Ann Oncol 2003; 14:1346–1363.
35. Slamon DJ, Godolphin W, Jones LA, et al. Studies of the HER-2/neu proto-oncogene in human breast and ovarian cancer. Science 1989; 244:707–712.
36. Ross JS, Fletcher JA. The HER-2/neu oncogene in breast cancer: prognostic factor, predicative factor, and target for therapy. Stem Cells 1998; 16:413–428.
37. Slamon DJ, Clark GM, Wong SG, et al. Human breast cancer: correlation of relapse and survival with amplification of the HER-2/neu oncogene. Science 1987; 235:177–182.
38. Tzahar E, Levkkowitz G, Karunagarano D, et al. ErbB-3 and ErbB-4 function as the respective low and high affinity receptors of all neu differentiation factor/heregulin isoforms. J Biol Chem 1994; 269:25226–25233.
39. Xue C, Liang F, Mahmood R, et al. ErbB-3 dependent motility and intravastion in breast cancer metastasis. Cancer Res 2006; 66:1418–1426.
40. Elenius K, Choi CJ, Paul S, et al. Characterization of a naturally occurring erbB4 isoform that does not bind or activate phosphatidylinositol 3 kinase. Oncogene 1999; 18:2607–2615.
41. Barnes NL, Khavari S, Boland GP, et al. Absence of HER4 expression predicts recurrence of ductal carcinoma in situ of the breast. Clin Cancer Res 2005; 11:2163–2168.
42. Yarden Y, Sliwkowski MX. Untangling the ErbB signaling network. Nat Rev Mol Cell Biol 2001; 2:127–137.
43. Olayioye MA, Graus-Porta D, Beerli RR, et al. ErbB-1 and ErbB-2 acquire distinct signal properties dependent upon their dimerization partner. Mol Cell Biol 1998; 18:5042–5051.
44. Ullrich A, Schlessinger J. Signal transduction by receptors with tyrosine kinase activity. Cell 1990; 61:203–212.
45. Hackel PO, Zwick E, Prenzel N, et al. Epidermal growth factor receptors: critical mediators of multiple receptor pathways. Curr Opin Cell Biol 1999; 11:184–189.
46. Bartlett JM, Langdon SP, Simpson BJ, et al. The prognostic value of epidermal growth factor mRNA expression in primary ovarian cancer. Br J Cancer 1996; 73:301–306.
47. Grandis JR, Melhem MF, Gooding WE, et al. Levels of TGF-alpha and EGFR protein in head and neck squamous cell carcinoma and patient survival. J Natl Cancer Inst 1998; 90:824–832.
48. Chow NH, Liu HS, Lee EI, et al. Significance of urinary epidermal growth factor and its receptor expression in human bladder cancer. Anticancer Res 1997; 17:1293–1296.
49. Eberhard DA, Huntzicker A, Anderson S, et al. Epidermal growth factor receptor immunochemistry (EGFR IHC): assay selection and amplification to breast cancers [abstr 1791]. Pro Am Soc Clin Oncol 2002; 21:448a.

50. Chung GG, Zerkowski MP, Ocal IT, et al. B-Catenin and p53 analysis of a breast carcinoma tissue microarray. Cancer 2004; 100:2084–2092.
51. Kersting C, Tidow N, Schmidt H, et al. Gene dosage PCR and fluorescence in situ hybridization reveal low frequency of EGFR amplifications despite overexpression in invasive breast carcinoma. Lab Invest 2004; 84:582–587.
52. Rampaul RS, Pinder SE, Paish C, et al. Quantitative analysis of breast cancer tissue microarray in the assessment of HER-2. Eur J Cancer 2003; 1:4–35.
53. Kumar RR, Meenakshi A, Sivakumar N, et al. Enzyme immunoassay of human epidermal growth factor receptor. Hum Antibodies 2001; 10:143–147.
54. Robertson KW, Reeves JR, Lannigan AK, et al. Radioimmunohistochemistry of epidermal growth factor in breast cancer. Arch Pathol Lab Med 2001; 126:177–181.
55. Pawlowski V, Revillion F, Hebbar M, et al. Prognostic value of the type 1 growth factor receptors in a large series of human primary breast cancers quantified with a real time RT-PCR assay. Clin Cancer Res 2000; 6:4217–4225.
56. Rampaul RS, Pinder SE, Nicholson RI, et al. Clinical value of epidermal growth factor receptor expression in primary breast cancer. Adv Anat Pathol 2005; 12:271–273.
57. Fox S, Smith K, Hollyer J, et al. The epidermal growth factor receptor as a prognostic marker: results of 370 patients and review of 3039 patients. Breast Cancer Res Treat 1994; 29:41–49.
58. Rampaul RS, Pinder SE, Robertson JF, et al. EGFR expression in operable breast cancer: is it of prognostic significance? Clin Cancer Res 1997; 3:1643–1651.
59. Slichenmyer WJ, Fry DW. Anticancer therapy targeting the ErbB family of receptor tyrosine kinases. Semin Oncol 2001; 28(suppl 16):67–79.
60. Wakeling AE, Guy SP, Woodburn JR, et al. ZD1839 (Iressa): an orally active inhibitor of epidermal growth factor signaling with potential for cancer therapy. Cancer Research 2002; 62:5749–5754.
61. Anderson NG, Ahmad T, Chan K, et al. ZD 1839 (Iressa), a novel epidermal growth factor receptor (EGFR) tyrosine kinase inhibitor, potentially inhibits the growth of EGFR positive cancer cell lines with or without erbB2 overexpression. Int J Cancer 2001; 94:774–782.
62. Moulder SL, Yakes FM, Muthuswamy SK, et al. Epidermal growth factor receptor (HER1) tyrosine kinase inhibitor ZD1839 (Iressa) inhibits Her2/neu (erbB2)-overexpressing breast cancer cells in vitro and in vivo. Cancer Res 2001; 61:8887–8895.
63. Moasser MM, Basso A, Averbach SD, et al. The tyrosine kinase inhibitor ZD1839 (Iressa) inhibits HER 2 driven signaling and suppresses the growth of HER 2 overexpressing tumor cells. Cancer Res 2001; 61:7184–7188.
64. Baselga J, Rischin D, Ranson M, et al. Phase I safety, pharmacokinetic, and pharmacodynamic trial of ZD1839, a selective oral epidermal growth factor receptor tyrosine kinase inhibitor, in patients with five selected solid tumor types. J Clin Oncol 2002; 20:4292–4302.
65. Herbst RS, Maddox AM, Rothenberg ML, et al. Selective oral epidermal growth factor receptor tyrosine kinase inhibitor ZD1839 is generally well tolerated and has activity in non small cell lung cancer and other solid tumors: results of a phase I trial. J Clin Oncol 2002; 20:3815–3825.
66. Nakagawa K, Tamura T, Negoro S, et al. Phase I pharmacokinetic trial of the selective oral epidermal growth factor receptor tyrosine kinase inhibitor gefitinib ("Iressa," ZD1839) in Japanese patients with solid malignant tumors. Ann Oncol 2003; 14:922–930.
67. Ranson M, Hammond LA, Ferry D, et al. ZD1839, a selective oral epidermal growth factor receptor tyrosine kinase inhibitor, is well tolerated and active in patients with solid, malignant tumors: results of a phase I trial. J Clin Oncol 2002; 20:2240–2250.
68. Albain K, Elledge R, Gradishar W, et al. Open label phase II multicenter trial of ZD1839 (Iressa) in patients with advanced breast cancer [abstr 20]. Breast Cancer Res Treat 2002; 76(S1):S33.

69. Von Minckwitz G, Jonat W, Beckman M, et al. A multicenter phase II trial to evaluate Gefitinib ('Iressa', ZD1839) (500 mg/day) in patients with metastatic breast cancer after previous chemotherapy. Eur J Cancer 2003; 1(suppl 1):S133.

70. Baselga J, Albanell J, Ruiz A, et al. Phase II and tumor pharmacodynamic study of Gefitinib (ZD 1839) in patients with advanced breast cancer. J Clin Oncol 2006; 23:5323–5333.

71. Robertson JFR, Gutteridge E, Cheung KL, et al. Gefitinib (ZD 1839) is active in acquire tamoxifen (TAM)-resistant oestrogen receptor (ER)-positive and ER-negative breast cancer: results from a phase II study [abstr 23]. Proc Am Soc Clin Oncol 2003; 22:7.

72. Levitt ML, Koty PP. Tyrosine kinase inhibitors in preclinical development. Invest New Drugs 1999; 17:213–226.

73. Huang SM, Harari PM. Epidermal growth factor receptor inhibition in cancer therapy: biology, rationale and preliminary clinical results. Invest New Drugs 1999; 17:259–269.

74. Karp PP, Silberman SL, Sudan R, et al. Phase I dose escalation study of anti-epidermal growth factor (EGFR) tyrosine kinase inhibitor CP-358, 774 in patients with advanced solid tumors [abstr 1499]. Proc Am Soc Clin Oncol 1999; 18:388a.

75. Hidalgo M, Siu LL, Nemunaitis J, et al. Phase I and pharmacological study of OSI-774, an epidermal growth factor tyrosine kinase inhibitor, in patients with advanced solid malignancies. J Clin Oncol 2001; 19:3267–3279.

76. Rowinsky EK, Hammond L, Siu L, et al. Dose–schedule-finding pharmacokinetic, biological and functional imaging studies of OSI-774, a selective epidermal growth factor receptor (EGFR) tyrosine kinase inhibitor [abstr 5]. Proc Am Soc Clin Oncol 2001; 20:2a.

77. Hammond LA, Denis LJ, Salman UA, et al. [18]FDG-PET evaluation of patients treated with the epidermal growth factor (EGFR) tyrosine kinase inhibitor, CP-358, 774 [abstr 385]. Clin Cancer Res 2000; 6(5):4543s.

78. Winer E, Cobleigh M, Dickler M, et al. Phase II multicenter study to evaluate the efficacy and safety of Tarceva (erlotinib, OSI-774) in women with previously treated locally advanced or metastatic breast cancer [abstr 445]. Breast Cancer Res Treat 2002; 76(suppl 1):S115.

79. Nanney LB, Stoscheck CM, King LE Jr, et al. Immunolocalization of epidermal growth factor receptors in normal developing human skin. J Invest Dermatol 1990; 94:742–748.

80. Jost M, Kari C, Rodeck U. The EGF receptor: an essential regulator of multiple epidermal functions. Eur J Dermatol 2000; 10:505–510.

81. Tan AR, Yang X, Hewitt SM. Evaluation of biological endpoints and pharmacokinetics in patients with metastatic breast cancer after treatment with erlotinib, an epidermal growth factor receptor tyrosine kinase inhibitor. J Clin Oncol 2004; 22:3080–3090.

82. Allen LF, Lenehan PF, Eiseman IA, et al. Potential benefits of the irreversible pan-erbB inhibitor, CI-1033, in the treatment of breast cancer. Semin Oncol 2002; 29:11–21.

83. Fry DW, Bridges AJ, Denny WA, et al. Specific, irreversible inactivation of the epidermal growth factor receptor and erbB2, by a new class of tyrosine kinase inhibitor. Proc Natl Acad Sci USA 1998; 95:12022–12027.

84. Gieseg MA, de Bock C, Ferguson LR, et al. Evidence for epidermal growth factor receptor-enhanced chemosensitivity in combinations for cisplatin and the new irreversible tyrosine kinase inhibitor CI-1033. Anticancer Drugs 2001; 12:681–682.

85. Fry DW. Site-directed irreversible inhibitors of the erbB family of receptor tyrosine kinases as novel chemotherapeutic agents for cancer. Anticancer Drug Des 2000; 15:3–16.

86. Shin DM, Nemunaitis J, Zinner RG, et al. A Phase 1 clinical and biomarker study of CI-1033, a novel pan erbB tyrosine kinase inhibitor in patients with solid tumors [abstr 324]. Proc Am Soc Oncol 2001; 20:82a.

87. Nemunaitis J, Eiseman I, Cunningham C, et al. Phase I clinical and pharmacokinetics evaluation of oral CI-1033 in patients with refractory cancer. Clin Cancer Res 2005; 11(10):3846–3853.

88. Rusnak DW, Lackey K, Affleck K, et al. The effects of the novel, reversible epidermal growth factor receptor/ErbB-2 tyrosine kinase inhibitor, GW572016, on the growth of human normal and tumor-derived cell lines in vitro and in vivo. Mol Cancer Ther 2001; 1:85–94.
89. Xia W, Mullin RJ, Keith BR, et al. Anti-tumor activity of GW572016: a dual kinase inhibitor blocks EGF activation of EGFR/erbB2 and downstream Erk1/2 and AKT pathways. Oncogene 2002; 21:6255–6263.
90. Burris HA III. Dual kinase inhibition in the treatment of breast cancer: initial experience with the EGFR/ErbB-2 inhibitor lapatinib. Oncologist 2004; 9(suppl 3):10–15.
91. Versola M, Burris H, Jones S, et al. Clinical activity of GW572016 in EGF 10003 in patients with solid tumors. J Clin Oncol 2004; 22:3047.
92. Burris HA, Hurwitz HI, Dees EC, et al. Phase I safety, pharmacokinetics, and clinical activity study of lapatinib (GW572016), a reversible dual inhibitor of epidermal growth factor receptor tyrosine kinases, in heavily pretreated patients with metastatic carcinomas. J Clin Oncol 2005; 23:5305–5313.
93. Blackwell K, Burstein H, Pegram M, et al. Determining relevant biomarkers from tissue and serum that may predict response to single agent lapatinib in trastuzumab refractory metastatic breast cancer. Proc Am Soc Oncol 2005; 23:3004.
94. Burstein H, Storniolo AM, Franco S, et al. A phase II trial, open label, multicenter study of lapatinib in two cohorts of patients with advanced or metastatic breast cancer who have progressed while receiving trastuzumab-containing regimens [abstr 1040]. Ann Oncol 2004; 15(suppl 3):iii27.
95. Gomez H, Chavez M, Doval D, et al. A Phase II, a randomized trial using the small molecule tyrosine inhibitor lapatinib as a first line treatment in patients with FISH positive advanced or metastatic breast cancer. Proc Am Soc Clin Oncol 2005; 23:3046.
96. Katz A, Zalewski P. Quality-of-life benefits and evidence of antitumor activity for patients with brain metastases treated with gefitinib. Br J Cancer 2003; 89(suppl 2); S15–S18.
97. Lin N, Carey LA, Liu MC, et al. Phase II trial of lapatinib for brain metastases in patients with HER2+ breast cancer [abstr 503]. Proc Soc Am Oncol 2006; 24:3S.
98. Lynch TJ, Bell DW, Sordella R, et al. Activating mutations in the epidermal growth factor receptor underlying responsiveness to non- small cell lung cancer to gefitinib. N Engl J Med 2004; 350:2129–2139.
99. Paez JG, Janne PA, Lee JC, et al. EGFR mutations in lung cancer: correlation with clinical response to gefitinib therapy. Science 2004; 304:1497–1500.
100. Lee JW, Soung YH, Seo SH, et al. Somatic mutations of ERBB2 kinase domain in gastric, colorectal and breast carcinomas. Clin Cancer Res 2006; 12:57–61.
101. Newby JC, Johnston SR, Smith IE, et al. Expression of epidermal growth factor receptor and c-erbB2 during the development of tamoxifen resistance in human breast cancer. Clin Cancer Res 1997; 3(9):1643–1651.
102. Nicholson RI, Gee JM. Oestrogen and growth factor cross-talk and endocrine sensitivity and acquired resistance in breast cancer. Br J Cancer 2000; 82:501–513.
103. Nicholson RI, McClelland RA, Finlay P, et al. Relationship between EGF-R, c-erbB-2 protein expression and Ki-67 immunostaining in breast cancer and hormonal sensitivity. Eur J Cancer 1993; 29A:1018–1023.
104. Nicholson RI, McClelland RA, Gee JM, et al. Epidermal growth factor receptor expression in breast cancer: association with response to endocrine therapy. Breast Cancer Res Treat 1994; 29:117–125.
105. Nicholson RI, Hutcheson IR, Knowlden J, et al. Modulation of epidermal growth factor receptor in endocrine resistance, oestrogen receptor positive breast cancer. Endocr Relat Cancer 2001; 8:175–182.
106. Nicholson RI, Hutcheson IR, Knowlden JM, et al. Nonendocrine pathways and endocrine resistance: observations with antiestrogens and signal transduction inhibitors in combination. Clin Cancer Res 2004a; 10:346S–354S.
107. Knowlden JM, Hutcheson IR, Jones HE, et al. Elevated levels of epidermal growth factor receptor/c-erbB2 heterodimers mediate an autocrine growth regulatory pathways in tamoxifen-resistant MCF-7 cells. Endocrinology 2003; 144:1032–1044.

108. Martin LA, Farmer I, Johnston SR, et al. Enhanced ER alpha ERBB2 and MAPK signal transduction pathways operate during the adaptation of MCF-7 cells to long term oestrogen deprivation. J Biol Chem 2003; 278:30458–30468.

109. McClelland RA, Barrow D, Madden TA, et al. Enhanced epidermal growth factor signaling in MCF7 breast cancer cells after long term culture in the presence of the pure antiestrogen ICI 182,780 (Faslodex). Endocrinology 2001; 142:2776–2788.

110. Agrawal A, Gutteridge E, Gee JW, et al. Overview of tyrosine kinase inhibitors in clinical breast cancer. Endocr Relat Cancer 2005; 12:S135–S144.

111. Jones HE, Goddard L, Gee JM, et al. Insulin-like growth factor-I receptor signaling and acquired resistance to gefitinib (ZD 1839;Iressa) in human breast and prostate cancer cells. Endocr Relat Cancer 2004; 11:793–811.

112. Gee M, Harper ME, Hutcheson IR, et al. The anti-epidermal growth factor receptor agent gefitinib (ZD1839/Iressa) improves antihormone response and prevents development of resistance in breast cancer in vitro. Endocrinology 2003; 144:5105–5117.

113. Cobleigh MA, Vogel CL, Tripathy D, et al. Multinational study of the efficacy and safety of humanized anti-HER 2 monoclonal antibody in women who have HER2 overexpressing metastatic breast cancer that has progressed after chemotherapy for metastatic disease. J Clin Oncol 1999; 17:2639–2648.

114. Vogel CL, Cobleigh MA, Tripathy D, et al. Efficacy and safety of trastuzumab as a single agent in first-line treatment of HER2 overexpressing metastatic breast cancer. J Clin Oncol 2002; 20:719–726.

115. Slamon DJ, Leyland-Jones B, Shak S, et al. Use of chemotherapy plus a monoclonal antibody against HER2 metastatic breast cancer that overexpresses HER2. N Engl J Med 2001; 344:783–792.

116. Robert N, Leyland-Jones B, Asmar L, et al. Updated results of a randomized phase III trial of trastuzumab, paclitaxel and carboplatin versus trastuzumab and paclitaxel in patients with HER2 overexpressing metastatic breast cancer (MBC): efficacy and safety [abstr 144]. Ann Oncol 2004; 15(suppl 3):39.

117. Burstein HJ, Harris LN, Marcom PK, et al. Trastuzumab and vinorelbine as first line therapy for HER 2-overexpressing breast cancer; multicenter phase II trial with clinical outcomes, analysis of serum tumor markers as predictive factors, and cardiac surveillance algorithm. J Clin Oncol 2003; 21:2889–2895.

118. Come SE, Buzdar AU, Arteaga CL, et al. Proceedings of the third international conference on recent advances and future directions in endocrine manipulation of breast cancer: conference summary statement. Clin Can Res 2004; 10:327S–330S.

119. Bharwani L, Schiff R, Mohsin SK, et al. Inhibiting the EGFR/HER2 pathway with gefitinib and/or trastuzumab restores tamoxifen sensitivity in HER 2 overexpressing tumors. Breast Cancer Res Treat 2003; 82:S13–14.

120. Normanno N, Campiglio M, DeLuca A, et al. The cooperative inhibitory effect of ZD 1839 (Iressa) in combination with trastuzumab (Herceptin) on human breast cancer cell growth. Ann Oncol 2002; 13:65–72.

121. Moulder SL, Arteaga CL. A Phase I/II trial of trastuzumab and gefitinib in patient with metastatic breast cancer that overexpresses HER2/neu (erbB-2). Clin Breast Cancer 2003; 4:142–145.

122. Arpino G, Weiss H, Wakeling AE, et al. Complete disappearance of ER+/HER2 + breast cancer xenografts with the combination of gefitinib, trastuzumab, and pertuzumab to block HER2 cross talk with ER and restore tamoxifen inhibition [abstr 23]. Breast Cancer Res Treat 2004; 88:S15.

123. Britten CD, Pegram M, Rosen P, et al. Targeting ErbB receptor interactions: a phase I trial of trastuzumab and erlotinib in metastatic Her2 + breast cancer [abstr 3045]. Proc Am Soc Clin Oncol 2004; 22:206.

124. Finn RS, Wilson CA, Sanders J, et al. Targeting the epidermal growth factor receptor (EGFR) and Her—2 with OSI-774 and trastuzumab, respectively, in HER—2 overexpressing human breast cancer cell lines results in a therapeutic advantage in vitro [abstr 940]. Proc Am Soc Clin Oncol 2003; 22:235.

125. Jones SF, Burris HA, Yardley DA, et al. Lapatinib (an oral dual kinase inhibitor) plus weekly or every 3 week paclitaxel. Breast Cancer Res Treat 2004; 88(suppl 1):S64.

126. Schwartz G, Chu QS-C, Hammond La, et al. Phase I clinical, biology, and pharmacokinetic study of the combination of GW 572016 and capecitabine in patients with advanced solid tumors [abstr 3070]. Proc Am Soc Oncol 2004; 23:212.
127. Chu Q, Cianfrocca ME, Murray N, et al. A phase I, open label study of the safety, tolerability and pharmacokinetics of lapatinib (GW 572016) in combination with letrozole in cancer patients [abstr 6044]. Breast Cancer Res Treat 2004; 88(suppl 1):S235.
128. Storniolo AM, Burris H, Pegram M, et al. A phase I, open label study of lapatinib (GW 572016) plus trastuzumab; a clinically active regimen [abstr 559]. J Clin Oncol 2005; 23(suppl):18s.
129. Geyer CE, Cameron D, Lindquist D, et al. A Phase II randomized, open-label international study comparing lapatinib and capecitabine vs. capecitabine in women with refractory advanced or metastatic breast cancer. Scientific Session: ASCO 2006.

19

Farnesyl Transferase Inhibitors

Tianhong Li and Joseph A. Sparano

Department of Oncology, Montefiore Medical Center, Albert Einstein Cancer Center,
New York, New York, U.S.A.

INTRODUCTION

Ras proteins belong to the small guanine triphosphate-binding protein (G protein) superfamily that is widely distributed in mammalian cells (1–3). The G protein superfamily consists of more than 100 members that are structurally classified into at least five families, including the Ras, Rho, Rab, Sar1/Arf, and Ran families. They all have consensus amino acid sequences for specific binding with guanosine diphosphate (GDP) and guanosine triphosphate (GTP), for GTPase activity (which hydrolyzes bound GTP to GDP and Pi) and for downstream effectors. G proteins regulate a wide variety of cellular functions, including gene expression in normal cell growth and differentiation (Ras), cytoskeletal reorganization and gene expression (Rho), vesicle trafficking (Rab and Sar1/Arf), nucleocytoplasmic transport (Ran), and microtubule organization (Ran). They are structurally similar and are physiologically regulated by many of the same signals. Multiple upstream regulators and downstream effectors have been identified, and their modes of activation and crosstalk have been extensively studied (4,5).

RAS PROTO-ONCOGENES

Ras proteins function as molecular switches linking receptor and nonreceptor-mediated tyrosine kinase activation to downstream cytoplasmic and nuclear events, in response to extracellular signals (4,5). They consist of four 21-kilodalton proteins (H-Ras, N-Ras, K-Ras4A, and K-Ras4B) that are encoded by three *ras* proto-oncogenes, including the *H-ras* (homologous to the oncogene of the Harvey murine sarcoma virus), *K-ras* (homologous to the oncogene of the Kirsten murine sarcoma virus), and *N-ras* genes (which does not have a retroviral homologue and was first isolated from a neuroblastoma cell line) (6). They contain 188 or 189 amino acids that have 50% to 55% sequence homology from various species. The first 86 amino acids are identical across the mammalian species, the next 78 amino acids have 79% homology, and the final 25 amino acids are highly variable but are important for post-translational modification.

POST-TRANSLATIONAL MODIFICATION OF RAS AND OTHER G PROTEINS

Small G proteins are synthesized in the cytosol of cells as an inactive precursor. Most of them require several post-translational modifications by proteolysis and addition of lipids at the "CAAX" tetrapeptide in their carboxyl termini that are crucial for their action (7). In the tetrapeptide "CAAX," "C" represents a cysteine residue, "A" represents an aliphatic amino acid (usually valine, leucine, or

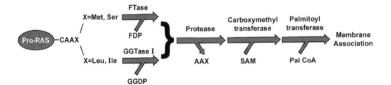

FIGURE 1 A simplified schema of post-translational modification of Ras. *Abbreviations*: AAX, a tripeptide of an aliphatic amino acid–an aliphatic amino acid–a different amino acid; FDP, farnesyl diphosphate; FTase, farnesyl trasferase; GGDP, geranylgeranyl diphosphate; GGTase I, type I geranylgeranyltransferase; Ile, isoleucine; Leu, leucine; Met, methionine; Pal CoA, palmitoyl coenzyme A; SAM, S-adenosyl-L-methionine; Ser, serine.

isoleucine), and "X" may represent different amino acids that influence the way in which the protein is modified. The first and most important post-translational modification is prenylation, which is the covalent addition of either a farnesyl (15-carbon) or a geranylgeranyl (20-carbon) isoprenoid group to the cysteine residue at the "CAAX" tetrapeptide (Fig. 1). Three classes of isoprenyltransferase enzymes have been identified in mammalian cells, including protein farnesyl transferase (FTase), type I protein geranylgeranyltransferase (GGTase-I), and type II protein geranylgeranyltransferase (GGTase-II). FTase is a heterodimeric zinc metalloenzyme composed of a 48-kilodalton alpha-subunit and 46-kilodalton beta-subunit. FTase catalyzes farnesylation of proteins in which X is methionine, serine, alanine, glutamine, or cysteine (e.g., Ras, Lamin B, Rho B) and GGTase-I catalyzes geranylgeranylation of proteins in which X is leucine, isoleucine, or phenylalanine (e.g., Rho, Rap, and Rac). GGTase-II catalyzes the geranylgeranylation of sequences CXC, CCX, or XXCC (e.g., Rab proteins). Both FTase and/or GGTase have been considered as potential therapeutic targets (8–12). FTase have many substrates in the mammalian cells, indicating that inhibition of this pathway is not specific in cancer cells and may result in unwanted toxicities.

THE RAS SIGNALING PATHWAY

Prenylated Ras proteins localize to the cytoplasmic membrane, where they serve to link activated surface receptors with downstream cytoplasmic signaling molecules, thereby regulating cytoplasmic and nuclear events, which is in response to extracellular stimuli (4,5). Typically, cell surface receptors for growth factors have tyrosine kinase activity that mediate downstream effects after ligand binding. After this binding occurs, there is receptor homodimerization and/or heterodimerization, autophosphorylation, and downstream signaling. The activity of Ras protein is tightly regulated in normal cells by guanine nucleotide exchange factors (GEFs), which positively regulate Ras signaling (by promoting formation of Ras-GDP), and GTPase-activating proteins (GAPs), which negatively regulate Ras signaling (by promoting formation of Ras-GTP). Ras-GTP activates several downstream effector pathways, including the cell survival (PI3K/AKT), proliferation (Raf/ERK/MAPK), stress kinase (SAPK/JNK, p38 MAPK), PLC/PKC/cyclin D1, and Rac/Rho pathways (Fig. 2). Ras signaling may be initiated by receptor-mediated and nonreceptor-mediated signaling, both of which are facilitated by binding with the *src*-homology 2 (SH2) and *src*-homology 3 (SH3) binding domains of growth factor receptor-binding protein (Grb2). GEFs catalyze the dissociation of GDP

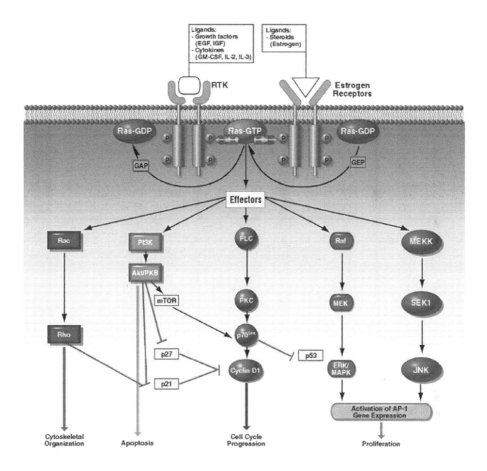

FIGURE 2   A simplified schema of normal ras signal pathway. *Abbreviations*: Akt, serine/threonine kinase (also known as protein kinase B, PKB); EGF, epidermal growth factor; ERK, extracellular signal-related kinases; GEF, guaninenucleotide-exchange factors; GM-CSF, granulocyte-macrophage colony stimulating factor; IGF, insulin-like growth factor; JNK, *c-jun* amino-terminal kinase; MAPK, mitogen-activated protein kinase; MEK, MAPK kinase; MEKK, MAPK kinase kinase; mTOR, mammalian target of rapamycin; P, phosphorylated tyrosine; p70^{S6K}, 70 kDa ribosomal S6 kinase; PI3K, phosphoinositol 3′-kinase; PKC, protein kinase C; PLC, phospholipase C; RTK, receptor tyrosine kinase; SEK, stress-activated protein kinase (SAPK)/ERK kinase.

from the inactive GTP-binding proteins; GTP can then bind and induce structural changes that allow interaction with effectors (13). GAPs, on the other hand, accelerate the rate of GTP hydrolysis by G-alpha subunits, converting active Ras-GTP to the inactive Ras-GDP (14).

ABERRANT RAS AND G PROTEIN SIGNALING IN CANCER

Oncogenic mutations of the three known human *ras* genes are found in 30% of all human cancers (15,16). Mutations are common in certain types of gastrointestinal cancers (e.g., pancreas 90%, colorectal 50%), uncommon in other cancer types (e.g., cervical 6%, breast 2%), and intermediate in other types (e.g., selective hematological malignancies 20–65%). Most of the mutations in *ras* genes are missense mutations at codons 12, 13, and 61 in exons 1 and 2. Each of these amino acid residues participates in GTP binding, and the amino acid substitutions result in the stabilization of the active GTP-bound form of Ras. These mutated Ras proteins have an intrinsic defect in GTP hydrolysis and are markedly resistant to degradation by GAPs. Although Ras mutations are rare observed in breast cancer (17,18), Ras protein overexpression or hyperactive Ras signaling frequently occurs in breast cancer (19,20). In addition to oncogenic Ras mutation, hyperactive Ras signaling may result from overexpression of upstream receptors, such as estrogen-receptor (21), HER2/neu (22), EGFR (23), or mutations in other Ras/Raf signaling molecules (24). Ras protein overexpression (not associated with *ras* mutations) is associated with poor prognosis of breast cancer (19,20). In addition, overexpression of RhoC protein, a downstream effector of Ras, is associated with local regional and/or distant metastases of breast cancer and inflammatory breast cancer (25–28).

STRATEGIES FOR TARGETING THE ABERRANT RAS/G PROTEIN PATHWAY

At least three different strategies have been developed to target the aberrant Ras/G protein pathway in cancers: (*i*) blocking upstream activation of Ras at the cell surface receptors (such as ER, HER2/neu, EGFR, or other receptor tyrosine kinases); (*ii*) targeting Ras itself by inhibiting either *Ras* gene expression (e.g., antisense molecules) or interrupting protein processing (e.g., farnesyl transferase or geranylgeranyl transferase inhibitors); and (*iii*) inhibiting downstream effector pathways (e.g., Raf kinase or MEK inhibitors)(8,29–32).

Most preclinical and clinical studies to date have been focused on inhibiting Ras/G protein prenylation with farnesyl transferase inhibitors (FTIs) (32–36). FTI s have been classified into three subclasses, including (*i*) farnesyl pyrophosphate analogs (nonpeptidomimetics), which compete with the isoprenoid substrates for FTase, (*ii*) peptidomimetic inhibitors, which mimic the structure of CAAX portion of Ras and compete with Ras for FTase, and (*iii*) bisubstrate analogs, which combine the properties of both. Two oral farnesyl transferase inhibitors that have been most extensively studied in clinical trials ranging from phase I to phase III trials, including the nonpeptidomimetic agents tipifarnib (R115777, Zarnestra™; Johnson & Johnson Pharmaceutical Research and Development, L.L.C., Raritan, New Jersey, U.S.A.) and lonafarnib (SCH66336, Sarasar®; Schering-Plough, Inc., Kenilworth, New Jersey, U.S.A.). However, only tipifarnib has been evaluated in breast cancer, both as a single agent (37), and in combination with hormonal therapy (38) and chemotherapy (39).

EFFECTS OF RAS INHIBITORS IN PRECLINICAL MODELS

There is considerable preclinical data demonstrating that FTIs have potent anti-tumor effects at clinical relevant concentrations in vitro and in vivo. Tipifarnib, significantly, inhibited the growth of all six cell lines (100%) harboring *H-ras* or *N-ras* mutations, 82% of 33 cell lines with wild type *ras* genes, and 50% of 14 cell lines with *K-ras* mutations (40). The relative resistance of cell lines harboring *K-ras* mutations may be due to prenylation mediated by GGTase-I or GGTase-II (10–12), and because Ras proteins may mediate some of their effects via alternative mechanisms that do not require prenylation (41). FTIs also inhibit the growth of MCF-7 human breast cancer xenografts (which have wild type Ras) in a dose-dependent fashion by causing cell-cycle arrest in the G2/M phase or G1 phase, and induce apoptosis in other human tumor solid tumor cell lines (42–44). In addition, FTIs also inhibit nuclear factor (NF)-kappaB (45), inhibit inflammation (46), induce reactive oxygen-mediated DNA damage (47), and inhibit angiogenesis (48). With regard to angiogenesis, Han et al. demonstrated that the FTI lonafarib inhibits the interaction between hypoxia inducible factor (HIF)-1 α and heat shock protein (hsp) 90, which promotes proteasomal degradation of the proangiogenic molecule HIF-1α (48). Resistance to FTIs has also been associated with reduced FTase activity (49), pharmacogenetic variation in FTI transport and metabolism (50), and variation in dependence on downstream signaling pathways for tumor cell growth and survival (51).

PRECLINICAL STUDIES OF RAS INHIBITORS IN COMBINATION WITH HORMONAL THERAPY

Signaling via the estrogen and progesterone receptor plays a key role in normal breast development and breast cancer progression. Both the estrogen receptor (ER) and progesterone receptor (PR) consist of ligand binding domain and DNA-binding domain, the latter of which is flanked by transcriptional activation domains (referred to as AF-1 and AF-2 for ER). Upon ligand binding, there is also binding of coactivator and corepressors that modulate chromatic structure to facilitate or repress ligand induced gene transcription upon ER binding to nuclear DNA. ER may also modulate gene expression, without the need for DNA binding, by modulating gene expression at other regulatory sequences. In addition to its effects as a nuclear transcription factor, ER may also modulate and mediate effects via membrane-associated steroid signaling that involve signaling pathways. Evidence suggests that dysregulation of growth factor signaling is an important mechanism of resistance to antiestrogen therapy (52,53). The Ras pathway and its associated downstream elements, such as mitogen-activated protein (MAP) kinase, may also activate the ER pathway independently of the ligand estrogen. For example, transcriptional activation of ER-alpha independent of estrogen is potentiated by overexpression of a dominant active Ras mutant (*c-Ki-ras*[Val 12]), constitutively active MAP kinase, or activated MAP kinase by growth factors (54). Conversely, expression of dominant negative Ras (Ras[N17]) or dominant negative MAP kinase inhibits epidermal growth factor (EGF)-induced transcriptional activation of ER, suggesting a potential means to dampen the effect of other mitogenic signals (23). FTIs may directly stimulate both ER-alpha transcriptional activity, through AF-1 and AF-2, and also ER-beta transcriptional activity (55), and enhance the antiproliferative effects of either selective estrogen receptor modulators (SERMs) such as tamoxifen by both estrogen-dependent and independent pathways (56).

PRECLINICAL STUDIES OF RAS INHIBITORS IN COMBINATION WITH CYTOTOXIC THERAPY

The Ras/Raf pathway has also been shown to play an important role in resistance to cytotoxic therapy. Increased Ras/Raf-1/MEK/MARK activity has been implicated in doxorubicin resistant MCF-7 cell line (57), paclitaxel-resistant cells (58), and the expression of the multidrug resistance (*MDR*) gene and multidrug resistance protein (MRP) (58–61). Combination of FTIs with doxorubicin (57) or paclitaxel (62–64) leads to additive or synergistic cytotoxicity in vitro. FTIs synergistically augment the antimitotic and pro-apoptotic effects of paclitaxel and other microtubule-stabilizing drugs, and result in increased tubulin acetylation (a marker of microtubule stability) (64,65); this effect appears to be a mediated FTI-induced inhibition of histone deacetylase 6 (HDAC6), the only known tubulin deacetylase (64).

MONOTHERAPY OF FARNESYL TRANSFERASE INHIBITORS IN BREAST CANCER AND OTHER DISEASES

Table 1 summarizes the results of a phase I–II trial of tipifarnib monotherapy in patients with ER-positive metastatic breast cancer who have failed second-line endocrine therapy, or with ER-negative disease (37). Seventy-six patients received either 400 mg ($N = 6$) or 300 mg ($N = 35$) twice daily on a continuous schedule, or 300 mg BID using a 3-week on, 1-week off intermittent schedule ($N = 35$). The clinical benefit rate (partial response or stable for at least 24 weeks) was comparable in the continuous (25%) and intermittent schedules (23%). There was no statistical association between response to tipifarnib and tumor characteristics, such as the status of ER, HER2, and mutation in three *ras* genes. Sites of response occurred in liver, lung, pleura, lymph nodes, breast, and skin nodules. There was significantly less toxicity associated with the intermittent compared with the continuous schedule, including neutropenia, anemia, thrombocytopenia, and neurotoxicity. Although there was high interpersonal variability in pharmacokinetics of tipifarnib, no significant differences were observed between the two dosing regimens. Daily area under the curve (AUC) plasma concentration was found to be a better predictor for severe neutropenia than the administered daily dose.

Hematologic improvement or remission has been reported in patients with acute leukemia or myelodysplastic syndrome (66–69). However, numerous phase II studies in patients with a variety of solid tumors other than breast cancer have not demonstrated any activity for FTIs when used as monotherapy (32). A phase

TABLE 1   Phase II Trial of Tipifarnib for Metastatic Breast Cancer

	Continuous dosing	Intermittent dosing
No.	41	35
Dose	400 mg BID ($N = 6$) or 300 mg BID ($N = 35$)	300 mg BID
Efficacy		
Objective response	10%	14%
Stable disease $\geq$24 weeks	15%	9%
Clinical benefit rate	25% (95% CI, 12%, 40%)	23% (95% CI, 10%, 40%)
Median duration of benefit	11.9 mo (95% CI, 4.5, 14.0 mo)	8.7 mo (95% CI, 5.6, 13.3 mo)
Median time to progression	3.2 mo (95% CI, 2.8, 4.5 mo)	2.9 mo (95% CI, 2.0, 4.0 mo)
Median overall survival	15.1 mo (95% CI, 10.3, 21.1 mo)	10.4 mo (95% CI, 7.9, 16.6 mo)
Toxicity (grade 3–4)	43%[a]	14%
Neutropenia	9%[a]	0%
Anemia	26%[a]	3%
Thrombocytopenia	12%[a]	0%

[a]Includes 300 mg BID dose only.
Source: From Ref. 37.

III trial compared tipifarnib (300 mg twice a day given for 21 consecutive days every 28 days) with a placebo in 368 patients with metastatic colorectal carcinoma who had progressive disease after two prior chemotherapy regimens. This disease and setting were chosen because of the high rate of *ras* mutations in this disease (~50%), and the lack of a standard third-line treatment regimen at the time that the trial was performed. There was no significant difference in median progression-free survival or overall survival (5.7 months vs. 6.1 months, $P = 0.396$) (70).

COMBINING FARNESYL TRANSFERASE INHIBITORS WITH HORMONAL THERAPY IN BREAST CANCER

The FTI tipifarnib has been evaluated in combination with the selective estrogen receptor modulators (i.e., tamoxifen), aromatase inhibitors (i.e., letrozole), and selective estrogen receptor down regulators (i.e., fulvestrant). Lebowitz et al. (71) reported the results of a phase I and pharmacokinetic trial evaluating tipifarnib in combination with tamoxifen in 12 patients with ER-positive metastatic breast cancer who previously had disease progression on hormonal therapy. Patients received tipifarnib (200 or 300 mg twice daily for 21 of 28 days) plus tamoxifen (20 mg once daily beginning one week of tipifarnib monotherapy). Minimal toxicity was observed at the 200-mg dose level of tipifarnib. At the 300-mg dose, all six patients required dose reduction of tipifarnib due to toxicities that included grade 2 nausea, rash and fatigue, and grade 3 diarrhea and neutropenia. Tipifarnib pharmacokinetic and pharmacodynamic variables were similar in the presence and absence of tamoxifen. Average FTase inhibition in peripheral blood mononuclear cells was 42% at 200 mg and 54% at 300 mg. Of the 12 patients treated, there were two partial responses and one stable disease for at least six months, giving an overall clinical benefit rate of 25%. Given the superiority demonstrated for aromatase inhibitor compared with tamoxifen for the treatment of advanced and early stage disease (72–74), this combination has not been explored further.

Table 2 summarizes the results of a multicenter, randomized phase II trial evaluating the efficacy of tipifarnib in combination with an aromatase inhibitor letrozole. One hundred and twenty-one postmenopausal patients with metastatic ER-positive breast cancer who had progressed after tamoxifen were randomized (1:2) to receive letrozole (2.5 mg daily) in combination with either a placebo ($N = 40$) or tipifarnib ($N = 81$) (38). The dose and schedule of tipifarnib was 300 mg BID given for 21 of 28 days. Seventy percent of patients relapsed while receiving adjuvant tamoxifen, and 30% patients progressed on tamoxifen therapy as first-line treatment for metastatic disease. The dominant site of metastasis was visceral in 57%, soft tissue in 36%, bone in 7% of patients. Objective response rate occurred in 38 % (95% CI, 23–55%) for the letrozole arm and 26% (95% CI,

TABLE 2 Randomized Phase II Trial of Letrozole vs. Letrozole Plus Tipifarnib

	Letrozole plus placebo	Letrozole plus tipifarnib
No.	40	81
Objective response	38% (95% CI, 23%, 55%)	26% (95% CI, 16%, 37%)
Stable disease >24 weeks	23%	23%
Clinical benefit rate	62% (95% CI, 45%, 77%)	49% (95% CI, 37%, 61%)

Source: From Ref. 38.

16–37%) in the tipifarnib-letrozole arm. The median duration of objective response was similar in the two treatment arms (16.0 months versus 14.8 months), and an equal proportion had stable disease for at least 24 weeks (23% in both groups). The clinical benefit rate was 62% (95% CI, 45–77%) in the letrozole alone arm, and 49% (95% CI, 37–61%) in the tipifarnib-letrozole arm. There was no difference in time to disease progression or overall survival. As expected, the incidence of grade 3/4 adverse events was higher in the tipifarnib-containing arm (45% vs. 30%, respectively), including asymptomatic neutropenia in 19%, and fatigue, nausea, and diarrhea. A randomized phase II trial of anastrazole with or without lonafarnib is accruing in metastatic breast cancer (75).

Fulvestrant more effectively inhibits the estrogen signaling pathway than either tamoxifen or aromatase inhibitors in vitro, and has been shown to be equally or more effective than tamoxifen or aromatase inhibitors (76–78). A phase II trial evaluating the combination of tipifarnib and fulvestrant is currently ongoing (79).

COMBINING FARNESYL TRANSFERASE INHIBITORS WITH CYTOTOXIC THERAPY IN BREAST CANCER AND OTHER DISEASES

Sparano et al. (39) performed a phase I trial of tipifarnib plus doxorubicin and cyclophosphamide (AC) in patients with metastatic breast cancer, followed by a phase II trial of four cycles of the tipifarnib-AC combination as preoperative therapy in patients with locally advanced breast cancer. The primary endpoint for the phase II trial was pathological complete response (pCR) in the breast at the time of definitive surgery; pCR has been used as a surrogate marker for identifying active combinations because it has been shown to predict improved disease-free survival in several prospective trials in patients with operable breast cancer (80,81) and retrospective studies in patients with locally advanced breast cancer (82). The objective of the study was to determine whether the addition of tipifarnib to standard AC chemotherapy would increase the breast pCR rate to at least 25%, a result comparable to administering sequential docetaxel following AC for a total of eight cycles (81). Eleven with metastatic breast cancer received AC [doxorubicin (60 mg/m^2) and cyclophosphamide (600 mg/m^2)] given intravenously on day 1 every three weeks ($N = 2$) or two weeks ($N = 9$) plus tipifarnib (100, 200, or 300 mg BID for 6–14 days). After excessive toxicity consisting of grade 4 febrile neutropenia was seen at the first dose level using AC every three weeks plus tipifarnib (100 mg BID) on days 1 to 14, the trial was modified to reduce the duration of tipifarnib administration (days 2–7), add filgrastim, and shorten the interval between AC cycles from every three to every two weeks. Providing further rationale for shortening the interval between AC cycles, dose-dense administration of sequential AC-paclitaxel every two weeks was shown to be more effective than the same regimen given every three weeks as adjuvant therapy (83). The recommended phase II dose of tipifarnib was 200 mg BID given on days 2 to 7 when combined with AC; dose-limiting toxicities were febrile neutropenia and grade 3 nausea and vomiting when tipifarnib was given at higher doses (300 mg BID) using the same schedule. Twenty-one patients with locally advanced breast cancer subsequently received dose-dense AC plus filgrastim and tipifarnib (200 mg BID on days 2–7) for up to four cycles, of whom seven patients (33%; 95% CI, 15–55%) had a breast pCR at surgery, and five patients (24%; 95% CI, 8–47%) had a pCR in the breast and lymph nodes. This exceeded the 10% pCR rate expected for AC treatment alone in this patient population, and met the prespecified endpoint for continuation accrual to a total of 50 patients in the second stage of the phase II trial (accrual has completed). In addition, five of 12 ER-positive cases (42%) and two of nine ER/PR-negative cases (22%) had a breast pCR. Previous studies have consistently demonstrated a lower breast pCR rate in patients with ER-positive disease (6%) compared with ER-negative disease (14%) (81), suggesting that adding tipifarnib to standard chemotherapy may be particularly effective in augmenting response to treatment in patients with ER-positive disease. Five patients had paired tumor biopsies performed before treatment and after the last tipifarnib dose during the first cycle of therapy. All patients demonstrated at least 50% (median 100%, range 55–100%) inhibition of FTase enzyme activity in the primary breast tumors in vivo, only one of whom had a breast pCR (who demonstrated 91% FTase inhibition). Additional studies are planned to confirm the effectiveness of preoperative tipifarnib combined with standard chemotherapy, particularly in patients with ER-positive disease. Nevertheless, the study provides proof of principle for inhibition of the target enzyme in humans treated with an oral FTI in a solid tumor, and suggests that integration of an FTI with standard therapy may improve the breast pCR rate. Should the clinical activity be confirmed, this may provide sufficient rationale for conducting a large-scale adjuvant trial comparing adjuvant chemotherapy with or without an FTI. However, it remains unclear what breast pCR rate should be established as a threshold for carrying forward with a larger, more definitive phase III adjuvant trial, and whether the trial should be restricted to populations that typically derive less benefit from adjuvant chemotherapy and more potentially benefit from the addition of tipifarnib (e.g., ER-positive disease).

Three other trials combining FTIs with other chemotherapy agents in patients with metastatic breast cancer are currently ongoing. In one trial (E1103), tipifarnib (300 mg BID) is being combined with capecitabine (1000 mg/m^2 BID) given for 14 of every 21-day schedule in patients who have had prior anthracycline therapy and progressive disease during taxane therapy (84). A second trial is a phase I–II trial evaluating the combination of tipifarnib (given BID for 14 days) with gemcitabine (given on days 1 and 18 every 21 days) in patients with metastatic breast cancer (85). A phase II trial evaluating the combination of lonafarnib with trastuzumab and paclitaxel in HER2/neu-positive metastatic breast cancer is also ongoing (86).

A phase III trial has been reported comparing gemcitabine given in combination with tipifarnib (200 mg twice a day continuously) or a placebo in 688 patients with untreated, locally advanced or metastatic pancreatic carcinoma, a disease that is associated with Ras mutations in about 90% of cases. There was no difference in median progression-free survival (112 days vs. 109 days, stratified log-rank $p = 0.72$) or overall survival (193 days vs. 182 days, $p = 0.75$) of providing unequivocal evidence that this is not a useful treatment strategy for this disease (87). Other ongoing studies include a randomized phase II trial of carboplatin/paclitaxel alone or in combination with lonafarnib in advanced ovarian carcinoma (88), and a phase III trial comparing lonafarnib versus placebo in patients with myelodysplastic syndrome (89). A phase III trial comparing carboplatin/paclitaxel used alone or in combination with lonafarnib in nonsmall cell lung cancer has completed accrual.

SURROGATE MARKERS FOR TARGET INHIBITION

A critical issue in evaluating the clinical efficacy of FTIs is whether the agent being utilized is effectively inhibiting farnelysation of targeted proteins. Surrogate markers that have been commonly used include measurement of prenylated G proteins in the peripheral blood mononuclear cells, including Ras, Rho, lamins A and B (90,91), centromere-binding proteins E and F (CNP-E and CNP-F), and HDJ-2 (92,93). However, there has not been a consistent association between clinical activity and the inhibition of surrogate markers (94,95). Recent microarray and proteomic studies have suggested several candidate genes and pathways for the effect of FTIs that require validation (96,97).

SUMMARY AND FUTURE DIRECTIONS

The FTIs are a novel class of agents that have been rationally designed to interrupt signaling transduction. Inhibition of the prenylation of Ras and other G proteins can alter downstream signaling pathways that regulate tumor proliferation, apoptosis, stress response, cytoskeletal organization, and membrane trafficking. Preclinical evidence suggests that these agents are active in breast cancer in vitro and in vivo, and that they can circumvent the resistance to endocrine therapy or cytotoxic chemotherapy. Some FTIs have demonstrated single agent activity in metastatic breast cancer, although it is unlikely that these agents will play an important therapeutic role when used as monotherapy. Clinical trials combining FTIs with aromatase inhibitors or tamoxifen have not produced impressive results, although trials evaluating the combination of FTIs with more potent inhibitors of the ER-signaling pathway such as fulvestrant are ongoing. One study in patients with locally advanced breast cancer demonstrated that FTIs significantly inhibit tumor FTase enzyme activity in vivo, and also suggested that adding the FTI to standard preoperative chemotherapy may significantly increase the breast pCR rate, particularly in patients with ER-positive disease; this observation merits further study. If the FTIs are to play a role in the management of breast cancer, they will need to be carefully evaluated in combination with standard therapies. Additional mechanistic studies are also required in order to identify predictive biomarkers to optimally select individuals who may benefit from FTI therapy.

REFERENCES

1. Burgoyne RD. Small GTP-binding proteins. Trends Biochem Sci 1989;14(10):394–396.
2. Chardin P. Small GTP-binding proteins of the ras family: a conserved functional mechanism? Cancer Cells 1991; 3(4):117–126.
3. Downward J. The ras superfamily of small GTP-binding proteins. Trends Biochem Sci 1990; 15(12):469-472.
4. Hall A. The cellular functions of small GTP-binding proteins. Science 1990; 249(4969):635–640.
5. Takai Y, Sasaki T, Matozaki T. Small GTP-binding proteins. Physiol Rev 2001; 81(1):153–208.
6. Takai Y, Kikuchi A, Kawata M, Yamamoto K, Hoshijima M. Purification, characterization, and possible functions of small molecular weight GTP-binding proteins. Am J Hypertens 1990; 3(8 Pt 2):220S–223S.
7. Basso AD, Kirschmeier P, Bishop WR. Thematic review series: lipid posttranslational modifications. Farnesyl transferase inhibitors. J Lipid Res 2006; 47(1):15–31.
8. Sebti SM, Hamilton AD. Inhibition of Ras prenylation: a novel approach to cancer chemotherapy. Pharmacol Ther 1997; 74(1):103–114.
9. Rowinsky EK, Windle JJ, Von Hoff DD. Ras protein farnesyltransferase: a strategic target for anticancer therapeutic development. J Clin Oncol 1999; 17(11):3631–3652.
10. Sebti SM, Hamilton AD. Farnesyltransferase and geranylgeranyltransferase I inhibitors and cancer therapy: lessons from mechanism and bench-to-bedside translational studies. Oncogene 2000; 19(56):6584–6593.

11. Thoma NH, Iakovenko A, Owen D, et al. Phosphoisoprenoid binding specificity of geranylgeranyltransferase type II. Biochemistry 2000; 39(39):12043–12052.

12. Lobell RB, Omer CA, Abrams MT, et al. Evaluation of farnesyl:protein transferase and geranylgeranyl:protein transferase inhibitor combinations in preclinical models. Cancer Res 2001; 61(24):8758–8768.

13. Cherfils J, Chardin P. GEFs: structural basis for their activation of small GTP-binding proteins. Trends Biochem Sci 1999; 24(8):306–311.

14. Paduch M, Jelen F, Otlewski J. Structure of small G proteins and their regulators. Acta Biochim Pol 2001; 48(4):829–850.

15. Feinberg AP, Vogelstein B, Droller MJ, Baylin SB, Nelkin BD. Mutation affecting the 12th amino acid of the c-Ha-ras oncogene product occurs infrequently in human cancer. Science 1983; 220(4602):1175–1177.

16. Fearon ER. K-ras gene mutation as a pathogenetic and diagnostic marker in human cancer. J Natl Cancer Inst 1993; 85(24):1978–1980.

17. Thor A, Ohuchi N, Hand PH, et al. Ras gene alterations and enhanced levels of ras p21 expression in a spectrum of benign and malignant human mammary tissues. Lab Invest 1986; 55(6):603–615.

18. Rochlitz CF, Scott GK, Dodson JM, et al. Incidence of activating ras oncogene mutations associated with primary and metastatic human breast cancer. Cancer Res 1989; 49(2):357–360.

19. Clark GJ, Der CJ. Aberrant function of the Ras signal transduction pathway in human breast cancer. Breast Cancer Res Treat 1995; 35(1):133–144.

20. Malaney S, Daly RJ. The ras signaling pathway in mammary tumorigenesis and metastasis. J Mammary Gland Biol Neoplasia 2001; 6(1):101–113.

21. Kato S, Masuhiro Y, Watanabe M, et al. Molecular mechanism of a cross-talk between oestrogen and growth factor signalling pathways. Genes Cells 2000; 5(8):593–601.

22. Smith CA, Pollice AA, Gu LP, et al. Correlations among p53, Her-2/neu, and ras overexpression and aneuploidy by multiparameter flow cytometry in human breast cancer: evidence for a common phenotypic evolutionary pattern in infiltrating ductal carcinomas. Clin Cancer Res 2000; 6(1):112–126.

23. Bunone G, Briand PA, Miksicek RJ, Picard D. Activation of the unliganded estrogen receptor by EGF involves the MAP kinase pathway and direct phosphorylation. Embo J 1996; 15(9):2174–2183.

24. Ikehara N, Semba S, Sakashita M, Aoyama N, Kasuga M, Yokozaki H. BRAF mutation associated with dysregulation of apoptosis in human colorectal neoplasms. Int J Cancer 2005; 115(6):943–950.

25. Kleer CG, Griffith KA, Sabel MS, et al. RhoC-GTPase is a novel tissue biomarker associated with biologically aggressive carcinomas of the breast. Breast Cancer Res Treat 2005; 93(2):101–110.

26. Kleer CG, van Golen KL, Zhang Y, Wu ZF, Rubin MA, Merajver SD. Characterization of RhoC expression in benign and malignant breast disease: a potential new marker for small breast carcinomas with metastatic ability. Am J Pathol 2002; 160(2):579–584.

27. Kleer CG, Zhang Y, Pan Q, et al. WISP3 and RhoC guanosine triphosphatase cooperate in the development of inflammatory breast cancer. Breast Cancer Res 2004; 6(2): R110–R115.

28. van Golen KL, Davies S, Wu ZF, et al. A novel putative low-affinity insulin-like growth factor-binding protein, LIBC (lost in inflammatory breast cancer), and RhoC GTPase correlate with the inflammatory breast cancer phenotype. Clin Cancer Res 1999; 5(9):2511–2519.

29. Gibbs JB, Oliff A, Kohl NE. Farnesyltransferase inhibitors: Ras research yields a potential cancer therapeutic. Cell 1994; 77(2):175–178.

30. Marshall CJ. Cell signalling. Raf gets it together. Nature 1996; 383(6596):127–128.

31. Adjei AA. Blocking oncogenic Ras signaling for cancer therapy. J Natl Cancer Inst 2001; 93(14):1062–1074.

32. Li T, Sparano JA. Inhibiting Ras signaling in the therapy of breast cancer. Clin Breast Cancer 2003; 3(6):405–416; discussion 17–20.

33. Wright JJ, Zerivitz K, Gravell AE, Cheson BD. Clinical trials referral resource. Current clinical trials of R115777 (Zarnestra). Oncology (Huntingt) 2002; 16(7):930–931.

34. Venet M, End D, Angibaud P. Farnesyl protein transferase inhibitor ZARNESTRA R115777—history of a discovery. Curr Top Med Chem 2003; 3(10):1095–1102.
35. Johnston SR. Farnesyl transferase inhibitors: a novel targeted therapy for cancer. Lancet Oncol 2001; 2(1):18–26.
36. Caraglia M, Budillon A, Tagliaferri P, Marra M, Abbruzzese A, Caponigro F. Isoprenylation of intracellular proteins as a new target for the therapy of human neoplasma: preclinical and clinical implications. Curr Drug Targets 2005; 6(3):301–323.
37. Johnston SR, Hickish T, Ellis P, et al. Phase II study of the efficacy and tolerability of two dosing regimens of the farnesyl transferase inhibitor, R115777, in advanced breast cancer. J Clin Oncol 2003; 21(13):2492–2499.
38. Johnston S, Semiglazov V, Manikhas G, et al. A randomised, blinded, phase II study of tipifarnib (Zarnestra) combined with letrozole in the treatment of advanced breast cancer after antiestrogen therapy. San Antonio Breast Cancer Symposium 2005:(Abstr#5087).
39. Sparano JA, Moulder S, Kazi A, et al. Targeted inhibition of farnesyltransferase in locally advanced breast cancer: a phase I and II trial of tipifarnib plus dose-dense doxorubicin and cyclophosphamide. J Clin Oncol 2006; 24:3013–3018.
40. End DW, Smets G, Todd AV, et al. Characterization of the antitumor effects of the selective farnesyl protein transferase inhibitor R115777 in vivo and in vitro. Cancer Res 2001; 61(1):131–137.
41. Pan J, Yeung SC. Recent advances in understanding the antineoplastic mechanisms of farnesyltransferase inhibitors. Cancer Res 2005; 65(20):9109–9112.
42. Sepp-Lorenzino L, Rosen N. A farnesyl-protein transferase inhibitor induces p21 expression and G1 block in p53 wild type tumor cells. J Biol Chem 1998; 273(32):20243–20251.
43. Ashar HR, James L, Gray K, et al. The farnesyl transferase inhibitor SCH 66336 induces a $G(2) \rightarrow M$ or $G(1)$ pause in sensitive human tumor cell lines. Exp Cell Res 2001; 262(1):17–27.
44. Le Gouill S, Pellat-Deceunynck C, Harousseau JL, et al. Farnesyl transferase inhibitor R115777 induces apoptosis of human myeloma cells. Leukemia 2002; 16(9): 1664–1667.
45. Takada Y, Khuri FR, Aggarwal BB. Protein farnesyltransferase inhibitor (SCH 66336) abolishes NF-kappaB activation induced by various carcinogens and inflammatory stimuli leading to suppression of NF-kappaB-regulated gene expression and up-regulation of apoptosis. J Biol Chem 2004; 279(25):26287–26299.
46. Xue X, Lai KT, Huang JF, Gu Y, Karlsson L, Fourie A. Anti-inflammatory activity in vitro and in vivo of the protein farnesyltransferase inhibitor tipifarnib. J Pharmacol Exp Ther 2006; 317:53–60.
47. Pan J, She M, Xu ZX, Sun L, Yeung SC. Farnesyltransferase inhibitors induce DNA damage via reactive oxygen species in human cancer cells. Cancer Res 2005; 65(9):3671–3681.
48. Han JY, Oh SH, Morgillo F, et al. Hypoxia-inducible factor 1 alpha and antiangiogenic activity of farnesyltransferase inhibitor SCH66336 in human aerodigestive tract cancer. J Natl Cancer Inst 2005; 97(17):1272–1286.
49. Smith V, Rowlands MG, Barrie E, Workman P, Kelland LR. Establishment and characterization of acquired resistance to the farnesyl protein transferase inhibitor R115777 in a human colon cancer cell line. Clin Cancer Res 2002; 8(6):2002–2009.
50. Sparreboom A, Marsh S, Mathijssen RH, Verweij J, McLeod HL. Pharmacogenetics of tipifarnib (R115777) transport and metabolism in cancer patients. Invest New Drugs 2004; 22(3):285–289.
51. Bruzek LM, Poynter JN, Kaufmann SH, Adjei AA. Characterization of a human carcinoma cell line selected for resistance to the farnesyl transferase inhibitor 4-(2-(4-(8-chloro-3, 10-dibromo-6,11-dihydro-5H-benzo-(5,6)-cyclohepta(1,2- b)-pyridin-11(R)-yl)-1-piperidinyl)-2-oxo-ethyl)-1-piperidinecarboxamide (SCH66336). Mol Pharmacol 2005; 68(2):477–486.
52. Nicholson RI, Gee JM. Oestrogen and growth factor cross-talk and endocrine insensitivity and acquired resistance in breast cancer. Br J Cancer 2000; 82(3):501–513.
53. Katzenellenbogen BS, Montano MM, Ekena K, Herman ME, McInerney EM. William L. McGuire Memorial Lecture. Antiestrogens: mechanisms of action and resistance in breast cancer. Breast Cancer Res Treat 1997; 44(1):23–38.
54. Kato S, Endoh H, Masuhiro Y, et al. Activation of the estrogen receptor through phosphorylation by mitogen-activated protein kinase. Science 1995; 270(5241):1491–1494.

55. Cestac P, Sarrabayrouse G, Medale-Giamarchi C, et al. Prenylation inhibitors stimulate both estrogen receptor alpha transcriptional activity through AF-1 and AF-2 and estrogen receptor beta transcriptional activity. Breast Cancer Res 2005; 7(1):R60–R70.

56. Dalenc F, Giamarchi C, Petit M, Poirot M, Favre G, Faye JC. Farnesyl-transferase inhibitor R115,777 enhances tamoxifen inhibition of MCF-7 cell growth through estrogen receptor dependent and independent pathways. Breast Cancer Res 2005; 7(6):R1159–R1167.

57. Weinstein-Oppenheimer CR, Henriquez-Roldan CF, Davis JM, et al. Role of the Raf signal transduction cascade in the in vitro resistance to the anticancer drug doxorubicin. Clin Cancer Res 2001; 7(9):2898–907.

58. Cornwell MM, Smith DE. A signal transduction pathway for activation of the mdr1 promoter involves the proto-oncogene c-raf kinase. J Biol Chem 1993; 268(21):15347–15350.

59. Kim SH, Lee SH, Kwak NH, Kang CD, Chung BS. Effect of the activated Raf protein kinase on the human multidrug resistance 1 (MDR1) gene promoter. Cancer Lett 1996; 98(2):199–205.

60. Wang E, Casciano CN, Clement RP, Johnson WW. The farnesyl protein transferase inhibitor SCH66336 is a potent inhibitor of MDR1 product P-glycoprotein. Cancer Res 2001; 61(20):7525–7529.

61. Wang EJ, Johnson WW. The farnesyl protein transferase inhibitor lonafarnib (SCH66336) is an inhibitor of multidrug resistance proteins 1 and 2. Chemotherapy 2003; 49(6): 303–308.

62. Rasouli-Nia A, Liu D, Perdue S, Britten RA. High Raf-1 kinase activity protects human tumor cells against paclitaxel-induced cytotoxicity. Clin Cancer Res 1998; 4(5):1111–1116.

63. Izbicka E, Campos D, Carrizales G, Patnaik A. Biomarkers of anticancer activity of R115777 (Tipifarnib, Zarnestra) in human breast cancer models in vitro. Anticancer Res 2005; 25(5):3215–3223.

64. Marcus AI, Zhou J, O'Brate A, et al. The synergistic combination of the farnesyl transferase inhibitor lonafarnib and paclitaxel enhances tubulin acetylation and requires a functional tubulin deacetylase. Cancer Res 2005; 65(9):3883–3893.

65. Zhu K, Gerbino E, Beaupre DM, et al. Farnesyltransferase inhibitor R115777 (Zarnestra, Tipifarnib) synergizes with paclitaxel to induce apoptosis and mitotic arrest and to inhibit tumor growth of multiple myeloma cells. Blood 2005; 105(12):4759–4766.

66. Zimmerman TM, Harlin H, Odenike OM, et al. Dose-ranging pharmacodynamic study of tipifarnib (R115777) in patients with relapsed and refractory hematologic malignancies. J Clin Oncol 2004; 22(23):4816–4822.

67. Cortes J. Farnesyl transferase inhibitor R115777 in myelodysplastic syndrome. Curr Hematol Rep 2004; 3(3):157–158.

68. Cortes J, Albitar M, Thomas D, et al. Efficacy of the farnesyl transferase inhibitor R115777 in chronic myeloid leukemia and other hematologic malignancies. Blood 2003; 101(5):1692–1697.

69. Gotlib J. Farnesyltransferase inhibitor therapy in acute myelogenous leukemia. Curr Hematol Rep 2005; 4(1):77–84.

70. Rao S, Cunningham D, de Gramont A, et al. Phase III double-blind placebo-controlled study of farnesyl transferase inhibitor R115777 in patients with refractory advanced colorectal cancer. J Clin Oncol 2004; 22(19):3950–3957.

71. Lebowitz PF, Eng-Wong J, Widemann BC, et al. A phase I trial and pharmacokinetic study of tipifarnib, a farnesyltransferase inhibitor, and tamoxifen in metastatic breast cancer. Clin Cancer Res 2005; 11(3):1247–1252.

72. Goss PE, Strasser K. Aromatase inhibitors in the treatment and prevention of breast cancer. J Clin Oncol 2001; 19(3):881–894.

73. Ariazi EA, Ariazi JL, Cordera F, Jordan VC. Estrogen receptors as therapeutic targets in breast cancer. Curr Top Med Chem 2006; 6(3):195–216.

74. Carlson RW, Brown E, Burstein HJ, et al. NCCN task force report: adjuvant therapy for breast cancer. J Natl Compr Canc Netw 2006; 4 (suppl 1):S1–S26.

75. John A. Glapsy. Phase II randomized study of Anastrazole with or without lonafarnib in postmenopausal women with hormone receptor-positive stage IIIB, IIIC or IV breast cancer. http://www.clinicaltrials.gov/ct/show/NCT00098904

76. Howell A, Robertson JF, Quaresma Albano J, et al. Fulvestrant, formerly ICI 182,780, is as effective as anastrozole in postmenopausal women with advanced breast cancer progressing after prior endocrine treatment. J Clin Oncol 2002; 20(16):3396–3403.

77. Osborne CK, Pippen J, Jones SE, et al. Double-blind, randomized trial comparing the efficacy and tolerability of fulvestrant versus anastrozole in postmenopausal women with advanced breast cancer progressing on prior endocrine therapy: results of a North American trial. J Clin Oncol 2002; 20(16):3386–3395.

78. Howell A, Robertson JF, Abram P, et al. Comparison of fulvestrant versus tamoxifen for the treatment of advanced breast cancer in postmenopausal women previously untreated with endocrine therapy: a multinational, double-blind, randomized trial. J Clin Oncol 2004; 22(9):1605–1613.

79. Vahdat LT. Phase II study of tipifarnib and fulvestrant as second-line therapy in postmenopausal women with hormone receptor-positive inoperable locally advanced or metastatic breast cancer with progressive disease after prior first-line endocrine therapy. http://www.clinicaltrials.gov/ct/show/NCT00082810

80. Fisher B, Brown A, Mamounas E, et al. Effect of preoperative chemotherapy on local-regional disease in women with operable breast cancer: findings from National Surgical Adjuvant Breast and Bowel Project B-18. J Clin Oncol 1997; 15(7):2483–2493.

81. Bear HD, Anderson S, Brown A, et al. The effect on tumor response of adding sequential preoperative docetaxel to preoperative doxorubicin and cyclophosphamide: preliminary results from National Surgical Adjuvant Breast and Bowel Project Protocol B–27. J Clin Oncol 2003; 21(22):4165–4174.

82. Guarneri V, Broglio K, Kau SW, et al. Prognostic value of pathologic complete response after primary chemotherapy in relation to hormone receptor status and other factors. J Clin Oncol 2006; 24(7):1037–1044.

83. Citron ML, Berry DA, Cirrincione C, et al. Randomized trial of dose-dense versus conventionally scheduled and sequential versus concurrent combination chemotherapy as postoperative adjuvant treatment of node-positive primary breast cancer: first report of Intergroup Trial C9741/Cancer and Leukemia Group B Trial 9741. J Clin Oncol 2003; 21(8):1431–1439.

84. William J. Gradishar. Phase II study of capecitabine and tipifarnib in women with taxane-resistant metastatic breast cancer. http://www.clinicaltrials.gov/ct/show/NCT00077363

85. Banu Arun. Phase I/II study of tipifarnib and gemcitabine in women with metastatic breast cancer. http://www.clinicaltrials.gov/ct/show/NCT00100750

86. Jan HM Schellens. Phase I study of lonafarnib, trastuzumab (herceptin®), and paclitaxel in patients with HER2/Neu-overexpressing stage IIIB, IIIC, or IV breast cancer. http://www.clinicaltrials.gov/ct/show/NCT00068757

87. Van Cutsem E, van de Velde H, Karasek P, et al. Phase III trial of gemcitabine plus tipifarnib compared with gemcitabine plus placebo in advanced pancreatic cancer. J Clin Oncol 2004; 22(8):1430–1438.

88. Werner Meier. An open-label, multicenter, randomized phase II study to compare the effects of paclitaxel/carboplatin and lonafarnib to those of paclitaxel/carboplatin for first-line treatment of patients with epithelial ovarian cancer FIGO stages IIB-IV. http://www.clinicaltrials.gov/ct/show/NCT00281515

89. Schering-Plough. A pivotal randomized study of lonafarnib versus placebo in the treatment of subjects with myelodysplastic syndrome (MDS) or chronic myelomonocytic leukemia (CMML) who are platelet transfusion dependent with or without anemia. http://www.clinicaltrials.gov/ct/show/NCT00109538

90. Adjei A, Croghan GA, Erlichman C, et al. A phase I trial of the farnesyltransferase inhibitor R115777, in combination with gemcitabine and cisplatin in patients with advanced cancer. Clin Cancer Res 2003; 9:2520–2526.

91. Kelland LR, Smith V, Valenti M, et al. Preclinical antitumor activity and pharmacodynamic studies with the farnesyl protein transferase inhibitor R115777 in human breast cancer. Clin Cancer Res 2001; 7(11):3544–3550.

92. Britten CD, Rowinsky EK, Soignet S, et al. A phase I and pharmacological study of the farnesyl protein transferase inhibitor L-778,123 in patients with solid malignancies. Clin Cancer Res 2001; 7(12):3894–3903.
93. Haas N, Peereboom D, Ranganathan S, Thistle A, Greenberg R, Ross E, Lewis N, Wright J, Hudes G. Phase II trial of R115777, an inhibitor of farnesyltransferase, in patients with hormone refractory prostate cancer. Proc Am Soc Clin Oncol 2002; 21:(abstract 271).
94. Adjei AA, Davis JN, Erlichman C, Svingen PA, Kaufmann SH. Comparison of potential markers of farnesyltransferase inhibition. Clin Cancer Res 2000; 6(6):2318–2325.
95. Moasser MM, Rosen N. The use of molecular markers in farnesyltransferase inhibitor (FTI) therapy of breast cancer. Breast Cancer Res Treat 2002; 73(2):135–144.
96. Hu W, Wu W, Verschraegen CF, et al. Proteomic identification of heat shock protein 70 as a candidate target for enhancing apoptosis induced by farnesyl transferase inhibitor. Proteomics 2003; 3(10):1904–1911.
97. Raponi M, Belly RT, Karp JE, Lancet JE, Atkins D, Wang Y. Microarray analysis reveals genetic pathways modulated by tipifarnib in acute myeloid leukemia. BMC Cancer 2004; 4(56):1–12. http://www.biomedcentral.com/1471-2407/4/56.

nab-Paclitaxel: Reducing Toxicity Using Albumin-Bound Particles as the Carrier for Paclitaxel

Joanne L. Blum

Baylor-Charles A. Sammons Cancer Center, Texas Oncology, P.A. and U.S. Oncology, Dallas, Texas, U.S.A.

INTRODUCTION

The taxanes, paclitaxel and docetaxel, are some of the most effective chemotherapeutic agents, and have an important role in the treatment of breast cancer. Because taxanes are not soluble in aqueous solution, they require a vehicle to solubilize them in an injectable form. Polyoxyethylated castor oil (Cremophor® EL; CrEL) and ethanol were used as vehicles for the first clinically available formulation of paclitaxel (solvent-based paclitaxel) (1). Docetaxel uses polysorbate 80 as its vehicle (2).

Solvent-based paclitaxel was found to be associated with severe hypersensitivity reactions in a review of reports of adverse drug reactions during phase 1 trials (3,4). On the basis of these observations, the National Cancer Institute recommended premedication with steroids and antihistamines to prevent paclitaxel-induced hypersensitivity reactions (4). Nonclinical and clinical evidence suggests that polyoxyethylated castor oil may contribute to these hypersensitivity reactions from solvent-based paclitaxel (5,6). These two solvents may also contribute to paclitaxel-associated neurotoxicity (7). Additionally, neutropenia was found to be the dose-limiting toxicity with solvent-based paclitaxel, with some reduction in severity after shortening the infusion time from 6 and 24 hours to 3 hours (4).

The reformulation of paclitaxel with albumin circumvents solvent-associated toxicity and utilizes the natural carrier role of albumin in the human circulation (8). Paclitaxel is homogenized with albumin using 130-nanometer albumin-bound (*nab*) technology to produce a colloidal suspension for intravenous infusion (*nab*-paclitaxel).

A nonclinical study of *nab*-paclitaxel and solvent-based paclitaxel compared mortality data at the 30 mg/kg/day doses of *nab*-paclitaxel and solvent-based paclitaxel (9). Toxicity was significantly less with *nab*-paclitaxel ($P = 0.0017$, Analysis of Variance). The maximum tolerated doses were 30 mg/kg/day for *nab*-paclitaxel and 13.4 mg/kg/day, which were considered to be equitoxic doses (4% for both). It has been reported that greater intratumoral accumulation was achieved with equal doses of *nab*-paclitaxel and solvent-based paclitaxel using models of five tumor types (breast, lung, ovarian, prostate, and colon). The study also showed that CrEL inhibits delivery of paclitaxel to tumor.

INITIAL CLINICAL STUDY OF *nab*-PACLITAXEL

The results of the first phase 1 study in patients with advanced solid tumors demonstrated that *nab*-paclitaxel could be given safely every three weeks without premedication (10). The first three patients were given infusions over three hours. Since no hypersensitivity reactions were observed, the remainder of the patients received treatment with a shorter infusion time (30 minutes). No acute hypersensitivity reactions occurred at either infusion rate at doses ranging from 135 to 375 mg/m².

Hematologic toxicity was dose dependent, but mild and not cumulative. The median absolute neutrophil count nadir ($\times 10^9$/L) ranged from 2.22 to 0.96. Febrile neutropenia was uncommon and no septic deaths were reported. The median platelet count nadir ($\times 10^9$/L) ranged from 173 to 204. One patient received a platelet transfusion. The investigators concluded that hematologic toxicity was less than expected and that it did not substantially effect dose and treatment decisions during the trial.

Most nonhematologic toxicities were grade 1 or 2, with no grade 4 toxicities. Nausea, vomiting, and muscle and joint aches were most common. The maximum tolerated dose of *nab*-paclitaxel was 300 mg/m² with dose-limiting toxicities (sensory neuropathy, stomatitis, and superficial keratopathy) occurring at 375 mg/m². The maximum tolerated dose was substantially higher (approximately 50%) than a typical solvent-based paclitaxel dose of 175 mg/m².

CLINICAL STUDIES IN PATIENTS WITH METASTATIC BREAST CANCER

Phase 2 Study

Because chemotherapy is typically given at the highest tolerated dose, the maximum tolerated dose achieved in the phase 1 trial (300 mg/m²) was chosen for further study in a phase 2, multicenter study (11). This trial included 63 women with histologically confirmed, measurable disease who had not received taxane therapy in the past six months. These women received a median of six cycles of *nab*-paclitaxel 300 mg/m² by intravenous infusion over 30 minutes every three weeks without antihistamine or corticosteroid premedication. Treatment was generally well tolerated with an acceptable level of dose interruptions and delays (Table 1). Dose reductions were primarily due to hematologic toxicities, and most delays were from four to eight days.

None of the women in this study experienced severe hypersensitivity reactions. The observed toxicity profile was similar to that which is typical for solvent-taxanes: grade 4 neutropenia occurred in 15 patients (24%) primarily during the first treatment cycle, grade 3 sensory neuropathy occurred in seven patients (11%), and grade 2 sensory neuropathy occurred in 12 patients (19%). Severe (grade 3 and 4) neutropenia and sensory neuropathy in this study were less frequent than reported for solvent-based paclitaxel at a lesser dose (250 mg/m² vs. 300 mg/m²) infused over three hours (73% and 22%, respectively) or 24 hours (81% and 13%, respectively) (12). Nausea, vomiting, fatigue, arthralgia, myalgia, and alopecia were reported to be easily managed, and are well recognized as taxane-associated toxicities (11).

The overall response rate for all patients was 48% (95% CI: 35.3–60.0%; complete response in two patients; partial response in 28 patients). For patients who received the drug as first-line therapy, the overall response rate was 64% (95% CI: 49.0–79.2%). Maximum confirmed responses were reported to occur most frequently at cycles 2 and 4. Median time to progression was 27 weeks for all patients and 48 weeks for responders. The median survival was 64 weeks.

TABLE 1 Summary of Dose Interruptions, Dose Delays, and Safety in a Phase 2 Trial of *nab*-Paclitaxel in 63 Patients with Metastatic Breast Cancer

Outcome measure	Number of patients (%)
Dose reductions	16 (25)
Dose delays	21 (7)
Treatment-related, severe (grades 3 and 4) hematologic toxicities (of either grade at ≥10%)	
Neutropenia	Grade 3: 17 (27)
	Grade 4: 15 (24)
Leukopenia	Grade 3: 12 (19)
	Grade 4: 3 (5)
Treatment-related, severe (grades 3 and 4) nonhematologic toxicities (of either grade at ≥10%)	
Fatigue	Grade 3: 8 (13)
	Grade 4: 0
Sensory neuropathy	Grade 3: 7 (11)
	Grade 4: 0

Source: Adapted from Ref. 11.

Phase 3 Study

A randomized, phase 3 clinical trial compared the safety and efficacy of *nab*-paclitaxel at $260 \, mg/m^2$ with those of solvent-based paclitaxel at the standard dose of $175 \, mg/m^2$ in patients with measurable metastatic breast cancer (13). The dose of solvent-based paclitaxel in this study was reduced from that used in the phase 2 study ($300 \, mg/m^2$) with the expectation that toxicity would not exceed that of the standard dose of standard (solvent-based) paclitaxel.

Patients were typically taxane-naive; three patients in each group had received taxane as part of adjuvant therapy more than a year before the study. Patients received either *nab*-paclitaxel $260 \, mg/m^2$ intravenously over 30 minutes without premedication ($n = 229$) or solvent-based paclitaxel $175 \, mg/m^2$ intravenously over three hours ($n = 225$) using standard premedication. Dosing cycles were every three weeks, and up to two dose reductions were allowed.

Dose modifications (interruptions, reductions, and delays) were reported to be infrequent (3% for *nab*-paclitaxel $260 \, mg/m^2$, and 7% for solvent-based paclitaxel $175 \, mg/m^2$) with no statistically significant difference reported. The incidence of hypersensitivity reactions also was reported to be low for both groups (<1% for *nab*-paclitaxel $260 \, mg/m^2$, and 2% for solvent-based paclitaxel $175 \, mg/m^2$). While no severe hypersensitivity was reported for the *nab*-paclitaxel 260-mg/m^2 cohort, five incidences of hypersensitivity were reported in the solvent-based paclitaxel 175-mg/m^2 cohort.

Of the adverse events of all grades reported in more than 20% of patients, neutropenia was more frequent in patients treated with solvent-based paclitaxel 175 mg/ m^2 compared with patients treated with *nab*-paclitaxel $260 \, mg/m^2$ ($P < 0.05$); sensory neuropathy, nausea, and diarrhea were more frequent in patients treated with *nab*-paclitaxel $260 \, mg/m^2$ compared with patients treated with solvent-based paclitaxel $175 \, mg/m^2$ ($P < 0.05$, Fig. 1). Grade 4 neutropenia was greater in patients treated with solvent-based paclitaxel $175 \, mg/m^2$ compared with patients treated with *nab*-paclitaxel (22% vs. 9%, $P < 0.001$). No episodes of grade 4 neuropathy were reported, and no treatment-related deaths occurred in the *nab*-paclitaxel $260 \, mg/m^2$ group. Grade 3 sensory neuropathy was greater in the *nab*-paclitaxel 260-mg/m^2 group than

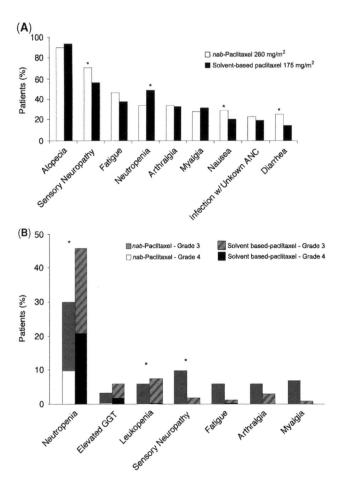

FIGURE 1 Adverse events in a phase 3 clinical trial of *nab*-paclitaxel or polyoxyethylated castor oil and ethanol-based (solvent-based) paclitaxel in 454 patients with metastatic breast cancer: (**A**) all grades reported in more than 20% of patients; (**B**) treatment-related adverse events (grade 3 and 4) reported in at least 5% of patients in either group. *P < 0.05, Cochran-Mantel-Haenszel test. *Abbreviations*: ANC, absolute neutrophil count; GGT, gamma glutamyl transferase. *Source*: Adapted from Ref. 13. Reprinted with permission from the American Society of Clinical Oncology.

in the solvent-based paclitaxel 175 mg/m² group (10% vs. 2%, P < 0.001) with a median time to improvement to grade 1 or 2 of 22 days (95% CI, 17–22).

   In a subgroup analysis, adverse events were reported to be similar in patients younger than 65 years (n = 392) compared with those who were at least 65 years of age (n = 62). In this analysis, however, patients who were at least 65 years old experienced notably fewer adverse events in the *nab*-paclitaxel group compared with those treated with solvent-based paclitaxel (Table 2). Neutropenia, leucopenia, nausea, hyperglycemia, and flushing were all reported to be more frequent in the solvent-based paclitaxel treated patients, but statistical significance was not reported. These results suggest no additional safety concerns for *nab*-paclitaxel treated women at least 65 years of age compared with younger women.

TABLE 2 Adverse Events in 62 Patients Aged 65 Years and Older in a Phase 3 Clinical Comparison of *nab*-Paclitaxel 260 mg/m^2 and Solvent-Based Paclitaxel 175 mg/m^2 in Patients with Metastatic Breast Cancer

Adverse event (any grade)	*nab*-Paclitaxel, 260 mg/m^2	Solvent-based paclitaxel, 175 mg/m^2	P value
Neutropenia	23	59	NR
Leukopenia	10	31	NR
Nausea	20	38	NR
Hyperglycemia	0	19	NR
Flushing	0	16	NR

Abbreviation: NR, not reported.
Source: Adapted from Ref. 13.

The efficacy results of *nab*-paclitaxel 260 mg/m^2 were generally favorable compared with solvent-based paclitaxel 175 mg/m^2 (Table 3). The overall response rate was greater for *nab*-paclitaxel 260 mg/m^2 compared with solvent-based paclitaxel 175 mg/m^2 in the overall population ($P = 0.001$) and in subset analyses. The overall response rates were greater for *nab*-paclitaxel 260 mg/m^2 compared with solvent-based paclitaxel 175 mg/m^2 in patients given first-line therapy for metastatic disease ($P = 0.029$), second-line or greater ($P = 0.006$), anthracycline-exposed patients in the adjuvant/metastatic setting ($P = 0.002$), metastatic setting only ($P = 0.010$), and patients with visceral-dominant disease ($P = 0.002$).

TABLE 3 Summary of Efficacy Outcomes of Phase 3 Clinical Comparison of *nab*-Paclitaxel and Solvent-Based Paclitaxel in 454 Patients with Metastatic Breast Cancer

	nab-Paclitaxel, 260 mg/m^2	Solvent-based paclitaxel, 175 mg/m^2	P value
Response [complete + partial response number of patients (%)]			
All patients	76 (33)	42 (19)	0.001
First-line therapy	41 (42)	24 (27)	0.029
Second- or greater-line therapy	35 (27)	18 (13)	0.006
Prior anthracycline therapy			
Adjuvant and/or metastatic	60 (34)	32 (18)	0.002
Metastatic only	31 (27)	18 (14)	0.010
Primary metastatic organ site			
Visceral	59 (34)	34 (19)	0.002
Age, years			
<65	68 (34)	36 (19)	<0.001
≥65	8 (27)	6 (19)	NS
Median time to progression (months)			
All patients	23.0	16.9	0.006
First-line therapy	24.0	19.7	NS
Second- or greater-line therapy	20.9	16.1	0.020
Median survival (months)[a]			
All patients	65.0	55.7	0.374
Second- or greater-line therapy	56.4	46.7	0.024

[a]At time of analysis.
Abbreviations: NS, not significant statistically; P value not reported.
Source: Adapted from Ref. 13.

Median time to progression was significantly longer with *nab*-paclitaxel 260 mg/m^2 than with solvent-based paclitaxel 175 mg/m^2 for all patients ($P = 0.006$) and for patients given second-line or greater therapy ($P = 0.020$). Time to progression in patients who received first-line therapy, however, was not statistically significant between groups (P value not reported). Patient survival (time from first dose of study drug until death) was not significantly different between the two groups ($P = 0.374$) except among those patients who received second-line or greater therapy, in which survival was significantly longer in the *nab*-paclitaxel 260 mg/m^2 population compared with the CrEL paclitaxel 175 mg/m^2 population ($P = 0.024$).

CONCLUSIONS

Safety data from the clinical trials of *nab*-paclitaxel support nonclinical findings that the albumin-bound formulation is more tolerable than the original CrEL formulation of paclitaxel, and that it may be administered at a higher dose (9,10,11,13). As a consequence, approximately a 50% higher dose of *nab*-paclitaxel than solvent-based paclitaxel was able to be administered in the phase 3 clinical comparison in patients with metastatic breast cancer (13). Owing to the different doses compared, it may not be concluded on the basis of this clinical trial alone that *nab*-paclitaxel intrinsically results in greater antitumor activity, although the nonclinical comparison of the two formulations of paclitaxel at equal doses suggests that albumin-binding may increase paclitaxel targeting of tumor (9,13). This hypothesis is further supported by evidence in the preclinical study supporting the idea that delivery of *nab*-paclitaxel to tumor occurs though active transport of albumin into tumor via an albumin-specific receptor (gp60) pathway (9).

The absence of CrEL in *nab*-paclitaxel is likely to be responsible for its improved hematologic safety profile in the phase 3 clinical trial in spite of the larger dose of paclitaxel. CrEL is known to sequester paclitaxel in the circulatory space as evidenced by the nonlinear pharmacokinetics of solvent-based paclitaxel in patients with solid tumors (14).

Overall, clinical data support that paclitaxel may be safely administered at a higher dose and a shorter infusion time without premedication using the *nab*-paclitaxel formulation than with the conventional solvent-based paclitaxel formulation in patients with breast cancer. Studies in patients with breast cancer in other settings, that is, adjuvant and neoadjuvant, at other dosing schedules, and in combination with other agents (e.g., capecitabine), are underway.

REFERENCES

1. Taxol® (paclitaxel) Injection [package insert]. Princeton, New Jersey: Bristol-Myers Squibb Co., 2003.
2. Taxotere® (docetaxel) Injection [package insert]. Bridgewater, New Jersey: Aventis Pharmaceutical Products, Inc., 2002.
3. Weiss RB, Donehower RC, Wiernik PH, et al. Hypersensitivity reactions from Taxol. J Clin Oncol 1990; 8(7):1263–1268.
4. Rowinsky EK, Eisenhauer EA, Chaudhry V, Arbuck SG, Donehower RC. Clinical toxicities encountered with paclitaxel (Taxol). Semin Oncol 1993; 20(4 suppl 3):1–15.
5. Price KS, Castells MC. Taxol reactions. Allergy Asthma Proc 2002; 23(3):205–208.
6. van Zuylen L, Verweij J, Sparreboom A. Role of formulation vehicles in taxane pharmacology. Invest New Drugs 2001; 19(2):125–141.

7. Windebank AJj, Blexrud MD, De Groen PC. Potential neurotoxicity of the solvent vehicle for cyclosporine. J Pharmacol Exp Ther 1994; 268(2):1051–1056.
8. Herve F, Urien S, Albengres E, et al. Drug binding in plasma. A summary of recent trends in the study of drug and hormone binding. Clin Pharmacokinet 1994; 26(1):44–58.
9. Desai N, Trieu V, Yao Z, et al. Increased antitumor activity, intratumoral paclitaxel concentrations, and endothelial cell transport of Cremophor-free, albumin-bound paclitaxel (ABI-007) compared with Cremophor-based paclitaxel. Clin Cancer Res 2006; 12(4):1317–1324.
10. Ibrahim NK, Desai N, Legha S, et al. Phase I and pharmacokinetic study of ABI-007, a Cremophor-free, protein-stabilized, nanoparticle formulation of paclitaxel. Clin Cancer Res 2002; 8(5):1038–1044.
11. Ibrahim NK, Samuels B, Page R, et al. Multicenter phase II trial of ABI-007, an albumin-bound paclitaxel, in women with metastatic breast cancer. J Clin Oncol 2005; 23(25):6019–6026.
12. Smith RE, Brown AM, Mamounas EP, et al. Randomized trial of 3-hour versus 24-hour infusion of high-dose paclitaxel in patients with metastatic or locally advanced breast cancer: National Surgical Adjuvant Breast and Bowel Project Protocol B-26. J Clin Oncol 1999; 17(11):3403–3411.
13. Gradishar WJ, Tjulandin S, Davidson N, et al. Phase III trial of nanoparticle albumin-bound paclitaxel compared with polyethylated castor oil-based paclitaxel in women with breast cancer. J Clin Oncol 2005; 23(31):7794–7803.
14. Sparreboom A, Scripture CD, Trieu V, et al. Comparative preclinical and clinical pharmacokinetics of a cremophor-free, nanoparticle albumin-bound paclitaxel (ABI-007) and paclitaxel formulated in Cremophor (Taxol). Clin Cancer Res 2005; 11(11):4136–4143.

21   The Epothilones

Craig A. Bunnell

Dana-Farber Cancer Institute, Harvard Medical School, Boston, Massachusetts, U.S.A.

INTRODUCTION

Microtubule-stabilizing agents are among the most effective and commonly used cytotoxic drugs in the treatment of breast cancer. Indeed, the taxanes, one class of microtubule-stabilizing agents, have become a standard treatment for patients with metastatic disease and, more recently, for those with high-risk, early-stage breast cancer. The main disadvantage of the taxanes is that tumors develop resistance to them. The epothilones, a promising new class of microtubule-stabilizing compounds, have commanded attention recently, as their mechanisms of action are similar to those of the taxanes, yet they have the potential to evade the known mechanisms of taxane resistance. This feature of the epothilones makes them valuable agents for the treatment of patients with taxane-resistant disease, an increasingly large population of patients with recurrent breast cancer.

BACKGROUND

The development of the epothilones exemplifies rational scientific drug development. This class of cytotoxic products was first isolated by Gerhard Höfle and Hans Reichenbach in 1991 from the fermentation of the myxobacterium *Sorangium cellulosum* (1,2). The name of these agents is derived from their molecular features: epoxide, thiazole, and ketone (3). Bollag et al. (4) demonstrated the microtubule-stabilizing mechanism of the epothilones.

Microtubule formation involves the polymerization of α- and β-tubulin heterodimer subunits. A dynamic equilibrium between microtubule polymerization and depolymerization is necessary for the appropriate function of the mitotic spindle. Microtubule-stabilizing agents that bind either tubulin subunits or polymerized microtubules disrupt this equilibrium by preventing depolymerization. As a result, normal spindle formation is altered, the cell cycle is arrested at the G2/M phase, and apoptosis occurs (5–9).

The epothilones and taxanes appear to have overlapping binding sites on the β-subunit of the tubulin protein heterodimer, based on studies showing that epothilones displace paclitaxel from tubulin polymers (10). In addition, epothilone-resistant cell lines contain β-tubulin mutations that map near the taxane-binding site of the docetaxel–tubulin complex, an observation that provides further support for the overlap in binding sites (11). Nevertheless, the absence of strict cross-resistance between taxanes and epothilones, as well as the unique tubulin mutational profiles of taxane-resistant cell lines, suggests that the two classes of agents interact differently with the amino acid residues that constitute their common binding site (3,12,13).

Modifications of the structure of naturally occurring epothilones have yielded multiple biologically active analogues with varying activity and toxicity profiles

(9,10,14–17). The three principal epothilone analogues under active development in breast cancer—ixabepilone (BMS-247550, aza-epothilone), patupilone (EPO906, epothilone B), and KOS-862 (epothilone D)—are reviewed here. The development of two other analogues, ZK-EPO and BMS-310705 (a water-soluble epothilone B analogue), has been put on hold.

PRECLINICAL STUDIES

Ixabepilone, patupilone, and KOS-862 all have broad-spectrum antitumor activity in cell culture and xenograft models (9). Each of the three analogues exhibits more potent tubulin-binding than paclitaxel, with tubulin polymerization induced and stabilized at lower concentrations. In addition, these epothilone analogues are generally 5 to 25 times more potent than paclitaxel in inhibiting cell growth in cultures (18). Furthermore, unlike the taxanes, the epothilones are cytotoxic against multi-drug resistant cell lines and against cells containing tubulin mutations that result in taxane-resistance (18). In vivo studies in xenograft models have corroborated the activity of epothilones against paclitaxel-sensitive and paclitaxel-resistant tumors (16).

CLINICAL STUDIES

The results of several clinical trials with epothilone analogues have been reported. Results of clinical trials with the three principal epothilone analogues under active development, ixabepilone (BMS-247550, aza-epothilone), patupilone (EPO906, epothilone B), and KOS-862 (epothilone D) are reported here. The trial with patupilone (EPO906) in patients with advanced breast cancer was halted in January 2006. Similarly, development of two other analogues, ZK-EPO and BMS310705 (a water-soluble epothilone B analogue) has, at the time of this writing, been put on hold.

IXABEPILONE (BMS-247550, AZA-EPOTHILONE)

Of the epothilone analogues in development, ixabepilone has been investigated most extensively. In vitro, ixabepilone's tubulin polymerization activity is more than twice that of paclitaxel (16). Phase I studies used four different treatment schedules: administration weekly, daily for five days every three weeks, daily for three days every three weeks, and once every three weeks. Responses were observed with each schedule in patients with a variety of cancers, including breast cancer. All the patients had drug-resistant tumors, and many had been treated previously with taxanes (19–24). Like paclitaxel, ixabepilone is administered in polyoxyethylated castor oil. Not surprisingly, hypersensitivity reactions were observed in the phase I studies, and oral histamine-1 and histamine-2 blocking agents have since been used as premedications (19). With both the once-every-three-weeks and the once-weekly dosing schedules, neutropenia, sensory neuropathy, and fatigue were dose-limiting (20,23). Interestingly, daily dosing for three or five days in a 21-day cycle altered the side-effect profile, with less neurotoxicity but more diarrhea observed (25,26).

Several phase II trials of ixabepilone in patients with advanced breast cancer have been reported. Low et al. (27) administered ixabepilone to patients with metastatic or locally advanced breast cancer who previously had received paclitaxel and/or docetaxel in the neoadjuvant, adjuvant, or metastatic setting. Patients were treated with ixabepilone at a dose of 6 mg/m^2/day given intravenously on days one through five every three weeks. Thirty-seven patients received a total of 153 cycles of ixabepilone treatment. Complete and partial responses were seen in 8 of the 37 patients (22%), and stable disease in 13 (35%). Grade-3 or -4 toxicities included neutropenia (in 35% of patients), febrile neutropenia (14%), fatigue (14%), diarrhea (11%), nausea or vomiting (5%), myalgias or arthralgias (3%), and sensory neuropathy (3%). Levels of glutamate-terminated and acetylated α-tubulin, which are markers of microtubule stabilization, were higher in tumor biopsy specimens obtained after treatment than in pretreatment specimens, corroborating the clinical activity suggested by the response rate.

Another phase II trial evaluated ixabepilone in patients with metastatic breast cancer who had previously received adjuvant treatment with an anthracycline. Nineteen patients received ixabepilone at a dose of 50 mg/m^2, given intravenously over a one-hour period every 21 days (28). The infusion time was subsequently increased to three hours because of neurotoxicity, observed in this study and in concomitant studies. After nine additional patients had been enrolled, the dose of the drug was decreased to 40 mg/m^2. Of the 65 patients who received the 40 mg/m^2 dose as a three-hour infusion every 21 days, 27 (42%) had a partial response, and 23 (35%) had stable disease. The median time to a response was six weeks (range: 5–17 weeks). The median duration of the response was 8.2 months (95% CI, 5.7–10.2 months). Of the 27 patients who responded, six did not have disease progression at for at least 12 months. Of the 23 patients with stable disease, 11 were progression-free for six or more months, and three for 12 or more months. Eleven (58%) of the 19 patients who received the 50 mg/m^2 dose as a one-hour infusion had a partial response, and six (32%) had stable disease.

With the 40 mg/m^2 dose given as a three-hour infusion, the most common hematologic toxicity was neutropenia, with grade-3 neutropenia occurring in 18 patients (27%) and grade-4 in 20 patients (31%). The median neutrophil nadir was 0.8×10^3/L (range: 0.1–4.6×10^3/L). Febrile neutropenia occurred in three (5%) patients. The most common non-hematologic treatment-related adverse event was sensory neuropathy. The neuropathy was generally mild to moderate in severity (grade-1 or -2), but 13 of the 65 (20%) patients developed grade-3 sensory neuropathy. Other grade-3 or -4 treatment-related adverse events occurring in 5% or more of the patients included myalgias (8%), vomiting (6%), and fatigue (6%).

A third phase II study of ixabepilone monotherapy was conducted in patients with prior anthracycline exposure and taxane-resistant disease, which was strictly defined (29). Patients were required to have received a paclitaxel- or docetaxel-based regimen as their most recent chemotherapy, with progression documented during or within four months after the last dose. Thirty-one percent of patients had received two or more taxane-containing regimens; 98% had received their most recent taxane regimen for metastatic disease. Objective responses were seen in 6 of 49 patients (12%), and an additional 20 (41%) patients had stable disease. The median duration of the response was 10.4 months. Treatment-related non-hematologic grade-3 adverse events were fatigue (in 27% of patients), sensory neuropathy (12%), myalgias (10%), nausea (6%), and vomiting (6%). The most common grade-3 or -4 hematologic toxicity was neutropenia (grade-3 in 33% of patients and grade-4 in 20%). Febrile neutropenia occurred in three patients. The sensory neuropathy was reported to be mostly mild to moderate in severity (grade-1 or -2), cumulative, and manageable with dose reductions. Three (6%) patients eventually discontinued treatment because of neuropathy (30).

The results of a phase II trial of ixabepilone monotherapy in patients with advanced breast cancer resistant to anthracyclines, taxanes, and capecitabine have recently become available (31). Patients in this trial had previously received at least 240 mg/m^2 of doxorubicin or at least 360 mg/m^2 of epirubicin or had developed recurrent disease less than six months after receiving an adjuvant anthracycline. They had also progressed within six months of receiving the last dose of a taxane given as adjuvant therapy or within eight weeks of the last doses of a taxane and capecitabine, if these agents were administered in the metastatic setting. A total of 113 patients could be evaluated. Ninety percent had received at least two prior chemotherapy regimens for metastatic disease and 50% had received three prior regimens; 31% percent had received a second taxane. The study investigators reported that 21 (19%) patients had a response, and an additional 16 (14%) patients had stable disease for more than six months; the clinical benefit rate (complete response, partial response, or stable disease greater than or equal to six months) was 33%.

As in other studies, the principal hematologic toxicity was neutropenia, which grade 3 or 4 in 54% of patients; febrile neutropenia was reported in only 3% of patients. Grade-3 or -4 non-hematologic toxicities included sensory neuropathy (in 14% of patients), fatigue (10%), myalgias (7%), and stomatitis (6%). The sensory neuropathy was generally managed with dose reductions; 6% of patients discontinued treatment because of neuropathy. Neuropathy improved by at lease one toxicity grade during follow-up in 82% of patients, with resolution to grade 1 or lower in 77%. The median time to improvement was 4.6 weeks, and the median time to resolution was 5.4 weeks.

The combination of ixabepilone and capecitabine was investigated in a phase I/II trial in patients with metastatic breast cancer that was resistant to anthracyclines and taxanes (32). Dose escalation was discontinued at a dose of 40 mg/m^2 for ixabepilone, given intravenously on day one of a 21-day cycle, and 2000 mg/m^2/day for capecitabine, given on days 1 through 14 of the cycle. Although these doses of the two drugs given in combination did not cause dose-limiting toxicity, the decision was made to stop the dose escalation because they are the respective, standard, single-agent doses. Of the 50 patients who received the 40 mg/m^2–2000 mg/m^2/day combination and who could be evaluated for a response, 15 (30%) had an objective response; the median duration of the response was 6.9 months.

The most common grade-3 or -4 hematologic toxicity was neutropenia (occurring in 79% of patients), with febrile neutropenia and septic shock each reported in one patient. The most common grade-3 or -4 non-hematologic toxicities were fatigue (in 34% of patients), myalgias (23%), nausea (16%), sensory neuropathy (13%), diarrhea (10%), and vomiting (10%).

Two, large, randomized studies are currently comparing ixabepilone monotherapy with ixabepilone plus capecitabine in patients with anthracycline- and taxane-resistant metastatic breast cancer. The study population for CA163-048 consists of patients who previously received anthracycline and taxane chemotherapy (33). The accrual goal is 1200 patients, and the primary endpoint is overall survival. This trial continues accrual. CA163-046, which used a strict definition of anthracycline and taxane resistance, had an enrollment goal of 750 patients and a primary endpoint of time to progression. This trial met its accrual goal and was recently closed (34).

Given the apparent synergy between trastuzumab and other microtubule-stabilizing agents (e.g., paclitaxel) in the treatment of HER2-positive breast cancer, two phase II trials of ixabepilone and trastuzumab are being conducted in women with HER2-positive metastatic disease. In one study, trastuzumab is being administered as an 8 mg/kg loading dose followed by 6 mg/kg every 21 days, with ixabepilone given at a dose of 40 mg/m^2 on day one of each cycle (35). Patients are stratified according to previous treatment, with one cohort having received no prior chemotherapy or trastuzumab for metastatic disease and another cohort having received prior chemotherapy and trastuzumab. In the second phase II trial, ixabepilone is being given in combination with weekly trastuzumab and carboplatin in a 28-day cycle (36). Trastuzumab is administered on days 1, 8, 15, and 22, with ixabepilone and carboplatin administered on days 1, 8, and 15 of a 28-day cycle.

PATUPILONE (EPO906)

Patupilone (EPO906) has been evaluated in the phase I setting, administered as a 5 to 10-minute bolus infusion either every three weeks or in a variety of weekly infusion schedules, including weekly for four weeks on/two weeks off, weekly for two weeks on/one week off, weekly for six weeks on/three weeks off, and weekly for three weeks on/one week off (37–40). The latter two weekly regimens have been the most extensively studied (38). Diarrhea was dose-limiting, regardless of the schedule, with a maximum tolerated dose of 6.0 mg/m^2 for the every three-week schedule and 2.5 mg/m^2 for the weekly schedule. Other, less common, grade-3 or -4 toxicities included nausea, vomiting, and fatigue. Serious neuropathy or myelosuppression was uncommon. Why patupilone and ixabepilone, which are structurally very similar, have such different toxicity profiles remains unclear, though differences in tissue metabolism may play a part (9). Unlike ixabepilone, patupilone can be inactivated by esterases, making tissue esterase activity a potentially important determinant of the drug's toxicity profile (41).

Several phase II trials of patupilone are being conducted in patients with a variety of cancers, including ovarian, colorectal, non-small cell lung cancer, gastric, prostate, and renal cell tumors (42–47). A phase II trial of patupilone in patients with advanced breast cancer was suspended in January 2006.

KOS-862 (EPOTHILONE D)

KOS-862 is at a relatively early stage of development in breast cancer treatment. It has been, and continues to be, investigated in several phase I studies using various dosing schedules including administration once every three weeks, fixed-rate dosing every three weeks, daily on the first three days of a three-week cycle, and weekly for three of every four weeks (48–51). Most of these phase I studies have not reported final results. Some patients who received the drug once every three weeks experienced neurologic toxicity (impaired gait, cognitive/perceptual abnormalities, and sensory neuropathies), fatigue, nausea, and vomiting (51). The neurotoxic effects generally occurred one to two days after infusion and resolved over a period of two to seven days, with no cumulative effect. A single dose given every three weeks caused more neurologic toxicity than dosing on days one, two, and three of a three-week cycle. Continuous infusions, given over a 24- or 72-hour period every two weeks, have also been investigated (50). Drug-related toxicities included fatigue, nausea, abdominal pain, dizziness, and neurosensory toxicity. Weekly dosing for three of every four weeks also caused fatigue and neurosensory toxicity (49). Final dose-limiting toxicity data have not yet been reported for any of these schedules.

In a phase II trial involving women with metastatic breast cancer who had previously received an anthracycline and a taxane, KOS-862 at a dose of 100 mg/m^2 was given intravenously as a weekly infusion for three weeks, followed by a week of rest (52). Of 29 patients who could be evaluated for a response, four (14%) had confirmed partial responses. Twenty-one of the 29 patients had peripheral sensory neuropathy, which was grade-3 in three of the patients. Grade-3 ataxia and dizziness were also reported. Overall, 18.5% of patients had grade-3 neurotoxicities. Other neurotoxicities (all grade-1 or -2) included cognitive disorder, confusion, or disorientation, memory impairment or amnesia, insomnia, hallucinations, and visual changes. The principal non-neurologic toxicities were fatigue (grade-3 in one patient), nausea (grade-3 in one patient), flushing, and anorexia. Accrual continues to the second Simon stage of this trial to determine the activity of KOS-862 in patients with anthracycline- and taxane-pretreated tumors.

SUMMARY

The epothilones are a novel class of anticancer agents that are active against taxane-sensitive and taxane-resistant breast cancer. Each of the epothilone analogues in development has demonstrated activity in women with anthracycline- and taxane-resistant metastatic breast cancer. Ixabepilone, the epothilone analogue that is furthest along in clinical development, shows promise both as monotherapy and in combination with other agents. The most common adverse events associated with ixabepilone are sensory neuropathy and neutropenia. Randomized phase III clinical trials are currently being conducted to evaluate its efficacy in combination with capecitabine for patients with advanced breast cancer. Patupilone and KOS-862, two other epothilone analogues, are currently in phase I and phase II clinical development. Despite their structural similarity to ixabepilone, these agents appear to have different toxicity profiles, with patupilone causing diarrhea rather than neurotoxicity or myelosuppression, and KOS-862 causing central nervous system and peripheral neurotoxicity. Though the therapeutic role of the epothilones has not yet been clearly defined, this new class of microtubule-targeting agents represent an important advance in the treatment of patients with breast cancer.

REFERENCES

1. Hofle G, Bedorf N, Gerth K, et al. Epothilone derivatives. Chem Abstr 1993; 120:52841.
2. Gerth K, Bedorf N, Hofle G, et al. Epothilones A and B: antifungal and cytotoxic compounds from *Sorangium cellulosum* (Myxobacteria): production, physico-chemical and biological properties. J Antibiot (Tokyo) 1996; 49:560–563.
3. Borzilleri R, Vite G. Epothilones: new tubulin polymerization agents in preclinical and clinical development. Drugs Future 2002; 27:1149–1163.
4. Bollag D, McQueney P, Zhu J, et al. Epothilones, a new class of microtubule-stabilizing agents with a taxol-like mechanism of action. Cancer Res 1995; 55:2325–2333.
5. Desai A, Mitchison T. Microtubule polymerization dynamics. Annu Rev Cell Dev Biol 1997; 13:83–117.
6. Jordan M, Toso R, Thrower D, et al. Mechanism of mitotic block and inhibition of cell proliferation by taxol at low concentrations. Proc Natl Acad Sci USA 1993; 90:9552–9556.
7. Trielli M, Andreassen P, Lacroix FB, et al. Differential taxol-dependent arrest of transformed and nontransformed cells in the G1 phase of the cell cycle, and specific-related mortality of transformed cells. J Cell Biol 1996; 135:689–700.

8. Wahl A, Donaldson K, Fairchild C, et al. Loss of normal p53 function confers sensitization to Taxol by increasing G2/M arrest and apoptosis. Nat Med 1996; 2:72–79.
9. Goodin S, Kane MP, Rubin EH. Epothilones: mechanism of action and biologic activity. J Clin Oncol 2004; 22:2015–2025.
10. Kowalski R, Giannakakou P, Hamel E. Activities of the microtubule-stabilizing agents epothilones A and B with purified tubulin and in cells resistant to paclitaxel (Taxol). J Biol Chem 1997; 272:2534–2541.
11. Nogales E, Wolf S, Khan I, et al. Structure of tubulin at 6.5 A and location of the taxol-binding site. Nature 1995; 375:424–427.
12. Giannakakou P, Sackett D, Kang Y, et al. Paclitaxel-resistant human ovarian cancer cells have mutant beta-tubulins that exhibit impaired paclitaxel-driven polymerization. J Biol Chem 1997; 272:17118–17125.
13. Giannakakou P, Gussio R, Nogales E, et al. A common pharmacophore for epothilone and taxanes: molecular basis for drug resistance conferred by tubulin mutations in human cancer cells. Proc Natl Acad Sci 2000; 97:2904–2909.
14. Borzilleri R, Zheng X, Schmidt R, et al. A novel application of a Pd(0)-catalyzed nucleophilic substitution reaction to the regio- and stereoselective synthesis of lactam analogues of the epothilone natural products. J Am Chem Soc 2000; 122:8890–8897.
15. Wartmann M, Altmann K-H. The biology and medicinal chemistry of the epothilones. Curr Med Chem Anti-Cancer Agents 2002; 2:123–148.
16. Lee F, Borzilleri R, Fairchild C, et al. BMS-247550: a novel epothilone analog with a mode of action similar to paclitaxel but possessing superior antitumor efficacy. Clin Cancer Res 2001; 7:1429–1437.
17. Chou T, Zhang X, Balog A. Desoxyepothilone B: an efficacious microtubule-targeted. Proc Natl Acad Sci 1998; 95(16):9642–9647.
18. de Jonge M, Verweij J. The epothilone dilemma. J Clin Oncol 2005; 23:9048–9050.
19. Spriggs D, Soignet S, Bienvenu B, et al. Phase I first-in-man study of the epothilone analog BMS-247550 in patients with advanced cancer [abstr]. Proc Am Soc Clin Oncol 2001; 20:428.
20. Mani S, McDaid H, Hamilton A, et al. Phase I clinical and pharmacokinetic study of BMS-247550, a novel derivative of epothilone B, in solid tumors. Clin Cancer Res 2004; 10:1289–1298.
21. Tripathi R, Gadgeel S, Wozniak A, et al. Phase I clinical trial of BMS-247550 (epothilone B derivative) in adult patients with advanced solid tumors [abstr]. Proc Am Soc Clin Oncol 2002; 21:407.
22. Awada A, Beeiberg H, de Valeriola D, et al. Phase I clinical and pharmacology study of the epothilone analog BMS-247550 given weekly in patients with advanced solid tumors [abstr]. Proc Am Soc Clin Oncol 2001; 20:427.
23. Hao D, Hammond L, deBono J, et al. Continuous weekly administration of the epothilone-B derivative, BMS-247550 (NSC710428): a phase I and pharmacokinetic (PK) study. Proc Am Soc Clin Oncol 2002; 21:411.
24. Thambi P, Edgerly M, Agarwal M, et al. A phase I trial of BMS-247550, an epothilone B derivative, given daily for 3 days on a 21 day cycle in patients with refractory neoplasms [abstr]. Proc Am Soc Clin Oncol 2003; 22:540.
25. Zhuang S, Agrawal M, Bakke S, et al. A phase I clinical trial of ixabepilone (BMS-247550), an epothilone B analog, administered intravenously on a daily schedule for 3 days. Cancer 2005; 103:1932–1938.
26. Abraham J, Agrawal M, Bakke S. Phase I trial and pharmacokinetic study of BMS-247550, an epothilone B analog, administered intravenously on a daily schedule for five days. J Clin Oncol 2003; 21:1866–1873.
27. Low J, Suparna B, Lee J, et al. Phase II clinical trial of ixabepilone (BMS-247550), an epothilone B analog, in metastatic and locally advanced breast cancer. J Clin Oncol 2005; 23:2726–2734.
28. Roche H, Cure H, Bunnell C, et al. A phase II study of epothilone analog BMS-247550 in patients (pts) with metastatic breast cancer (MBC) previously treated with an anthracycline [abstr]. Proc Am Soc Clin Oncol 2003; 22:69.

29. Conte P, Thomas E, Martin M, et al. Phase II study of ixabepilone in patients (pts) with taxane-resistant metastatic breast cancer (MBC): final report [abstr]. Proc Am Soc Clin Oncol 2006; 24:10505.

30. Fornier M, Martin M, Klimovsky J, et al. Manageable safety profile in patients with taxane-resistant metastatic breast cancer (MBC) treated with ixabepilone: final report [abstr]. Proc Am Soc Clin Oncol 2006; 24:10587.

31. Thomas E, Perez E, Mukhopadhyay P, et al. Phase II trial of ixabepilone in patients with metastatic breast cancer (MBC) who are resistant to an anthracycline, a taxane and capecitabine [abstr]. Proc Am Soc Clin Oncol 2006; 24:660.

32. Bunnell C, Klimovsky J, Thomas E. Final efficacy results of a phase I/II trial of ixabepilone in combination with capecitabine in patients with metastatic breast cancer (MBC) previously treated with a taxane and an anthracycline [abstr]. Proc Am Soc Clin Oncol 2006; 24:10511.

33. Epothilone (ixabepilone) plus capecitabine versus capecitabine alone in patients with advanced breast cancer. http://ww.clinicaltrials.gov/ct/show/CNT00082433?order=4.

34. Novel epothilone plus capecitabine versus capecitabine alone in patients with advanced breast cancer. http://www.clinicaltrials.gov/ct/show/NCT000803017order=1.

35. Trastuzumab and ixabepilone in treating women with HER2-positive metastatic breast cancer. http://www.clinicaltrials.gov/ct//gui/show/NCT00079326.

36. Trastuzumab, ixabepilone, and carboplatin in treating patients with HER2/neu-positive metastatic breast cancer. http://www.clinicaltrials.gov/ct//gui/show/NCT00077376.

37. Rubin EH, Siu L, Beers S, et al. A phase I and pharmacologic trial of weekly epothilone B in patients with advanced malignancies [abstr]. Proc Am Soc Clin Oncol 2001; 20:270.

38. Rubin EH, Rothermel J, Tesfaye F, et al. Phase I dose-finding study of weekly single-agent patupilone in patients with advanced solid tumors. J Clin Oncol 2005; 23: 9120–9129.

39. Altaha R, Fojo T, Reed E, et al. Epothilones: a novel class of non-taxane microtubule-stabilizing agents. Curr Pharm Des 2002; 8:1707–1712.

40. Calvert P, O'Neill V, Twelves C, et al. A phase I and pharmacokinetic study of EPO906 (epothilone B), given every three weeks, in patients with advanced solid tumors [abstr]. Proc Am Soc Clin Oncol 2001; 20:429.

41. Rothermel J, Wartmann M, Chen T, et al. EPO906 (epothilone B): a promising novel microtubule stabilizer. Semin Oncol 2003; 30(suppl 3):51–55.

42. Hsin K, Boyer M, Ducreux M, et al. Efficacy of patupilone in advanced local or metastatic gastric cancer: a phase IIa trial [abstr]. Proc Am Soc Clin Oncol 2006; 24:4069.

43. Osterlind K, Sanchez J, Zatloukal P, et al. Phase I/II dose escalation trial of patupilone every 3 weeks in patients with non-small cell lung cancer. Proc Am Soc Clin Oncol 2005; 23:647.

44. Sánchez J, Mellemgaard A, Perry M, et al. Efficacy and safety of patupilone in non-small cell lung cancer (NSCLC): a phase I/II trial [abstr]. Proc Am Soc Clin Oncol 2006; 24:7104.

45. Smit W, Sufliarsky J, Spanik S, et al. Phase I/II dose-escalation trial of patupilone every 3 weeks in patients with relapsed/refractory ovarian cancer [abstr]. Proc Am Soc Clin Oncol 2005; 23:5056.

46. Poplin E, Moore M, O'Dwyer P, et al. Safety and efficacy of EPO906 in patients with advanced colorectal cancer: a review of 2 phase II trials [abstr]. Proc Am Soc Clin Oncol 2003; 22:1135.

47. Thompson J, Swerdloff J, Escudier B, et al. Phase II trial evaluating the safety and efficacy of EPO906 in patients with advanced renal cancer [abstr]. Proc Am Soc Clin Oncol 2003; 22:1628.

48. Rosen P, Rosen L, Britten C, et al. KOS-862 (epothilone D): results of a phase I dose-escalating trial in patients with advanced malignancies [abstr]. Proc Am Soc Clin Oncol 2002; 21:413.

49. Spriggs D, Dupont J, Pezzulli S. KOS-862 (Epothilone D): phase I dose-escalating and pharmacokinetic (PK) study in patients with advanced malignancies [abstr]. Proc Am Soc Clin Oncol 2003; 22:894.

50. Holen K, Syed S, Hannah L, et al. Phase I study using continuous intravenous (CI) KOS-862 (Epothilone D) in patients with solid tumors [abstr]. Proc Am Soc Clin Oncol 2004; 22:2024.
51. Piro L, Rosen L, Parson G, et al. KOS-862 (epothilone D): a comparison of two schedules in patients with advanced malignancies [abstr]. Proc Am Soc Clin Oncol 2003; 22:539.
52. Buzdar A, Silverman P, Kaufman P, et al. A phase II study of KOS-862 (epothilone D) in anthracycline and taxane pretreated metastatic breast cancer: updated results [abstr]. Breast Cancer Res Treat 2005; 94S1:1087.

22 Antiangiogenic Agents in Breast Cancer

John T. Salter and Kathy D. Miller

Division of Hematology/Oncology, Indiana University, Indianapolis, Indiana, U.S.A.

INTRODUCTION

Angiogenesis represents a complex mechanism of finely regulated mediators that act to promote new blood vessel growth and migration. This physiologic process is typically active only under specific circumstances where new blood vessels are recruited to aid in wound healing, promote overall growth of an organism (e.g., developing embryo), or in unique events, such as female menstruation (1). In 1971, Folkman (2) described the association between angiogenesis and the malignant potential of solid neoplasms, and proposed that without neovascularization, tumors would reach a maximum diameter of 2 to 3 mm (the maximum distance for the adequate diffusion of oxygen), and then enter a dormant state. He went on to hypothesize that by releasing a soluble chemical signal, tumors could effectively "activate" new blood vessel formation and growth, providing the necessary supply of oxygen and nutrients for continued growth and malignant transformation. By attempting to block this "tumor-angiogenesis factor" he hoped to one day be able to arrest neoplastic growth in this early stage, providing a powerful tool in the fight against cancer. In the 30 years since Folkman's initial work, much has been elucidated about the regulation of angiogenesis and the potential targets within these pathways that might be exploited to halt malignant growth. Breast cancer research has recently seen a flood of work aimed at these very specific targets, many of which seem promising in a disease that continues to affect thousands of women every year. If Folkman's predictions hold true, one means for arresting breast cancer in its early stages and preventing its malignant course may lie in the elegant controls of angiogenesis.

EVIDENCE SUPPORTING THE ROLE OF ANGIOGENESIS IN BREAST CANCER

Angiogenesis has been shown to be critical in the growth and development of many solid tumors, including breast cancer (3). Many tumors also rely on this process for malignant transformation and the development of distant metastases (4). Translational work has confirmed these mechanisms in breast cancer, lending merit to the pursuit of antiangiogenesis targets in the treatment of this disease. Both hyperplastic murine breast papillomas and normal breast lobules develop new blood vessels when adjacent to malignant breast tissue (5,6). Studies such as these suggest that angiogenesis may in fact precede the transformation from mammary hyperplasia to malignancy. Further support for the role of angiogenesis in breast cancer has been shown in the correlative studies linking micro-vessel density (MVD) and the risk of malignant transformation. Fibrocystic lesions with the highest MVD have an increased risk for the development of invasive breast cancers (7). High MVD has also been linked to more aggressive ductal carcinoma in situ lesions (8), higher risk of metastatic disease (9), and shorter relapse-free and overall survival (OS) in node-negative breast cancers (10). Finally, there have been studies linking increased MVD to increased expression of vascular endothelial growth factor (VEGF) (8). This finding may hold one of the critical links in the targeting of angiogenesis, as VEGF has been found to hold a pivotal role in the formation of new blood vessels under both physiologic and pathologic conditions.

VASCULAR ENDOTHELIAL GROWTH FACTOR AND THE "ANGIOGENIC SWITCH"

Under normal physiologic conditions, pro-angiogenic and antiangiogenic mediators exist in a delicate balance (11). With appropriate stimulus (e.g., hypoxia, metabolic stress, and inflammation) the balance is "tipped" in favor of angiogenesis, and the switch promoting new vessel growth and recruitment is activated (12,13). Hypoxia is the characteristic event, which leads to the expression of hypoxia induced factor-1α (HIF-1α), triggering a cascade of events that culminates in the transcription of mRNA and the resultant increased expression of VEGF. Upon binding to its receptors, VEGF activates crucial signaling pathways leading to cell proliferation, increased vasopermeability, inhibition of apoptosis, and ultimately angiogenesis (11). Hypoxia is not the only stimulus for VEGF expression, and increased transcription of VEGF has been associated with a variety oncogenes, including mutant ras, erbB-2/HER2, activated epidermal growth factor receptor (EGFR), and bcr−abl (14,15). Many solid tumors produce VEGF as means of promoting pathologic angiogenesis, and up-regulation of VGEF mRNA has been found in the vast majority of human malignancies, including breast cancer (11,16). Researchers have identified high degrees of VEGF expression in invasive ductal cell carcinomas, metastatic ductal cell carcinomas, and comedo-type ductal carcinomas, whereas lobular carcinomas seem to have relatively lower expression (17). Elevated serum VEGF levels have been observed in patients with invasive breast cancers, predominantly in ductal cell carcinomas and those tumors expressing positivity for estrogen receptors (18). While still the subject of much debate, higher levels of VEGF in the serum have been linked to higher rates of recurrence and distant metastasis (19). Further studies have shown a correlation between increased tumor VEGF expression and poorer outcomes (including worsened relapse-free and OS in patients with resected primary breast cancers (20−22). In addition, other work has demonstrated resistance to both tamoxifen and chemotherapy in advanced breast cancers expressing increased VEGF (23). With such mounting evidence suggesting the key pathogenic role of VEGF in breast cancer, efforts to target this mediator were initiated with a variety of settings. If successful, we may develop, as Folkman (2) stated, "a powerful adjunct to present methods of cancer therapy."

Targeting Vascular Endothelial Growth Factor

In a study examining 64 resected breast cancer specimens, researchers looked at the degree of expression of various pro-angiogenic factors (24). While it was found that all specimens expressed at least six of the factors considered, the expression of VEGF in these tumors exceeded all other factors in the majority of specimens. On the basis of these and similar findings in translational work, many have concluded that VEGF may in fact be the key regulatory factor in angiogenesis, and perhaps by specifically targeting this pathway one could "turn-off" the angiogenic switch (1,11). This has launched a series of efforts aimed at potentially targeting the VEGF ligand, its receptors, intracellular receptor tyrosine-kinase domains, or the associated downstream signaling mediators, all with the hope of halting pathologic angiogenesis. While many approaches are still under investigation, the most studied and successful to date involves the development of a monoclonal antibody directed against the VEGF-A isoform, the most predominant and active ligand in this pathway. Initial efforts yielded promising results with demonstrable in vivo inhibition of tumor growth by the administration of an anti-VEGF monoclonal antibody (25). Subsequent studies confirmed these findings in a variety of cell lines, each showing that the addition of anti-VEGF antibodies could successfully block angiogenesis and inhibit in vivo tumor growth (26–28). This work has lead to the development of a humanized, monoclonal antibody directed at the VEGF-A ligand that has gained considerable attention in recent years, particularly in the treatment of breast cancer. Bevacizumab (Avastin®, Genentech, San Francisco, CA) is currently the only FDA-approved monoclonal antibody aimed at specifically inhibiting angiogenesis in solid tumors (29). Bevacizumab has been shown to effectively bind the soluble VEGF-A ligand, preventing binding to its receptors (*Flt-1 and KDR/Flk-1*), and essentially disrupting the initial signal in the angiogenic cascade. While bevacizumab is currently only approved for use with bolus IFL (irinotecan, 5-FU and leucovorin) in first-line therapy for metastatic colorectal cancer (30), it has shown potential in early trials investigating its use in nonsmall lung cancer (31), renal cell carcinoma (32), and breast cancer. In breast cancer studies, the benefits of adding this agent are still being evaluated, but much of the preliminary data suggests a role in both the metastatic and adjuvant settings.

Bevacizumab and Breast Cancer

Following initial phase I trials evaluating dosing and tolerability in a variety of advanced solid tumors, investigators looked at the safety and efficacy of single agent bevacizumab in a phase II trial (33). In this study, 75 women with previously treated, metastatic breast cancer (70% receiving two or more prior chemotherapy regimens) were assigned to receive single-agent bevacizumab at escalating doses starting at 3 mg/kg IV every other week, up to 20 mg/kg every other week. The overall response rate in this pretreated population was 9.3% (confirmed response rate 6.7%), with a median duration of confirmed response of 5.5 months, and a reported 17% of patients with stable disease or better after five months of therapy. The drug was well tolerated at all doses, with increased incidence of headache, nausea, and vomiting at the 20 mg/kg dose. The most substantial toxicity was hypertension (seen in 23% of participants, 18.6% requiring treatment) and proteinuria (1+ in 12.5%, 2+ in 2.7%, and 3+ in 8.3). Four patients (5.3%) discontinued the drug because of adverse events (AEs) (one patient with hypertensive encephalopathy, one with proteinuria, one with nephritic syndrome, and one with headache, nausea, and vomiting) (Table 1). There were no reported episodes of significant bleeding in these patients. Axillary/subclavian venous thrombosis was seen in two patients with indwelling central catheters, but no episodes of lower extremity venous thrombosis or pulmonary embolus were observed. On the basis of these findings, the authors concluded that bevacizumab was active as monotherapy in metastatic breast cancer, with an acceptable toxicity profile,

TABLE 1 Serious Adverse Events Seen with Bevacizumab[a]

Hypertension, including hypertensive crisis
Proteinuria including nephrotic syndrome
Thrombosis (venous and arterial)-including cerebral and myocardial infarction, transient ischemic attacks (TIA), and deep venous thrombosis
Bleeding and hemorrhage
Impaired wound healing
Congestive heart failure[b]

[a]Results from multiple clinical trials including studies in colorectal cancer, non-small cell lung cancer, renal cell carcinoma, and breast cancer.
[b]Seen only in patients receiving anthracyclines and/or left chest-wall irradiation.

supporting the initiation of trials investigating its use in combination with other chemotherapy agents in similar patients.

Combination of Chemotherapy with Bevacizumab
The theory that targeting angiogenesis could improve the efficacy of traditional chemotherapy has been proposed for several years, based largely on preclinical studies demonstrating a synergistic effect when these two approaches are combined (34,35). There are various theories as to how combining these agents could promote increased efficacy of one another when used in vivo. Anti-VEGF treatments may help to "normalize" the chaotic architecture of blood vessels associated with tumors, reducing vascular permeability and interstitial fluid pressure within the tumor itself, potentially improving drug delivery (i.e., cytotoxic agents) to the cancer (36). The fact that antiangiogenesis agents and traditional chemotherapy agents work by very different mechanisms to arrest tumor growth also argues in favor of combining these approaches to achieve maximum disease control. The first large trial investigating combined antiangiogenic and cytotoxic agents in breast cancer patients was a randomized phase III, study comparing responses with capecitabine plus bevacizumab to capecitabine alone (37). This study reported by Miller et al. enrolled 462 women with metastatic breast cancer, all receiving prior chemotherapy, and randomized them to receive either single-agent capecitabine (2500 mg/m^2/day twice daily for 14 days, followed by a seven day rest period) or the combination of capecitabine plus bevacizumab (15 mg/kg IV every three weeks). Patients continued therapy for a maximum of 35 cycles or until disease progression or toxicity warranted their withdrawal from the study. Patients in the combination arm could continue bevacizumab alone at disease progression—those on capecitabine monotherapy were not permitted to crossover to receive bevacizumab at any time during the trial. There was a reported doubling in the objective response rate (ORR) from 9.1% in the single-agent arm to 19.8% in the combination arm, which reached statistical significance ($P = 0.001$). Unfortunately, the results for progression-free survival (PFS) and OS were not similarly impacted. They reported a PFS of 4.86 months versus 4.17 months [hazard ration = 0.98, (95% CI 0.77–1.25), $P = 0.857$] and OS of 15.1 months versus 14.5 months. The addition of bevacizumab did not impact the frequency or severity of capecitabine-related toxicities, but was related to several AEs by itself. Hypertension and proteinuria were reported at higher frequency in the combination arm; there were no reported grade 4 events for either. Four patients discontinued bevacizumab due to hypertension, and two discontinued the treatment due to grade 3 proteinuria. Bevacizumab was associated

with an increase in minor mucosal bleeding, with significantly higher numbers of grades 1 and 2 epistaxis occurring in the combination arm. There were no reported grade 4 bleeding events, and each arm reported only one grade 3 event. The incidence of thrombosis and thromboembolic events was infrequent and similar in both treatment arms. There was an apparent increase in congestive heart failure in the combination arm (nine patients developed grade 3 or 4 events) versus the control arm (two similar events), the significance of which was uncertain, but did warrant further evaluation. These findings clearly indicate that the addition of bevacizumab to capecitabine does increase response rates in this population of pre-treated patients with a reasonable profile for both safety and tolerability. However, there was no survival benefit derived from the combination in this study a finding that left doubt in the minds of many as to the exact role for bevacizumab in this setting. Timing may be a crucial issue in these patients, as many received multiple lines of prior chemotherapy before receiving bevacizumab in this study. If this is true, then earlier treatment in the first-line metastatic or even the adjuvant settings may hold greater potential for angiogenesis-inhibitors to truly make an impact in disease-free and survival outcomes.

Fortunately, the disappointing results in the initial phase III study did not discourage researchers from looking to answer this very question. If timing were an essential element of the angiogenesis cascade, then perhaps blocking this pathway in first-line metastatic disease may show improvements in ORR, PFS, and OS compared to the patients in the prior phase III study who had received prior therapy for their disease. This lead to a second phase III trial (E2100) investigating the role of bevacizumab in metastatic breast cancer (38). This intergroup study enrolled 722 women with locally recurrent or metastatic breast cancer and randomized them to receive either single agent, weekly paclitaxel (90 mg/m^2 intravenously days 1, 8, and 15 every four weeks) or the same dose/schedule of paclitaxel plus bevacizumab (10 mg/kg days 1 and 8). At the time of first interim analysis (with updates), the authors were able to report a stunning benefit not only in overall response rates, but now for the first time in PFS and in OS (39). Overall response rates were significantly improved in the combination arm (29.9% vs. 13.8%; $P < 0.0001$) and in the subset of patients with measurable disease (34.3% vs. 16.4%; $P < 0.0001$). With an interim reporting of 484 events, PFS was also improved (11.4 months vs. 6.11 months; HR = 0.51, $P < 0.001$). The current data regarding OS is still immature and will require further observation before a trend is identified. Toxicity and tolerability data reported are consistent with prior studies, showing higher rates of hypertension and proteinuria in those patients receiving bevacizumab. These findings now support the role of bevacizumab in the treatment of advanced breast cancer, providing the impetus for further studies to investigate and hopefully refine the use of this potentially powerful agent.

While data from E2100 continue to accumulate, work on exploring the role of bevacizumab in the adjuvant setting is already under way. Many have held that if Folkman's theories were true, then the most beneficial use of antiangiogenesis agents would take place in adjuvant treatment. There is concern, however, regarding potential cardiac-toxicities that could develop in the adjuvant setting, particularly in patients receiving anthracyclines with bevacizumab (Table 2). An Eastern Cooperative Oncology Group (ECOG) pilot trial (E2104) will look specifically at this issue in patients with lymph node-positive, resected primary breast cancers. By design the study will look to evaluate the incidence of clinical congestive heart failure in the adjuvant setting with the use of these agents, with secondary

TABLE 2 Reported Incidence of Congestive Heart Failure with Bevacizumab

Study/regimen	Observed incidence of congestive heart failure
Bevacizumab monotherapy in breast cancer	2/75 patients (2.7%)—both received prior doxorubicin
Capecitabine +/− bevacizumab in breast cancer	2 (0.9%) vs. 7 (3.1%)
E2100—bevacizumab + paclitaxel in breast cancer	Preliminary data showing 1/342 (0.3%)
AML (1-beta-d-arabinofuranosylcytosine, mitoxantrone, and bevacizumab)	6% incidence of CHF
Neoadjuvant AT + bevacizumab inflammatory breast	2/21 (9.5%)
Doxorubicin + bevacizumab metastatic sarcomas	2/17 (11.8%) CHF + 4/17 (23.5%) decrease LVEF

Note: AT, doxorubicin and docetaxel.
Abbreviations: AML, acute myeloid leukemia; CHF, congestive heart failure; LVEF, left-ventricular ejection fraction.
Source: Adapted from Refs. 29, 38, 40, 62, 63, 82, 83.

endpoints looking at changes in left ventricular ejection fraction (LVEF) and non-cardiac toxicity. Patients will be assigned to either standard dose–dense combination doxorubicin/cyclophosphamide plus initial bevacizumab (10 mg/kg IV days every two weeks) or the dose–dense combination doxorubicin/cyclophosphamide without the addition of bevacizumab. Both arms will then go on to receive paclitaxel (175 mg/m^2 IV every two weeks) with bevacizumab (10 mg/kg IV every two weeks) for four cycles, followed by single-agent bevacizumab (10 mg/kg IV every two weeks) for an additional 18 cycles in the up-front arm, and/or additional 22 cycles in the remaining arm. Interim data from this trial has not yet been reported.

A definitive adjuvant trial has also been proposed and is currently awaiting final approval and activation from advisory committees. E5103 is a similarly designed adjuvant trial that will look at the impact of bevacizumab in combination with every three-week doxorubicin plus cyclophosphamide (AC), followed by weekly paclitaxel (T) in women with earlier stages of breast cancer. Once this study is initiated, the data on up-front bevacizumab will accumulate, providing the much needed answer to the critical questions of timing in the application of antiangiogenesis therapies in breast cancer. While these studies continue to collect data, several other phase II trials have looked at combining bevacizumab with other agents, including docetaxel in neoadjuvant (40) and advanced disease (41) vinorelibine (42), and letrozole (43). Investigators have also looked at the role of bevacizumab in combination with doxorubicin and docetaxel in the treatment of inflammatory and locally advanced breast cancer with promising findings based on several surrogate markers (44). Trials such as these will continue to provide data, hopefully determining the right combinations and schedules of agents that work best in conjunction with bevacizumab in breast cancer patients.

Combining Bevacizumab with Other Targeted Therapies
Angiogenesis is a complex process comprised of multiple signaling pathways. Many of these pathways are redundant, with several ligand–receptor combinations

resulting in the same eventual down-stream cascade of events. This observation has lead many to speculate that simultaneous blockade of multiple pathways might have an even greater impact on halting angiogenesis and slowing tumor growth and progression. Early work in this area discovered a link between the expression of human epidermal growth factor receptor 2 (HER2) and increased transcriptional regulation of VEGF (45). With the known impact of HER2 overexpression in breast cancer, efforts turned to evaluate not only the role of this receptor in angiogenesis, but also the possible additional effect on this process if blocked. The addition of a specific neutralizing anti-erbB2/neu monoclonal antibody in vitro to human breast cancer cell lines overexpressing this receptor resulted in the dose-dependent reduction of VEGF protein expression (46). This, combined with evidence that HER2 gene amplification correlated with higher levels of angiogenesis in breast cancer (47), and the development of a more malignant phenotype in breast cancer patients (48) lead to the proposed combination of anti-HER2 and anti-VEGF antibodies. Pegram et al. (49) first proposed this combined modality approach in 2002, and followed with a phase I trial employing bevacizumab and the anti-HER2 antibody trastuzumab (Herceptin®; Genentech, San Francisco, California, U.S.A.) (50). In this study, nine patients with HER2 overexpressing, metastatic or recurrent breast cancer received trastuzumab (4 mg/kg loading dose, then 2 mg/kg IV weekly) plus bevacizumab (10 mg/kg IV every 14 days) until progression. The authors reported one complete response (CR) and four partial reponses (PRs) and two patients with stable disease. There were no grade III/IV AEs observed, and pharmacokinetic studies did not reveal the alteration of levels of either antibodies with co-administration. Thus, this combination appears safe, well tolerated, and active in breast cancer patients over-expressing HER2. Phase II trials are currently ongoing to provide additional data in this area.

There is similar preclinical evidence suggesting an interaction between EGFR and VEGF in the angiogenesis signaling cascade. EGFR may transcriptionally up-regulate VEGF expression (51), and subsequent blockade of these receptors with antibodies (4,46), or blocking their associated tyrosine kinase signaling mechanisms (52) has been showed to decrease VEGF transcription and expression. Combined blockade of EGFR and VEGF has been evaluated in several solid malignancies with mixed results reported thus far. ZD6474, a dual inhibitor of the VEGF-receptor 2-tyrosine kinase and EGFR-associated tyrosine kinase, has shown impressive preclinical efficacy in blocking the formation of atypical ductal hyperplasia and carcinoma-in-situ in laboratory rats treated with 7,12-dimethylbenz[a]anthracene (53). In a phase II trial, single-agent ZD6474 was administered to 46 women with previously treated metastatic breast cancer (54). While this agent was well-tolerated with minimal reported toxicity, there were no objective responses seen in any of the dosing cohorts evaluated. Current studies are now evaluating the tyrosine kinase inhibitor erlotinib in combination with bevacizumab in patients with metastatic breast cancer (55). More work will obviously need to be done in this area before any definitive conclusions can be drawn about the synergy or efficacy of these agents in combination.

METRONOMIC CHEMOTHERAPY

Agents directed at VEGF may not be the only effective means of addressing neoplastic angiogenesis. In fact, many commonly employed cytotoxic agents appear to possess antiangiogenic capabilities both in vitro and in vivo (56,57). On the basis of several preclinical studies, the notion of "metronomic" chemotherapy as an antiangiogenic strategy was proposed (58), and the idea has received renewed interest in light of the success of other angiogenesis inhibitors in the treatment of cancer. Metronomics is based on the premise that continuous delivery of low-dose cytotoxic agents without a prolonged drug-free interval will selectively inhibit proliferating endothelial cells in the tumor, thus disrupting the blood supply and arresting malignant growth (59). In addition, this technique has also been shown to decrease circulating endothelial progenitor cells (CEPs) that would otherwise be incorporated into forming tumor vasculature (60). There are several potential advantages to this strategy over the more traditional method of administering higher dose cytotoxic regimens (34). This strategy reduces treatment related toxicity as drug efficacy will not require administering the maximally-tolerated dose of a single agent in order to achieve a clinical benefit. Metronomics could also conceivably be combined with other treatment modalities, such as targeted monoclonal antibodies, with a potential synergy that would not pose significant additive side effects. This type of treatment could also be administered for a prolonged duration, possibly maintaining a state of durable remission or stable disease. The most promising agents evaluated with this technique are methotrexate, cyclophosphamide, vinblastine, paclitaxel, and docetaxel. Preclinical data have also shown possible synergy combining metronomic therapy with the thrombospondin peptide ABT-510, a combination in the lab that seems to slow tumor take in metastasis, and stabilize tumor growth via increased endothelial cell apoptosis and angio-suppression (61). In immunodeficient mice with widespread human breast cancer xenografts, employing metronomic schedules of drug administration resulted in a marked prolongation of survival with minimal observed toxicity (62).

Several phase II trials have looked at using metronomic treatments in patients with advanced breast cancer, including a nonrandomized trial of 64 women with metastatic breast cancer treated with a combination of low-dose oral methotrexate and cyclophosphamide (63). This relatively small study revealed an overall response rate of 19%, with two CRs, 10 PRs, and an overall clinical benefit (CR + PR + stable disease >24 weeks) of 31.7%. The regimen was well tolerated, and may offer an alternative to more toxic regimens in patients with metastatic disease. More recently, a group from Dana Farber/Harvard Cancer Center reported results from a phase II, randomized study comparing metronomic-scheduled, oral cyclophosphamide and methotrexate with and without the addition of bevacizumab in patients with advanced breast cancer (64). Results presented at the 2005 San Antonio Breast Cancer Symposium demonstrated clear improvements in response rates for the combination arm compared with metronomic therapy alone. The group reported two PRs for the chemotherapy alone group (10%), compared with 10 PRs for the chemotherapy plus bevacizumab arm (29%). Median time-to-progression was also increased in the combined arm (5.5 months vs. 2.0 months), and toxicities appear minimal between the two arms. An adjuvant pilot trial comparing metronomic therapy with and without bevacizumab in postoperative breast cancer patients with residual disease has been proposed as a follow-up to this study. Trials such as this may lead the way to a new approach to patients for whom traditional cytotoxic agents cannot be used due to limiting comorbidities.

OTHER ANTIANGIOGENIC AGENTS IN INVESTIGATION

While bevacizumab has lead the efforts in antiangiogenesis studies, several other agents have shown promise in early clinical investigation. A second class of agents specifically targeting the VEGF receptor tyrosine kinase has seen a few compounds reach phase II trials with varying success. SU11248 (sunitinib, Sutent®, Pfizer, New York, NY), a multi-targeted tyrosine-kinase inhibitor which blocks not only the VEGF-receptors, but also platelet-derived growth factor receptor (PDGFR), c-kit and Flt-3, has recently been approved for the treatment of gastrointestinal stromal tumors and renal cell carcinoma. Since breast cancer has been shown to express several of these receptors, SU11248 should be effective in blocking several pathways regulating angiogenesis in breast carcinomas. In fact, preclinical data support this notion (65) leading to a recently reported phase II trial where single agent SU11248 demonstrated activity in heavily pretreated patients with refractory metastatic breast cancer (66). Toxicity in this trial did prompt dose-reductions in several patients, and future studies should look to explore alternative dosing schedules in patients with less refractory disease.

The matrix metalloproteinase inhibitors are agents designed to block the action of naturally occurring enzymes whose overexpression in cancer leads to the degradation of the basement membrane and extracellular matrix, promoting conditions favorable for angiogenesis and metastasis (67). The ECOG performed a randomized, placebo-controlled, phase III trial looking at the use of marimastat, an oral MMPI, versus placebo in patients with metastatic breast cancer following first-line chemotherapy (68). This study (E2196) evaluated 190 patients with responding or stable disease following six to eight cycles of prior first-line treatment. The findings revealed no significant difference in median PFS or OS between the groups, and in fact higher plasma marimastat levels were associated with an increased risk of death in the treatment arm. Additional studies looking at MMPIs in other cancers have similarly failed to show any treatment benefit with these agents, and one agent (BAY12-9566) has even shown diminished survival in treated patients with pancreatic cancer (vs. gemcitabine) (69). Thus these agents have largely been abandoned in active clinical investigation.

Two-methoxyestradiol (2-ME), a naturally occurring metabolite of estradiol that disrupts microtubule function, has been shown to inhibit proliferating cells and inhibit angiogenesis in vitro. Human breast cancer cells have shown particular sensitivity to this agent, making it an intriguing choice for clinical study. In fact, preclinical studies with breast cancer xenografts in mice showed a 60% suppression in growth in these tumors after one month of treatment with 2-ME with minimal toxicity (70). In addition, this same group showed that treatment with 2-ME could reduce VEGF-induced neovascularization by 54%. Studies combining 2-ME with other microtubule inhibitors (vinorelbine and paclitaxel) demonstrated superior tumor control in breast cancer xenografts in nude mice, with little additional toxicity (71). Early clinical work with 2-ME in patients with metastatic breast cancer, both as a single-agent (72) or combined with docetaxel (73), showed a reasonable response rate with most patients tolerating the drug quite well. Further studies looking at a newer preparation of 2-ME are currently underway.

ISSUES REGARDING THE FUTURE OF ANTIANGIOGENESIS THERAPY

As the blockade of angiogenesis comes to the forefront of cancer therapy, a number of new and compelling issues arise as a consequence. Defining clinical response to these agents poses a significant problem in many regards. Traditional cytotoxic chemotherapy uses objective indicators for tumor response that may not be applicable in settings where angiogenesis inhibition may be most effective (i.e., in earlier stages of disease). If the efficacy of these drugs is truly inversely related to tumor burden, then it may turn out that their use will be most beneficial in patients with limited measurable disease (74). Thus, there is a need to identify alternative surrogate markers by which angiogenesis inhibition can be followed, and tumor response can be monitored. Noninvasive assessment of tumor vasculature by various methods, including computed tomography (CT), dynamic contrast-enhanced magnetic resonance imaging (DCE-MRI), and positron emission tomography (PET), have all been evaluated for this application (75,76). Many clinical trials evaluating angiogenesis agents alone or in combination with other drugs are now employing these imaging techniques as an additional means of objectively evaluating responses in their study patients (44). In the adjuvant setting, however, imaging may have little role when primary tumors have been resected completely. This has lead researchers to seek measurable markers in blood and urine specimens, which could potentially mirror treatment response. Among the possible surrogate markers that are currently being evaluated are serum and urine VEGF levels, CEPs, soluble vascular cell adhesion molecule-1 (VCAM-1), and others. While intuition would suggest that declining circulating VEGF would correlate with clinical response, several studies have refuted this notion (59,75), where others have shown declining serum VEGF levels to be a marker of response (78). Further prospective studies are needed to validate these markers as potential surrogate indicators of biologic response.

Studying agents designed to be targeted therapy can be difficult when trials cannot select patients for the presence of specific markers of drug activity. We have learned that agents, such as trastuzumab, are very effective in a carefully selected patient population, but may offer no benefit if studied in all patients with breast cancer. Similarly, we may find that properly identifying molecular markers that correlate with efficacy will make angiogenesis therapy more effective, by identifying those patients who stand to benefit the most from the treatment (79). The difficulty thus far lies in identifying which sub-group of patients who will ultimately be most responsive to treatment. Immunohistochemistry for VEGF expression is being evaluated both retrospectively (80) (although not all tumor blocks in previous studies will be available) and now prospectively in on-going clinical trials with bevacizumab. Still, there is no consensus or standardization for measuring VEGF tissue expression at present—an issue that makes sub-group analysis more difficult should a response be identified. Perhaps a future goal should be to develop a clearly defined system of stratifying tumor marker expression for angiogenesis inhibitors. With these criteria, one could begin to perform prospective studies with patients selected for a cut-off threshold of expression, theoretically choosing those patients most likely to respond to the experimental treatment.

The timing of antiangiogenesis therapy also leaves significant open questions for clinicians and researchers to address. The optimal sequence of such therapies is an important issue, with obvious implications for both patients and doctors. As mentioned earlier, many studies suggest that earlier blockade of angiogenesis may hold the most treatment potential for patients with cancer. Studies also now suggest that combining antiangiogenesis drugs with cytotoxic chemotherapy or other targeted agents will increase the efficacy through synergistic means. The sequence of how these various agents are best administered to patients will prove to be another important question for research in this area. This also leads to the obvious question of the duration of therapy as well. Since antiangiogenesis agents are potentially useful in preventing early angiogenesis and halting metastasis, will this effect be reversed after withdrawal of the drug? How long must these drugs be administered to achieve the desired effects on tumor burden and metastatic arrest? Questions like these may ultimately drive researchers to seek out alternative end-points for patients receiving these drugs on study (as opposed to maximum, measurable tumor reduction) (34,81). While prolonged "maintenance" therapy may offer a benefit to patients with stable disease, the costs associated with long-term administration of these newer agents may make this an extremely expensive treatment approach, one that may make this sort of treatment more difficult to justify without definite survival advantages.

CONCLUSION

Thirty years following Dr. Folkman's initial hypothesis research has finally proven the significant role of angiogenesis in the development of malignant disease. What is more promising is the clinical impact now derived from agents specifically designed to inhibit this process. The difficulty now lies making a sound transition from drugs active in the lab to those that are effective in controlling cancer in actual patients. Early preclinical success was met with discouraging preliminary results in clinical trials with many of these new, developmental drugs. Still enough evidence exists to continue this approach, now fueled by exciting results in phase III studies demonstrating a definite response to treatment and a minimal toxicity profile compared to current, standard-of-care drugs. With on-going studies looking to answer many of the lingering questions in this field, we are getting closer to developing the ideal combination of targeted therapies directed against a multitude of aspects in neoplastic cell differentiation and malignant transformation. These approaches may one day replace the indiscriminate methods of cell-kill with cytotoxic agents, providing patients with durable responses with potentially much less toxicity. Whether blocking angiogenesis holds one of the keys to achieving this goal will take time and patience to answer, but it seems a worthwhile endeavor for the patients and clinicians who must confront breast cancer and its impact in their daily lives.

REFERENCES

1. Yancopoulos G. Vascular-specific growth factors and blood vessel formation. Nature 2000; 407:242–248.
2. Folkman J. Tumor angiogenesis: therapeutic implications. New Engl J Med 1971; 285:1182–1186.
3. Fidler IJ, Ellis LM. The implications of angiogenesis for the biology and therapy of cancer metastasis. Cell 1994; 79:185–188.
4. Carmeliet P, Jain R. Angiogenesis in cancer and other diseases. Nature 2000; 407: 249–257.
5. Brem SS, Gullino PM, et al. Angiogenesis: a marker for neoplastic transformation of mammary papillary hyperplasia. Science 1977; 195:880–882.
6. Jensen HM, Chen I, et al. Angiogenesis induced by "normal" human breast tissue: a probable marker for precancer. Science 1982; 218:293–295.
7. Guinbretiere JM, Le Monique G, et al. Angiogenesis and risk of breast cancer in women with fibrocystic disease. J Natl Cancer Inst 1994; 86:635–636.
8. Guidi AJ, Schnitt SJ, Fischer L, et al. Vascular permeability factor (vascular endothelial growth factor) expression and angiogenesis in patients with ductal carcinoma in situ of the breast. Cancer 1997; 80:1945–1953.

9. Weidner N, Semple JP, Welch WR, et al. Tumor angiogenesis and metastasis–correlation in invasive breast carcinoma. N Engl J Med 1991; 324:1–8.

10. Weidner N, Folkman J, Pozza F, et al. Tumor angiogenesis: a new significant and independent prognostic indicator in early-stage breast carcinoma. J Natl Cancer Inst 1992; 84:1875–1887.

11. Ferrara N, Davis-Smith T. The biology of vascular endothelial growth factor. Endocrine Rev 1997; 18:4–25.

12. Bouck N, Stellmach V, Hsu SC. How tumors become angiogenic. Adv Cancer Res 1996; 69:135–174.

13. Hanahan D, Weinberg RA. The hallmarks of cancer. Cell 2000; 100:57–70.

14. Kerbel R, Folkman J. Clinical translation of angiogenesis inhibitors. Nature Rev Cancer 2002; 2:727–739.

15. Rak J, Mitsuhashi Y, Bayko L, et al. Mutant ras oncogenes upregulate VEGF/VPF expression: implications for induction and inhibition of tumor angiogenesis. Cancer Res 1995; 55:4575–4580.

16. Dvorak HF. Vascular permeability factor/vascular endothelial growth factor: a critical cytokine in tumor angiogenesis and a potential target for diagnosis and therapy. J Clin Oncol 2002; 20:4368–4380.

17. Brown LF, Berse B, Jackman RW, et al. Expression of vascular permeability factor (vascular endothelial growth factor) and its receptors in breast cancer. Hum Pathol 1995; 26:86–91.

18. Heer K, Kumar H, Read JR, et al. Serum vascular endothelial growth factor in breast cancer: its relation with cancer type and estrogen receptor status. Clin Cancer Res 2001; 11:3491–3494.

19. Nishimura R, Nagao K, Miyayama H, et al. Higher plasma vascular endothelial growth factor levels correlate with menopause, overexpression of p53, and recurrence of breast cancer. Breast Cancer 2003; 2:120–128.

20. Toi M, Hoshima S, Takayanagi T, et al. Association of vascular endothelial growth factor expression with tumor angiogenesis and with early relapse in primary breast cancer. Jpn J Cancer Res 1994; 85:1045–1049.

21. Linderholm B, Grankvist K, Wilking N, et al. Correlation of vascular endothelial growth factor content with recurrences, survival, and first relapse site in primary node-positive breast carcinoma after adjuvant treatment. J Clin Oncol 2000; 18:1423–1431.

22. Linderholm B, Tavelin B, Grankvist K, et al. Vascular endothelial growth factor is of high prognostic value in node-negative breast carcinoma. J Clin Oncol 1998; 16:3121–3128.

23. Foekens JA, Peters HA, Grebenchtchikov N, et al. High tumor levels of vascular endothelial growth factor predict poor response to systemic therapy in advanced breast cancer. Cancer Res 2001; 61:5407–5414.

24. Relf M, LeJune S, Scott PA, et al. Expression of the angiogenic factors vascular endothelial growth factor, acidic and basic fibroblast growth factor, tumor growth factor beta-1, platelet derived endothelial cell growth factor, placenta growth factor, and pleiotrophin in human primary breast cancer and its relation to angiogenesis. Cancer Res 1997; 57:963–969.

25. Kim KJ, Li B, Winer J, et al. Inhibition of vascular endothelial growth factor-induced angiogenesis suppresses tumor growth in vivo. Nature 1993; 362:841–844.

26. Borgstrom P, Hillan KJ, Sriramarao P, Ferrara N. Complete inhibition of angiogenesis and growth of microtumors by anti-vascular endothelial growth factor neutralizing antibodies. Novel concepts of angiostatic therapy from intravital videomicroscopy. Cancer Res 1996; 56:4032–4039.

27. Asano M, Yukita A, Matsumoto T, et al. Inhibition of tumor growth and metastasis by an immunoneutralizing monoclonal antibody to vascular endothelial growth factor/vascular permeability factor. Cancer Res 1995; 55:5296–5301.

28. Yuan F, Chen Y, Dellian M, et al. Time-dependent vascular regression and vascular permeability changes in established xenografts induced by anti-vascular endothelial growth factor/vascular permeability factor antibody. Proc Natl Acad Sci USA 1996; 93:14,765–14,770.

29. Presta LG, Chen H, O'Connor SJ, et al. Humanization of an anti-vascular endothelial growth factor monoclonal antibody for the therapy of solid tumors and other disorders. Cancer Res 1997; 57:4593–4599.
30. Hurwitz H, Fehrenbacher L, Novotny W, et al. Bevacizumab plus irinotecan, fluorouracil, and leucovorin for metastatic colorectal cancer. N Engl J Med 2004; 350:2335–2342.
31. Johnson DH, Fehrenbacher L, Novotny WF, et al. Randomized phase II trial comparing bevacizumab plus carboplatin and paclitaxel with carboplatin and paclitaxel alone in previously untreated locally advanced or metastatic non-small cell lung cancer. J Clin Oncol 2004; 22:2184–2191.
32. Yang J, Haworth L, Sherry RM, et al. Randomized trial of bevacizumab, an anti-VEGF antibody, for metastatic renal cell cancer. N Engl J Med 2003; 349:427–434.
33. Cobleigh M, Langmuir V, Sledge G, et al. A phase I/II dose-escalation trial of bevacizumab in previously treated metastatic breast cancer. Sem Oncol 2003; 5(suppl 16):117–124.
34. Gasparini G, Longo R, Fanelli M, Teicher B. Combination of antiangiogenic therapy with other anticancer therapies: results, challenges, and open questions. J Clin Oncol 2005; 23:1295–1311.
35. Kakeji Y, Teicher BA. Preclinical studies of the combination of angiogenic inhibitors with cytotoxic agents. Invest New Drugs 1997; 15:39–48.
36. Jain RK. Normalization of tumor vasculature: an emerging concept in antiangiogenic therapy. Science 2005; 307:58–62.
37. Miller KD, Chap L, Holmes F, et al. Randomized phase III trial of capecitabine compared with bevacizumab plus capecitabine in patients with previously treated metastatic breast cancer. J Clin Oncol 2005; 23:792–799.
38. Miller KD, Wang M, Gralow J, et al. A randomized phase III trial of paclitaxel versus paclitaxel plus bevacizumab as first line therapy for locally recurrent or metastatic breast cancer: a trial coordinated by the Eastern Cooperative Oncology Group (E2100). Breast Cancer Res Treat 2005; 94(suppl 1):(abstract 3). www.sabcs.org
39. Miller KD, Wang M, Gralow J, et al. A randomized phase III trial of paclitaxel versus paclitaxel plus bevacizumab as first line therapy for locally recurrent or metastatic breast cancer: a trial coordinated by the Eastern Cooperative Oncology Group (E2100). Data presented at San Antonio Breast Cancer Symposium—obtained through personal correspondence (2005).
40. Overmoyer B, Silverman P, Leeming R, et al. Phase II trial of neodjeuvant docetaxel with or without bevacizumab in patients with locally advanced breast cancer. Proc Am Soc Clin Oncol 2004; 23:(abstract 727). www.asco.org
41. Ramaswamy B, Shapiro CL. Phase II trial of bevacizumab in combination with docetaxel in women with advanced breast cancer. Clin Breast Cancer 2003; 4:292–294.
42. Burstein H, Parker L, Savoie J, et al. Phase II trial of the anti-VEGF antibody bevacizumab in combination with vinorelbine for refractory advanced breast cancer. Breast Cancer Res Treat 2002; 76:S115 (abstract 446).
43. Traina TA, Dickler MN, Caravelli JF, et al. A phase II trial of letrozole in combination with bevacizumab, an anti-VEGF antibody, in patients with hormone receptor-positive metastatic breast cancer. Breast Cancer Res Treat 2005; 94(suppl 1): (abstract 2030).
44. Bonthala Wedam S, Low JA, Yang, SX, et al. Antiangiogenic and antitumor effects of bevacizumab in patients with inflammatory and locally advanced breast cancer. J Clin Oncol 2005; 24:769–776.
45. Koukourakis MI, Giatromanolaki A, O'Byrne KJ, et al. bcl-2 and c-erbB-2 proteins are involved in the regulation of VEGF and thymidine phosphorylase angiogenic activity in non-small cell lung cancer. Clin Exp Metastasis 1999; 17:545–554.
46. Petit AM, Rak J, Hung MC, et al. Neutralizing antibodies against epidermal growth factor and ErbB-2/neu receptor tyrosine kinases down-regulate vascular endothelial growth factor production by tumor cells in vitro: angiogenic implications for signal transduction therapy of solid tumors. Am J Pathol 1997; 151:1523–1530.
47. Blackwell KL, Dewhirst MW, Liotcheva V, et al. HER-2 gene amplification correlates with higher levels of angiogenesis and lower levels of hypoxia in primary breast tumors. Clin Cancer Res 2004; 10(12 pt 1):4083–4088.

48. Konecny GE, Meng YG, Untch M, et al. Association between HER-2/neu and vascular endothelial growth factor expression predicts clinical outcome in primary breast cancer patients. Clin Cancer Res 2004; 10:1706–1716.

49. Pegram MD, Reese DM. Combined biologic therapy of breast cancer using monoclonal antibodies directed against HER2/neu protein and vascular endothelial growth factor. Semin Oncol 2002; 3(suppl 11):29–37.

50. Pegram MD, Yeon C, Ku NC, et al. Phase I combined biological therapy of breast cancer using two humanized monoclonal antibodies directed against HER2 proto-oncogene and vascular endothelial growth factor (VEGF). Breast Cancer Res Treat 2004; 88(suppl 1): (abstract 3039). www.sabcs.org

51. Maity A, Pore N, Lee J, et al. Epidermal growth factor receptor transcriptionally up-regulates vascular endothelial growth factor expression in human glioblastoma cells via a pathway involving phosphatidylinositol 3'-kinase and distinct from that induced by hypoxia. Cancer Res 2000; 60:5879–5886.

52. Sini P, Wyder L, Schnell C, et al. The antitumor and antiangiogenic activity of vascular endothelial growth factor receptor inhibition is potentiated by erbB1 blockade. Clin Cancer Res 2005; 11:4521–4532.

53. Heffelfinger SC, Yan M, Gear RB, et al. Inhibition of VEFR2 prevents DMBA-induced mammary tumor formation. Lab Invest 2004; 84:989–998.

54. Miller K, Trigo J, Stone A, et al. A phase II trial of ZD6474, a vascular endothelial growth factor receptor-2 (VEGFR-2) and epidermal growth factor receptor (EGFR) tyrosine kinase inhibitor, in patients with previously treated metastatic breast cancer (MBC). Breast Cancer Res Treat 2004; 88:S240 (abstract 6060).

55. Rugo HS, Dickler MN, Scott JH, et al. Circulating endothelial cell (CEC) and tumor cell (CTC) analysis in patients (pts) receiving bevacizumab and erlotinib for metastatic breast cancer (MBC). Breast Cancer Res Treat 2004; 88(suppl 1): (abstract 3088).

56. Gasparini G. Metronomic scheduling: the future of chemotherapy? Lancet Oncol 2001; 2:733–740.

57. Miller KD, Sweeney CJ, Sledge GW. Redefining the target: chemotherapeutics as anti-angiogenics. J Clin Oncol 2001; 19:1195–1206.

58. Hanahan D, Bergers G, Bergsland E. Less is more, regularly: Metronomic dosing of cyto-toxic drugs can target tumor angiogenesis in mice. J Clin Invest 2000; 105:1045–1047.

59. Gately S, Kerbel R. Antiangiogenic scheduling of lower dose cancer chemo-therapy. Cancer J 2001; 7:427–436.

60. Bertolini F, Paul S, Mancuso P, et al. Maximum tolerable dose and low-dose chemother-apy have opposite effects on the mobilization and viability of circulating endothelial progenitor cells. Cancer Res 2003; 63:4342–4346.

61. Yap R, Veliceasa D, Emmenegger U, et al. Metronomic low-dose chemotherapy boosts CD95-dependent antiangiogenic effect of the thrombospondin peptide ABT-510: a com-plementation to antiangiogenic strategy. Clin Cancer Res 2005; 11:6678–6685.

62. Munoz R, Shaked Y, Bertolinin F, et al. Anti-angiogenic treatment of breast cancer using metronomic low-dose chemotherapy. Breast 2005; 14:466–479.

63. Colleoni M, Rocca A, Sandri T, et al. Low-dose oral methotrexate and cyclophosphamide in metastatic breast cancer: antitumor activity and correlation with vascular endothelial growth factor levels. Annal Oncol 2002; 13:73–80.

64. Burstein HJ, Spigel D, Kindsvogel K, et al. Metronomic chemotherapy with and without bevacizumab for advanced breast cancer: a randomized phase II study. Breast Cancer Res Treat 2005; 94(suppl 1): (abstract 4). www.sabcs.org

65. Abrams TJ, Murray LJ, Pesenti E, et al. Preclinical evaluation of the tyrosine kinase inhibitor SU11248 as a single agent and in combination with "standard of care" therapeutic agents for the treatment of breast cancer. Mol Cancer Ther 2003; 2:1011–1021.

66. Miller KD, Burstein HJ, Elias AD, et al. Phase II study of SU11248, a multitargeted tyro-sine kinase inhibitor (TKI) in patients (pts) with previously treated metastatic breast cancer (MBC). Breast Cancer Res Treat 2005; 94(suppl 1): (abstract 1066).

67. Hidalgo M, Eckhardt SG. Development of matrix metalloproteinase inhibitors in cancer therapy. J Natl Cancer Inst (Bethesda) 2001; 93:178–193.

68. Sparano JA, Bernardo P, Gradishar WJ, et al. Randomized phase III trial of marimastat versus placebo in patients with metastatic breast cancer who have responding or stable disease after first line chemotherapy: an Eastern Cooperative Oncology Group Trial (E2196). Proc Am Soc Clin Oncol 2002; 21:44a.

69. Moore M, Hamm J, Eisenberg P, et al. A comparison between gemcitabine (GEM) and the matrix metalloproteinase (MMP) inhibitor BAY12-9566 in patients with advanced pancreatic cancer. Proc Am Soc Clin Oncol 2000; 19:240a.

70. Klauber N, Parangi S, Flynn E. Inhibition of angiogenesis and breast cancer in mice by the microtubule inhibitors 2-methoxyestradiol and taxol. Cancer Res 1997; 57:81–86.

71. Han GZ, Liu ZJ, Shimoi K, et al. Synergism between the anticancer actions of 2-methoxyestradiol and microtubule-disrupting agents in human breast cancer. Cancer Res 2005; 65:387–393.

72. Sledge G, Miller K, Haney L, et al. A phase I study of 2-methoxyestradiol (2ME2) in patients with refractory metastatic breast cancer. Proc Am Soc Clin Oncol 2002; 21:111a (abstract 441).

73. Miller K, Murry D, Curry E, et al. A phase I study of 2-methoxyestradiol (2ME2) plus docetaxel in patients with metastatic breast cancer. Proc Am Soc Clin Oncol 2002; 21:11a (abstract 442).

74. Longo R, Sarmiento R, Fanelli M, et al. Anti-angiogenic therapy: rationale, challenges, and clinical studies. Angiogenesis 2002; 5:237–256.

75. Pearlman JD, Laham RJ, Post M, et al. Medical imaging techniques in the evaluation of strategies for therapeutic angiogenesis. Curr Pharm Des 2002; 8:1467–1496.

76. Costouros NG, Diehn FE, Libutti SK. Molecular imaging of tumor angiogenesis. J Cell Biochem 2002; 39(suppl):72–78.

77. Gasparini G, Gion M. Molecular-targeted anticancer therapy: challenges related to study design and choice of proper end-points. Cancer J 2000; 6:117–131.

78. Lissoni P, Fugamalli E, Malugani F, et al. Chemotherapy and angiogenesis in advanced cancer: vascular endothelial growth factor (VEGF) decline as predictor of disease control during taxol therapy in metastatic breast cancer. Int J Biol Markers 2000; 15:308–311.

79. Bergsland E, Dickler M. Maximizing the potential of bevacizumab in cancer treatment. The Oncologist 2002; 9(suppl):36–42.

80. Hillan KJ, Koeppen HKW, Tobin P, et al. The role of VEGF expression in response to bevacizumab plus capecitabine in metastatic breast cancer (MBC). Proc Am Soc Clin Oncol 2003; 22:191.

81. Schneider BP, Miller KD. Angiogenesis of breast cancer. J Clin Oncol 2005; 23: 1782–1790.

82. Karp JE, Gojo I, Pili R, et al. Targeting vascular endothelial growth factor for relapsed and refractory adult acute myelogenous leukemias: therapy with sequential 1-beta-d-arabinofuranosylcytosine, mitoxantrone, and bevacizumab. Clin Cancer Res 2004; 10:3577–3585.

83. D'Adamo DR, Anderson SE, Albritton K, et al. Phase II study of doxorubicin and bevacizumab for patients with metastatic soft-tissue sarcomas. J Clin Oncol 2005; 23:7135–7142.

23 Epigenetic Regulation as a New Target for Breast Cancer Therapy

Vered Stearns, Qun Zhou, and Nancy E. Davidson
Department of Oncology, Johns Hopkins University, Baltimore, Maryland, U.S.A.

INTRODUCTION

Most cancers in humans occur as a result of a multi-step process that generally consists of initiation and progression. As a result of repeated insults, malignancy occurs. Mutations are clearly implicated in carcinogenesis. Most mutations are sporadic and their prevalence increases with age. Other mutations are inherited. Regardless, a mutation may result in activation of oncogenes or inactivation of tumor suppressor genes.

Gene silencing or inactivation of a tumor suppressor gene may be not only due to a mutation, but also a result of a translocation or inhibition of transcription. Inactivation of genes that regulate cell proliferation and death is a critical part of the neoplastic process. One important mechanism that may lead to inhibition of transcription is gene silencing through epigenetic alterations like acquisition of promoter methylation and changes in chromatin structure. Activation of oncogenes may also be a result of epigenetic changes through post-translational modifications in histone acetylation or DNA conformation.

Epigenetic changes can be implicated both in cancer initiation and progression. In this chapter, we will review the hallmarks of epigenetic regulation in cancer and will briefly describe the role of epigenetic alterations as biomarkers of breast cancer risk, detection, prognosis, or response to treatment. Because epigenetic changes may be reversible, they represent an active area for new drug investigation and are promising targets for cancer therapy.

EPIGENETIC REGULATION AND CANCER: OVERVIEW

Epigenetics is a process by which gene expression may be modulated without an alteration in the primary nucleotide sequence of a gene (1). Epigenetic regulation is critical in normal growth and development and provides a layer of transcriptional control of gene expression. Stability of DNA structure requires faithful replication of DNA, and alterations may lead to abnormal processes, such as autoimmune disease, genetic disorders, and cancer. Key components of epigenetic regulation of transcription include faithful management of gene methylation and maintenance of chromatin structure.

DNA methylation patterns are profoundly deranged in human cancer and include both losses and gains. In some cases, epigenetic modification may lead to loss of gene expression analogous to that seen with classic mutations or deletions. Epigenetic changes may be inherited or result from environmental exposures. Epigenetic changes may include alterations in the methylation state of the DNA in promoter regions of genes, or may be a result of alterations in proteins that wrap the DNA into chromosomes or in proteins that regulate the process.

DNA Methylation

The normal DNA is a collection of four bases, adenine, guanine, cytosine, and thymine, which provide our genetic code. In replicating DNA (i.e., in dividing cells), enzymes called DNA methyltransferases (DNMTs) add a methyl group to the cytosine ring to form methyl cytosine. This modification takes place only on a cytosine that precedes a guanosine in the DNA sequence, called the CpG dinucleotide. During evolution, the number of CpG dinucleotides in the genome has been depleted because of mutations, resulting in only a small number of such sites compared to a mathematically expected number. However, several small regions of DNA contain the expected number of CpG dinucleotides, the so-called CpG islands. CpG islands are generally present at the promoter region of most genes. CpG dinucleotides that are not in CpG islands are usually methylated, resulting in suppression of transcription. In contrast, most CpG dinucleotides in CpG islands in gene promoter regions are unmethylated and allow for active gene transcription (1).

In cancer cells, CpG islands that are normally unmethylated may become methylated, resulting in silencing of important genes, such as inactivation of tumor suppressor genes. At the same time, CpG dinucleotides in other regions may become unmethylated, leading to diminished transcriptional repression of normally silenced genes such as oncogenes.

DNA methylation is mediated by several proteins. As noted, DNMTs add methyl groups to the cytosines in CpG dinucleotides. Three active DNMTs have been recognized in humans and are designated DNMT1, DNMT3a, and DNMT3b. Each DNMT may have a specific role in the methylation process, or may act in association with another methyltransferase. DNMTs are also responsible for the recruitment of histone deacetylases (HDACs) to the sites of gene promoters, and may bind to other proteins with a goal of maintaining a repressed transcriptional status. Several DNMT inhibitors are under investigation for cancer treatment. The identification of methylated genes is also under investigation.

Histone Modifications and Chromatin Structure

The human chromatin is comprised of nucleosomes of DNA and histones. Each nucleosome consists of 146 base pairs of DNA wrapped around a core of histone octamers (Fig. 1) (2). The chromatin structure is determined in part by post-translational modifications of histones. Changes in the histone proteins or other components required for DNA structure may alter the normal interaction between DNA and histones and modify the recruitment of other proteins. Chromatin remodeling could result in abnormal transcription. The histone acetylation status is maintained by the balance in the activity of histone acetyltransferases (HATs) and HDACs. The HATs and HDACs are recruited by sequence-specific DNA binding proteins. The HATs are responsible for the addition of acetyl groups that stabilize open chromatin structures, while the HDACs deacetylate histones, and are thus responsible for resetting chromatin into a close conformation. Open chromatin is transcriptionally active, whereas condensed chromatin is transcriptionally inactive. Reduced or abnormal histone acetylation has been found in many types of cancer. As we will discuss, HDAC inhibition can restore the normal histone acetylation status in cancer cells.

Other important proteins that contribute to the normal chromatin structure include primary transcription factors, transcriptional coactivators, transcriptional

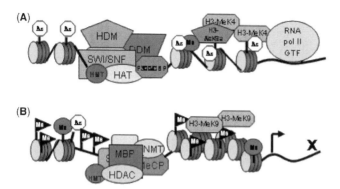

FIGURE 1 Epigenetic regulation of chromatin. Each nucleosome consists of 146 base pairs of DNA wrapped around a core of histone octamers (⬛). (**A**) Euchromatin: An unmethylated promoter and a normal balance between histone deacetylases (HDAC) and histone acetyltransferases (HAT) allows for acetylation of histone tails, creating a chromatin that is open and transcriptionally active. Aceylated histones associate preferentially with transcriptionally active chromatin. Histone acetylation as well as methylation of histone H3 at lysine 4 may also facilitate binding of transcription factors to promote or disrupt higher order chromosome structure. (⬡) A histone H3 methylated at lysine 4. (**B**) Heterochromatin: Promoter methylation (▶) and hypoacetylation of histones create a chromatin that is condensed and transcriptionally inactive. Methylation of lysine 9 on histone H3 (H3-MeK9) is associated with gene transcription. *Abbreviations*: DNMT, DNA methyltransferases; HAT, histone acetyltransferases; HDAC, histone deacetylases; HDM, histone demethylase; HMT, histone methyltransferase; MB, MeCP, methyl binding proteins; SWI/SNF, chromatin remodeling complex (switching defective and sucrose nonfermenting). These remodeling factor subunits can regulate both transcriptional activation and repression.

corepressors, and methylcytosine–binding proteins. A change in the balance of proteins that regulate histone modification may result in a change in chromatin structure and, subsequently, abnormal transcription.

In general, active chromatin is comprised of unmethylated DNA with high levels of acetylated histones (Fig. 1A), whereas methylated DNA and deacetylated histones characterize inactive chromatin (Fig. 1B). The status of methylation or histone acetylation may change during different stages of development or due to environmental factors, such as hormone levels, diet, or exposure to drugs or chemicals (3). Epigenetic changes that result from such exposures may interact with genetic factors leading to cancer. Thus, epigenetic modifications can explain in part why one identical twin may develop an illness like cancer while the other does not, or why family members carrying the same germ-line mutation in a tumor suppressor gene may or may not develop cancer, or why some cancers may appear earlier in life compared to a previous generation.

EPIGENETIC REGULATION AND CANCER: CLINICAL IMPLICATIONS

Normal and altered epigenetic regulation may play an important role in several aspects of cancer progression. Changes in gene methylation or histone acetylation may serve as biomarkers of cancer risk, assist in cancer detection, provide molecular staging, or predict prognosis or response to treatment (4). Importantly, epigenetic changes represent an exciting target for therapy.

Assays to Assess Abnormal Methylation

A review of therapeutic strategies targeting epigenetic changes cannot be complete without an overview of assays that can assess the methylation status of target genes. Recent advances in high throughput technologies may provide robust ability to detect epigenetic changes in tissues of interest. Moreover, the technologies allow for evaluation of very few cells or small tissue samples without complex processing. Recently, several methylation-specific polymerase chain reaction (PCR)-based techniques, designated methylation-specific PCR (MSP) have been developed to better characterize CpG dinucleotide hypermethylation. In these techniques, sodium bisulfite-treated DNA is amplified with primers specific to the sequences of unmethylated and methylated DNA within the gene of interest. The MSP techniques have been further modified to include real-time quantitative multiplex MSP (QM-MSP) techniques. The method allows for accurate assessment of promoter hypermethylation for many genes simultaneously in small samples. QM-MSP is highly sensitive (1 in 10^4–10^5 copies of DNA) and linear over five orders of magnitude (5).

Gene array technologies may also allow for DNA methylation profiling of large genomic regions (6). In this method, unmethylated and methylated DNA fractions are enriched using a series of treatments with methylation-sensitive restriction enzymes, and interrogated on microarrays. Early reports are promising that such methods may be useful for epigenetic profiling of the entire human genome.

These techniques can now be applied to small specimens obtained from patients and have the potential for use as markers of risk of future cancer, as molecular diagnostic tools, or as markers of response to treatment. Other assays can be applied to evaluate functionality of a specific gene of interest. Such techniques may include assessment of transcription to RNA or expression of the protein product. Other assays can determine transcription of downstream genes or function. Ultimately, of course, the value of methylated marker measurement needs to be ascertained in a clinical setting.

Epigenetics and Breast Cancer Progression

In breast cancer, multiple genes are methylated compared to noncancerous tissue. DNA methylation, acquired over time, leads to silencing of genes that are critical in several pathways. For example, genes involved in growth (estrogen receptor, progesterone receptor) evasion of apoptosis (*HOXA5, DAPK, Twist*), tissue invasion and metastasis (E-cadherin), and limitless replicative potential (*cyclin D2, p16, BRCA1, GSTP1, 14.3.3 sigma,* and *RAR-beta*) can be methylated in breast cancers (7).

The prevalence of methylation in specific genes in normal and malignant breast tissue has been evaluated. Some investigations have focused on a single candidate gene, whereas others evaluated methylation status of several genes. Using a panel of seven genes with the MSP assay in a variety of breast cancers, investigators have demonstrated that virtually all invasive breast carcinomas examined contained at least one hypermethylated gene, 80% contained two, and 60% contained three or more methylated genes (8,9). Similarly, 95% of ductal carcinoma in situ (DCIS) specimens contained at least one methylated gene. In contrast, the percentage of women with benign breast disease having one or more methylated genes was only 15%, and only one of eight reduction mammoplasty specimens contained hypermethylated genes. It is indeed possible that early epigenetic changes may indicate future risk of breast cancer. Researchers evaluated human mammary epithelial cells from healthy individuals and have noted that hypermethylation of the *p16INK4a* promoter sequences may precede the clonal outgrowth of premalignant lesions (10,11).

Taken together, these early reports suggest that candidate gene hypermethylation can be seen in virtually all malignant breast neoplasms and in some premalignant tissues. Additional studies are required to assess the role of gene methylation as a marker of risk or a molecular diagnostic for breast cancer.

INHIBITION OF DNA METHYLATION AND HISTONE ACETYLATION AS THERAPEUTIC STRATEGIES IN CANCER

As noted, in contrast to gene mutations, epigenetic changes may be reversible. Therefore, targeting epigenetic changes in an attempt to relieve transcriptional repression has been an attractive therapeutic strategy. Agents that have been extensively studied include DNMT inhibitors and HDAC inhibitors. While several HDAC and DNMT inhibitors have been investigated in preclinical models of breast cancer, the clinical experience remains limited.

Demethylating Agents

DNMT inhibitors do not remove methyl groups from methylated chromatin, but rather prevent methylation of daughter DNA in CpG islands during DNA replication (12). DNMT expression and activity are highly variable across tumor types, and thus it would be expected that the activity of the agents may vary across tumor types and across individual tumors.

Methyltransferase inhibitors include the nucleoside inhibitors 5-azacitydine (azacitidine), 5-aza-2′-deoxycytidine (decitabine), and zebularine. These agents are incorporated into DNA and the end result is depletion of methyltransferase and demethylation of DNA. Other agents are the nonnucleoside inhibitors procainamide, epigallocatechin-3-gallate (EGCG), and RG108, which block DNA directly (12). Azacitidine (Vidaza, Pharmion) is a pyrimide nucleoside analog of cytidine. It has been approved by the FDA for treatment of myelodysplastic syndromes of all subtypes. Decitabine (Dacogen, MGI Pharma) is a deoxycytidine analog prodrug activated by deoxycytidine kinase, and was recently FDA-approved for myledysplastic syndrome. Few studies have evaluated the efficacy of DNMT inhibitors in solid tumors, including breast cancer, although anecdotal responses were seen in the early phase I trials. Recent studies in leukemia suggest that the dose of DNMT inhibitor required to re-express epigenetically silenced gene is far less than maximal tolerated dose.

Histone Deacetylase Inhibitors

Several HDAC inhibitors have been developed and investigated in preclinical models of solid and hematological malignancies, and a few are in early phase clinical trials. The HDAC inhibitors are generally divided into four groups including hydroxamic acids, cyclic peptides, aliphatic acids, and benzamides (13). The most common HDAC inhibitors that are currently in clinical investigations are listed in Table 1. Several HDAC isoenzymes have been identified and are designated HDAC 1 through 11. The isoenzymes are classified to type I, which includes HDAC1, HDAC2, HDAC3, HDAC8, and HDAC11, and type II, which includes HDAC4, HDAC5, HDAC6, HDAC7, HDAC9, and HDAC10. HDAC inhibitors may target several HDAC isoenzymes. Several HDAC inhibitors have been

TABLE 1 Histone Deacetylase Inhibitors in Clinical Investigation

Class	Compound
Hydroxamate	TSA
	SAHA
	CBHA
	LBH-589
	PXD-101
Cyclic peptide	Depsipeptide (FK-228)
Aliphatic acid	Valproic acid
	Phenylbutyrate
Benzamide	MS-275
	p-N-Acetyl dinaline (CI-994)
	MGC0103

Abbreviations: CBHA, M-carboxycinnamic acid bis-hydroxamide; SAHA, sub-eroylanilide hydroxamic acid; TSA, trichostatin A.

studied in phase I trials in hematological and nonhematological malignancies. Sub-eroylanilide hydroxamic acid (SAHA), depsipeptide, phenyl butyrate, MS-275, and LBH589 are currently in or nearing phase II investigations or in phase I studies testing combinations with other agents. Other agents, such as PXD-101 and MGO0103, are in early phase development. SAHA is currently under evaluation in several trials targeting breast cancer patients.

The HDAC inhibitors have demonstrated multiple effects in cancer cell lines. These effects include alteration of gene expression and differentiation, induction of cell death, reduced proliferation, and/or cell cycle arrest and are summarized in Table 2.

TABLE 2 Multiple Biologic Effects of Deacetylase Inhibition

Pathway	Effect
Induction of apoptosis	↑ p53
	↑ DR4
	↑ Bax, Bak
	↓ FLIP
	↓ IAPs
	↓ Bcl-2, Bcl-x_L
Induction of cell-cycle arrest	↑ p21
	↑ p27
	↓ Cyclin D
	↓ CDK4
	↓ Thymidylate synthetase
Oncogene destabilization	↓ BCR/abl
	↓ HER2/neu
	↓ EGFR
	↓ FLT-3
	↓ pAKT
	↓ ER-alpha
Antiangiogenesis	↓ VEGF
	↓ Ang2
	↓ Tie2
	↓ HIF1-alpha

Abbreviations: FLIP, FLICE-inhibitory protein; IAP, inhibitor of apoptosis protein; HER2, human epidermal growth factor receptor 2; EGFR, epidermal growth factor receptor; FLT, Fms-like tyrosine kinase; VEGF, vascular endo-thelial growth factor.

INHIBITION OF DNA METHYLATION AND HISTONE ACETYLATION IN BREAST CANCER

Promoter methylation has been identified in several key genes that are important in breast cancer initiation and progression. Among others, p16, retinoic acid receptor, BRCA1, APC, E-cadherin, GSTP1, and RASSF1A are frequently methylated. Several HDAC inhibitors and DNMT inhibitors have been investigated in preclinical models in breast cancer and are reviewed subsequently; however, the clinical experience is limited. Preclinical studies suggest that agents that modulate epigenetic changes may have single agent activity or may have synergy in combination with standard treatments.

Reactivation of Estrogen Receptor Alpha

Estrogen receptor alpha (ER) is one of the most important targets for the treatment and prevention of breast cancer. The ER gene has a CpG island in its A and B promoters and first exon. Absence of ER protein expression is frequently associated with loss of ER transcript in human breast cancer cell lines and cancers. In contrast, the ER gene is unmethylated at its CpG island in normal tissues and in several ER-positive human breast cancer cell lines. In a small study, 72% of tumors that are ER-positive but PR-negative and 100% of tumors that are both ER- and progesterone receptor (PR)-negative are methylated at the ER promoter (14). Because hormone treatments such as tamoxifen are most effective in tumors that express ER and PR, it is possible that reversal of methylation at the ER promoter will sensitize the tumors to the hormone treatment.

The effects of HDAC inhibitors and/or demethylating agents on ER re-expression in breast cancer cell lines have been examined. The administration of trichostatin A (TSA) to ER-negative breast cancer cell lines was associated with ER mRNA and protein re-expression. When administered in combination with the DNMT 5-aza-2'-deoxycytidine, further enhancement in ER mRNA and protein re-expression was observed (15). The novel HDAC inhibitor scriptaid administered to ER-negative breast cancer cell lines has also induced the expression of a functional ER (16). Scriptaid was also associated with significant growth inhibition and increased acetylation of histone tails. The combination of scriptaid and 5-aza-2'-deoxycytidine was more effective in inducing ER than either agent alone.

Similarly, treatment of ER-positive MCF-7 cells or ER-negative MDA-MB-231 cells for 48 hours with trichostatin, LAQ824, or LBH589 resulted in accumulation of acetylated histones at the ER promoter. Re-expression of ER mRNA was confirmed by real-time PCR. Further, the PR, an ER-responsive gene, was also shown to be re-expressed in both MCF-7 and MDA-MB-231 cells by real-time PCR, indicating that the re-expressed ER is functional. Treatment of MDA-MB-231 cells with trichostatin, LAQ824, LBH589, or SAHA sensitized the cells to concomitant treatment with 4-hydroxy tamoxifen, providing further evidence that ER function is restored (17). Tamoxifen inhibition of cell growth in these cells is mediated by the tamoxifen-bound ER (18). Tamoxifen-bound reactivated ER induces transcriptional repression of estrogen responsive genes by recruitment of multiple distinct chromatin- modifying complexes, including NCoR (nuclear receptor corepressor), HDAC3 and NuRD (nucleosome remodeling and histone deacetylation) (18). These results suggest that multiple HDAC inhibitors can indeed induce ER in ER-negative human breast cancer cells, restoring sensitivity to 4-hydroxy tamoxifen, thereby providing strong evidence that the re-expressed gene is indeed active and can be targeted by standard agents.

Reactivation of the Retinoid Acid Receptor Beta

Retinoid acid receptor beta (RARβ) resides in the nucleus and acts as a ligand-dependent transcriptional factor. Binding of retinoids to RARβ triggers RARβ dimerization and subsequently activates retioniod-responsive target genes, which induce cellular differentiation and apoptosis. Therefore, expression of functional RARβ is critical for antitumor activity of retinoids. The RARβ has been recognized as a tumor suppressor gene. The RARβ is expressed as β1, β2 and β4 (19). The biological activity of β2 is regulated by the P2 promoter containing a high affinity RA-responsive element (RARE) (20). Loss of the RARβ2 occurs early during carcinogenesis and correlates with the malignant phenotype. The progressive decrease in RARβ2 mRNA is mediated, at least in part, by epigenetic mechanisms. Hypermethylation in the RARβ2 promoter has been found in 48 of 50 invasive breast cancers and in 8 of 14 ductal carcinomas in situ, but was not detected in normal breast tissue (21). Histone deacetylation at the RARβ2 P2 promoter can reinforce DNA methylation status, ultimately resulting in stable RAR gene silencing. RARβ2 P2 methylation or deacetylation therefore appears to be a predictor of retinoic acid response, and reactivation of RARβ2 could restore RARβ anticancer effects in breast cancer.

Treatment of T47D and MCF-7 cells with 5-aza-2′-deoxycytidine leads to demethylation within RARβ2 P2 promoter and re-expression of RARβ2 (22,23). In the retinoic acid-resistant MDA-MB-231 cell line, TSA can also restore retinoic acid RARβ2 transcription activity (23). The combination of TSA and retinoic acid for four weeks reactivates RARβ2 gene expression in MCF-7 xenografts that contain a methylated RARβ P2. These data suggest that drugs that result in chromatin-remodeling may provide a strategy to restore RARβ2 gene re-expression and overcome the retinoic acid resistance in breast cancer.

Combination Strategies of Epigenetic Modifiers

Although preclinical results with HDAC inhibitors are promising, the effects they exert on cancer cells in vitro are incomplete and reversible upon discontinuation of the agent. Thus, it is possible that HDAC inhibitors may be most efficacious if combined with other agents. One strategy is a combination of the HDAC inhibitor with an agent that targets the re-expressed gene, such as tamoxifen or retinoic acid, as described earlier. Other promising combinations include HDAC inhibitors and DNMT inhibitors, or other novel drugs like trastuzumab.

The HDAC inhibitors were combined with chemotherapeutic agents or novel compounds in preclinical investigations. Treatment of breast cancer cells with HER2/neu amplification or overexpression (SKBR-3 and BT-474) with the HDAC inhibitor, LAQ824, induced p21(WAF1) and p27(KIP1) leading to growth arrest and apoptosis. The treatment was associated with depletion of mRNA and protein levels of HER2/neu. The addition of trastuzumab to LAQ824 was associated with a significant increase in apoptosis in the same cell lines (24). These results suggested that HDAC inhibitors may be associated with down-regulation of oncogenes. Similarly, treatment with SAHA was associated with up-regulation of p21 and p27 levels, growth arrest, and apoptosis (25). Clinical trials to test the combination of trastuzumab and SAHA are planned. LAQ824 and SAHA also enhanced apoptosis induced by several common chemotherapy agents used for the treatment of breast cancer, such as docetaxel and gemcitabine (24,25). These results provide a strong rationale for clinical trials with HDAC inhibitor combined with standard chemotherapy agents.

Another promising combination may be a demethylating agent and an HDAC inhibitor based on preclinical results that dual treatment re-expresses epigenetically silenced genes to a greater extent than either agent alone. Clinical studies evaluating combinations are ongoing mostly in hematologic malignancies.

Suberoylanilide Hydroxamic Acid (Vorinostat)

Much work in breast cancer is focused on suberoylanilide hydroxamic acid (SAHA), a small molecule that binds to the catalytic site of HDACs, preventing them from interacting with its substrate. SAHA targets class I and II HDACs. SAHA affects transcription of cell-cycle regulators as well as other specific transcriptional programs and also has nontranscriptional cellular effects that are not HDAC-mediated. It promotes cell differentiation, cell cycle arrest, and apoptosis and induces histone acetylation. In breast cancer cell lines, SAHA inhibits clonogenic growth by inducing G1 and G2/M cell cycle arrest and apoptosis (26). Effects are seen within 24 to 72 hours following drug administration. Importantly, SAHA induces morphological changes consistent with differentiation in tumor cells with different properties, such as the ER-negative or HER2/neu or EGFR-amplified cell lines. In the MCF-7 cell line, SAHA enhances the activity of cytotoxic agents, such as cisplatin, epirubicin, paclitaxel, and docetaxel (27,28).

SAHA has been investigated in phase I clinical trials in hematological and non-hematological malignancies. The most common toxicities include fatigue, gastrointestinal symptoms, hyperglycemia, hypokalemia, anemia, and thrombocytopenia (29,30). Doses and schedules recommended for phase II studies include 300 mg po bid daily for 3 days a week, 400 mg po daily continuous, or 200 mg po bid daily continuous. The SAHA-related adverse events are generally rapidly reversible after study drug cessation. Inhibition of HDAC activity was achieved in peripheral blood mononuclear cells at the 200 mg dose level. At dose levels of 400 and 600 mg, the duration of HDAC inhibition lasted 10 or more hours. Tumor responses have been documented in patients with diffuse large B-cell lymphoma, laryngeal cancer, thyroid cancer, and mesothelioma. The FDA has recently approved SAHA (Zolinza, Mesck & Co., Inc.) for the treatment of cutaneous manifestations of cutaneous T-cell lymphoma (CTCL) in patients with progressive, persistent, or recurrent disease on or following two systemic therapies.

Several phase II studies of SAHA are ongoing in breast and other solid malignancies. Other studies are designed to understand modulation in breast cancer tissue. For example, in one study, women with primary breast cancer receive short-term administration of SAHA prior to definitive breast surgery, and baseline and change in markers of proliferation, apoptosis, as well as modulation of gene methylation and histone acetylation are evaluated. In addition, phase I and II clinical trials under investigation include combination therapy of SAHA and cytotoxic agents, biologic modulators, such as trastuzumab, bevacizumab, and novel agents. Other HDAC inhibitors have shown preliminary activity in the clinic, but an urgent need remains to identify optimal dose, schedule and duration of therapy for future clinical trials.

POTENTIAL LIMITATIONS AND FUTURE DIRECTIONS

While epigenetic changes may be reversible and thus represent an exciting area for new drug investigation, many unknowns remain. For example, the gene re-expression and other changes induced by HDAC inhibitors appear to be reversible upon drug discontinuation, suggesting a need for prolonged continuous treatment with the agent that may be associated with frequent symptoms that can interfere with quality of life. Ongoing and new clinical trials are addressing questions of proper dose and schedule of several HDAC inhibitors. The goal of dose-finding studies is to optimize treatment schedules for maximal biologic effectiveness.

Another gap in the current knowledge is that HDAC inhibitors likely induce expression of many genes, but current work has focused mainly on one or very few target genes. Ongoing research is focusing on epigenetic and expression profiling of multiple genes. It is also important to note that HDAC inhibitors may not work solely by epigenetic modulation and may have other important cellular actions. In addition, understanding of HDAC class and enzyme specificity is currently limited. Work to understand the mechanism of action of individual HDAC inhibitors is essential. At the same time, other efforts are focused on designing new agents that may be gene or target specific, and identifying the optimal targets.

Other research questions include identification of optimal correlative assays for clinical trials, or assays that will allow identification of either global acetylation patterns or specific promoter acetylation. Novel bioanalytical tools for DNA methylation analysis and other functional assays are also under investigation. Taken together, preclinical and early clinical data suggest that epigenetic changes are a hallmark of many cancers, including breast cancer, and epigenetic modulators alone or in combination with targeted agents should be evaluated in women with breast cancer.

REFERENCES

1. Herman J.G, Baylin SB. Gene silencing in cancer in association with promoter hypermethylation. N Engl J Med 2003; 349:2042–2054.
2. Luo RX, Dean DC. Chromatin remodeling and transcriptional regulation. J Natl Cancer Inst 1999; 91:1288–1294.
3. Bjornsson HT, Fallin MD, Feinberg AP. An integrated epigenetic and genetic approach to common human disease. Trends Genet 2004; 20:350–358.
4. Jones PA. Epigenetics in carcinogenesis and cancer prevention. Ann NY Acad Sci 2003; 983:213–219.
5. Fackler MJ, McVeigh M, Mehrotra J, et al. Quantitative multiplex methylation-specific PCR assay for the detection of promoter hypermethylation in multiple genes in breast cancer. Cancer Res 2004; 64:4442–4452.
6. Schumacher A, Kapranov P, Kaminsky Z, et al. Microarray-based DNA methylation profiling: technology and applications. Nucleic Acids Res 2006; 34:528–542.
7. Widschwendter M, Jones PA. DNA methylation and breast carcinogenesis. Oncogene 2002; 21:5462–5482.
8. Pu RT, Laitala LE, Alli PM, Fackler MJ, Sukumar S, Clark DP. Methylation profiling of benign and malignant breast lesions and its application to cytopathology. Mod Pathol 2003; 16:1095–1101.
9. Fackler MJ, McVeigh M, Evron E, et al. DNA methylation of RASSF1A, HIN-1, RAR-beta, Cyclin D2 and Twist in in situ and invasive lobular breast carcinoma. Int J Cancer 2003; 107:970–975.
10. Romanov SR, Kozakiewicz BK, Holst CR, Stampfer MR, Haupt LM, Tlsty TD. Normal human mammary epithelial cells spontaneously escape senescence and acquire genomic changes. Nature 2001; 409:633–637.
11. Tlsty TD, Romanov SR, Kozakiewicz BK, Holst CR, Haupt LM, Crawford YG. Loss of chromosomal integrity in human mammary epithelial cells subsequent to escape from senescence. J Mammary Gland Biol Neoplasia 2001; 6:235–243.

12. Lyko F, Brown R. DNA methyltransferase inhibitors and the development of epigenetic cancer therapies. J Natl Cancer Inst 2005; 97:1498–1506.
13. Dokmanovic M, Marks PA. Prospects: histone deacetylase inhibitors. J Cell Biochem 2005; 96:293–304.
14. Lapidus RG, Nass SJ, Butash KA, et al. Mapping of ER gene CpG island methylation-specific polymerase chain reaction. Cancer Res 1998; 58:2515–2519.
15. Yang X, Phillips DL, Ferguson AT, Nelson WG, Herman JG, Davidson NE. Synergistic activation of functional estrogen receptor (ER)-alpha by DNA methyltransferase and histone deacetylase inhibition in human ER-alpha-negative breast cancer cells. Cancer Res 2001; 61:7025–7029.
16. Keen JC, Yan L, Mack KM, et al. A novel histone deacetylase inhibitor, scriptaid, enhances expression of functional estrogen receptor alpha (ER) in ER negative human breast cancer cells in combination with 5-aza 2'-deoxycytidine. Breast Cancer Res Treat 2003; 81:177–186.
17. Zhou Q, Agoston AT, Blum J, Atadja P, Nelson WG, Davidson NE. Histone Deacetylase Inhibition Restores Estrogen Receptor Alpha Gene Expression and Tamoxifen Sensitivity in ER-negative Human Breast Cancer Cells. Proceedings of the American Association of Cancer Research, 97th annual meeting, Washington, DC, April 1–5, 2006; American Association for Cancer Research, abstract 2280.
18. Sharma S, Saxena NK, Davidson NE, Vertino PM. Restoration of tamoxifen sensitivity in ER-negative breast cancer cells: Tamoxifen-bound reactivated estrogen receptor recruits distinctive corepressor complexes. Cancer Res 2006; 66:6370–6378.
19. Toulouse A, Morin J, Pelletier M, Bradley WE. Structure of the human retinoic acid receptor beta 1 gene. Biochim Biophys Acta 1996; 1309:1–4.
20. de The H, Vivanco-Ruiz MM, Tiollais P, Stunnenberg H, Dejean A. Identification of a retinoic acid responsive element in the retinoic acid receptor beta gene. Nature 1990; 343:177–180.
21. Evron E, Dooley WC, Umbricht CB, et al. Detection of breast cancer cells in ductal lavage fluid by methylation-specific PCR. Lancet 2001; 357:1335–1336.
22. Sirchia SM, Ferguson AT, Sironi E, et al. Evidence of epigenetic changes affecting the chromatin state of the retinoic acid receptor beta2 promoter in breast cancer cells. Oncogene 2000; 19:1556–1563.
23. Sirchia SM, Ren M, Pili R, et al. Endogenous reactivation of the RARbeta2 tumor suppressor gene epigenetically silenced in breast cancer. Cancer Res 2002; 62:2455–2461.
24. Fuino L, Bali P, Wittmann S, et al. Histone deacetylase inhibitor LAQ824 down-regulates Her-2 and sensitizes human breast cancer cells to trastuzumab, taxotere, gemcitabine, and epothilone B. Mol Cancer Ther 2003; 2:971–984.
25. Bali P, Pranpat M, Swaby R, et al. Activity of suberoylanilide hydroxamic Acid against human breast cancer cells with amplification of her-2. Clin Cancer Res 2005; 11:6382–6389.
26. Munster PN, Troso-Sandoval T, Rosen N, Rifkind R, Marks PA, Richon VM. The histone deacetylase inhibitor suberoylanilide hydroxamic acid induces differentiation of human breast cancer cells. Cancer Res 2001; 61:8492–8497.
27. Kim MS, Blake M, Baek JH, et al. Inhibition of histone deacetylase increases cytotoxicity to anticancer drugs targeting DNA. Proc Am Assoc Cancer Res 2003; 44:A790.
28. Marchion DC, Bicaku E, Daud AI, Richon V, Sullivan DM, Munster PN. Sequence-specific potentiation of topoisomerase II inhibitors by the histone deacetylase inhibitor suberoylanilide hydroxamic acid. J Cell Biochem 2004; 92:223–237.
29. Kelly WK, O'Connor OA, Krug LM, et al. Phase I study of an oral histone deacetylase inhibitor, suberoylanilide hydroxamic acid, in patients with advanced cancer. J Clin Oncol 2005; 23:3923–3931.
30. Kelly WK, Richon VM, O'Connor O, et al. Phase I clinical trial of histone deacetylase inhibitor: suberoylanilide hydroxamic acid administered intravenously. Clin Cancer Res 2003; 9:3578–3588.

24 | Tumor Vaccines for Breast Cancer

Karen S. Anderson

Cancer Vaccine Center, Dana-Farber Cancer Institute, Harvard Medical School, Boston, Massachusetts, U.S.A.

CANCER AND THE IMMUNE RESPONSE

The immune system is a complex multi-cellular network, which can quickly accommodate or combat novel pathogens. This network of activating and inhibitory cells and molecules result in a tight balance between immunity and autoimmunity. It is the ability of the immune system to distinguish self from non-self that results in effective clearance of pathogens and immunologic memory. The primary challenge facing the field of tumor immunology is that, unlike infections, all tumor cells contain self-antigens that vary from normal tissue, primarily by mutation or by expression level. Many of these self-antigens are critical for biologic processes, such as DNA replication, or are expressed at some level on normal tissues. Thus, effective tumor immunity carries the risk of clinically significant autoimmunity.

There are several lines of evidence suggesting that breast cancer is subject to immunosurveillance. A case–control study of 176 women with breast cancer showed a genetic association with protective human leukocyte antigen (HLA) class II alleles (1). MHC molecules are down regulated in 20% to 50% of primary breast tumors and cell lines, and class II molecules have been detected in around 30% of breast carcinoma lesions (2,3), but this is of unclear clinical significance. As with ovarian cancer, melanoma, and colon cancer, lymphocytic infiltrates have been shown to be associated with improved overall survival in breast cancer (4,5). T-cells recognizing MUC-1 and HER2/neu-derived antigens have been isolated from the blood of breast cancer patients (6,7). Evidence that T-lymphocytes can effectively target breast cancer tumor cells is demonstrated by the small, but measurable graft-versus-tumor effects that have been shown in patients, undergoing donor-lymphocyte infusion after allogeneic stem-cell transplantation (8–10).

Innate Immunity

The identification of the molecular pathways involved in the innate immune response has led to numerous clinical trials of immune adjuvants. The innate immune response represents the first line of defense against pathogens, and includes natural barriers (skin, mucosa, and the blood–brain barrier), cytokines, complement, and cellular immunity including natural killer cells (NK cells), neutrophils, and macrophages (11). This response is primarily mediated by activation of the family of toll-like receptors (TLRs) on macrophages. There are at least 10 known human TLRs, each of which is stimulated by specific molecular structures. These agonists are potent immunostimulants and include double-stranded RNA (which activates TLR3), lipo-polysaccharide (which activates TLR4), and CpG

DNA (which activates TLR9). TLR stimulation leads to the destruction of pathogens by means of activated macrophages or natural killer (NK) cells as well as cytokine release for immune amplification and dendritic cell maturation (12). As a result, TLR agonists are being developed as adjuvants in both infectious and cancer vaccine trials. For example, CpGs are synthetic 8 to 30 base-long oligonucleotides that mimic pathogenic DNA, and activate TLR9 on dendritic cells to augment T-cell responses to vaccination (13,14).

In addition to TLRs, NKG2D is an activating receptor expressed on NK cells and macrophages. NKG2D can interact with ligands expressed by tumor cells, causing alteration of innate immunity (15). In animal models, NKG2D ligand expression early in tumor development protects the host from tumor initiation (16). These ligands include major histocompatibility complex (MHC) class I chain-related protein A and B (MICA and MICB). MIC proteins are overexpressed in most epithelial cancers, including breast tumors (17,18), and soluble major histo-computibility complex (MHC) antigens secreted by tumors down regulate T-cell activity (19). In addition, the inhibitory NK cell ligands HLA-E and -F have been detected on a subset of breast tumor cell lines (3), and soluble HLA-G, which induces apoptosis of T-cells that has been detected in malignant ascites (20). The mechanisms used by tumor cells to regulate the innate immune response are all potential targets for therapeutic intervention.

Adaptive Immunity
The adaptive immune response, which involves T- and B-lymphocytes, is required for immunologic memory. This response is initially slower than the innate response but leads to rapid and highly specific memory responses on subsequent challenge. Antigens may be either directly presented by tumor cells, or cross-presented by

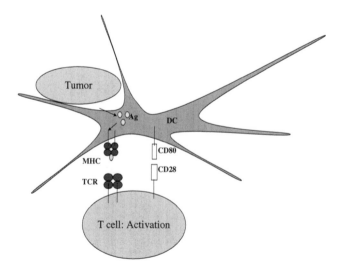

FIGURE 1 Induction of T-cell immunity. Tumor antigens are endocytosed by immature dendritic cells, processed by proteases, and presented as peptides by MHC molecules to T cells. Expression of costimulatory molecules such as CD80 and CD86 are required for efficient priming of T cells via activation of CD28. *Abbreviations*: DC, dendritic cells; MHC, major histocompatibility complex; TCR, T-cell receptor.

antigen-presenting cells (APCs). Either way, the antigens are degraded to peptide epitopes, which are then bound to MHC molecules, for presentation to T-cells (Fig. 1). MHC class I peptide epitopes that are created by proteasomal cleavage are structurally limited by the size of the MHC peptide-binding groove. Therefore, for a given antigenic sequence, potential MHC class I-binding epitopes, such as the E75 peptide of HER2/neu (21) or the I540 peptide of telomerase (22), can be predicted with some accuracy using algorithms based on the primary sequence of the protein. A limited number of tumor antigenic epitopes have been directly sequenced from purified class I MHC molecules (23,24), but the low concentration of specific peptides has made direct identification of tumor antigenic sequences by mass spectrometry difficult.

In contrast, MHC class II molecules primarily bind peptides derived from exogenous antigen that is endocytosed by APCs for presentation to CD4+ T-cells. Since the peptide-binding groove of class II molecules is structurally more flexible than that of class I molecules, prediction of antigenic peptides is more difficult and requires systematic empirical identification with the use of overlapping peptide sets. As a result, fewer class II peptide epitopes from tumor antigens have been identified and tested in clinical trials (25,26).

Antibody Immunity

The natural development of B cell antibody responses to tumor antigens is dependent on antigen overexpression, mutation, apoptosis, changes structural, and aberrant glycosylation (27). Aberrently glycosylated carbohydrate antigens, such as Tn, are expressed by tumor cells and have been used in clinical vaccine trials in breast cancer (28–31) with evidence of immunogenicity. Serologic expression cloning has been used to detect antibodies to multiple breast cancer protein antigens, including HER2/neu, p53, MUC1, and NY-ESO-1 (32–35). In prostate cancer, patterns of autoantibody production correlate with disease outcome (36), suggesting that autoantibodies may be useful as proteomic biomarkers both for diagnosis and prognosis (27). Similarly, antibodies to HER2/neu have been detected in serum samples from 20% of patients with HER2+ early-stage of breast cancer (32). Although HER2 antibody titers of exceeding 1:5000 have been reported, it is unclear whether they confer a protective immune response. Since B-cell immunity often correlates with T-cell immunity, autoantigen identification has led to the identification of T-cell antigens for vaccine development (37,38). Since tumor antigen-specific antibodies can enhance tumor antigen cross-presentation, combined vaccine and antibody therapy, such as HER2-vaccines and trastuzumab, may augment anti-tumor immunity.

Cytokine Dysregulation

In the tumor microenvironment, tumor cells both actively down regulate the immune function and co-opt the immune molecules for tumor activation, invasion, and metastasis (39–41). Molecules such as vascular endothelial growth factor (VEGF), interleukin-6, macrophage-colony stimulating factor (M-CSF), cyclo-oxygenase 2 (COX-2), interleukin-10, stem cell factor-1, and transforming growth factor (TGF β) are abundant in the tumor microenvironment, resulting in altered dendritic cell and T-cell function (Fig. 2) (39). In addition to secreted molecules, transmembrane molecules such as FasL (CD95L), B7-H1/PD-L1 and B7-H4 are potent inhibitors of T-lymphocyte function (42). FasL (43), B7-H1 (44), and B7-H4 (45) are

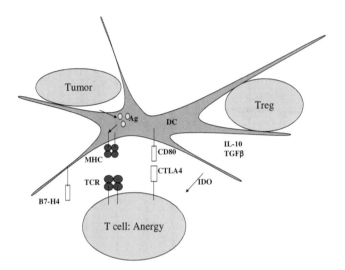

FIGURE 2 Regulation of T-cell immunity. CD4+CD25+ regulatory T cells and cytokines in the tumor microenvironment such as IL-10 and TGF-β result in altered dendritic cell and effector T-cell function. This includes overexpression of inhibitory molecules, such as B7-H4 and indoleamine 2,3-dioxygenase, and activation of the T-cell inhibitory molecule, CTLA-4. These pathways result in T-cell anergy or tolerance. *Abbreviations*: CTLA4, cytotoxic T-lymphocyte-associated antigen; DC, dendritic cell; IDO, indoleamine 2,3-dioxygenase; MHC, major histocompatibility complex; TCR, T-cell receptor; TGFβ, transforming growth factor.

all expressed by subsets of breast tumors and are potential targets of immune intervention.

Antigen Presentation and Dendritic Cells

Although tumor antigenic peptides can be presented directly from tumor cells, professional APCs, in particular dendritic cells, are essential for priming naïve T-cells and activating the immune response (46). Tumors of epithelial origin generally do not express costimulatory signals, such as B7, CD40, 4-1BBL (47), and OX40L (48) that are required for activation of effective T-cell responses. Immature DC's may actively endocytose necrotic, apoptotic, or antibody-coated tumor cells ("cross-presentation"), and then undergo maturation upon activation of TLRs, CD40 ligand, or cytokine signals such as TNF-alpha (Fig. 1). Upon maturation, dendritic cells upregulate MHC molecules and costimulatory molecules, secrete cytokines and chemokines to enhance the migration of lymphocytes, and express chemokine receptors for migration to lymph nodes (49).

There is mounting evidence that dendritic cells have abnormal function in cancer patients (Fig. 2) (50). Indoleamine 2,3-dioxygenase (IDO) is involved in tryptophan catabolism and is thought to play a role in placental-based maternal immune tolerance. Accumulation of IDO in dendritic cells correlates with impairment of T-cell function in vitro and has been observed in lymph nodes of patients with melanoma and breast cancer, and other tumors (51,52). IDO accumulation in dendritic cells can predate the development of overt lymph-node metastases. Inhibitors of IDO are now being developed as potential immune adjuvants.

TABLE 1 Breast Cancer Vaccination Strategies

Antigen	Antigen delivery	Adjuvant
HER2/neu	Peptide	GM-CSF
MUC-1	Protein	CpG
CEA	RNA	TRICOM™
Survivin	DNA	Dendritic cells
Telomerase	Vaccinia virus	QS-21
NY-ESO-1	Fowlpox virus	
Cyp1B1	Nanoparticles	
Cyclin B1	Expanded T cells	
Mammaglobin A	Cell fusion	
Carbohydrate antigens		
Autologous cells		
Allogeneic cells		

There have been multiple clinical trials of vaccine delivery with the use of dendritic cells. The cells are usually isolated from peripheral blood by means of leukapheresis. They are cultured in vitro with the cytokines GM-CSF and interleukin-4, loaded with antigen, and matured ex vivo to enhance antigen presentation and costimulation of T-cells before being injected into patients. Antigen may be delivered as peptide, protein, RNA (53), or tumor lysates (54) (Table 1). In addition, dendritic cells have been directly fused with autologous breast cancer tumor cells, which allows for the presentation of multiple tumor antigens (55). Although dendritic cell-based vaccines have had minimal side effects and have induced measurable T-cell immunity, few durable clinical responses have been reported (55–57). However, a dendritic cell-based vaccine was shown to confer a modest survival benefit in hormone-refractory prostate cancer (58). Because dendritic cell production must be performed in specialized clinical laboratories, alternative strategies, including using artificial APCs or targeting antigen directly to dendritic cells in vivo using DC-targeted antibodies, microparticles, electroporation, or nanotechnology are being explored.

TARGETING TUMOR ANTIGENS
Antigen-Specific Vaccines
The ideal breast cancer vaccine would induce broadly reactive immunity to multiple types of breast cancer without causing clinically significant autoimmunity and, most important, be clinically effective. One approach to minimize autoimmunity and enhance specificity of vaccines is to target them to specific protein antigens that are overexpressed on the tumor cells but that have limited distribution in normal tissue. Many breast cancer tumor antigens are also expressed on tumor cells in other epithelial-derived cancers, such as ovarian cancer and colon cancer, and have been targeted in early-phase clinical trials in breast cancer and other solid tumors. In addition to MUC-1, HER2/neu, and telomerase (see subsequently), target antigens include CEA (59,60), cyp1B1 (61), survivin (62,63), and others (Table 1).

MUC-1
Overexpression and aberrant glycosylation of mucin-1 (MUC-1) antigen by epithelial tumors results in endogenous antibody responses in cancer patients to

MUC-1 antigen (64). This finding has led to the identification of MUC-1-derived peptide epitopes that induce T-cell responses. MUC-1-based clinical trials have used peptides (65–69), protein (70), pulsed dendritic cells (61), or keyhole limpet hemocyanin (KLH) adjuvant (31).

HER2/neu

The HER2/neu antigen is a well-known target of antibody-mediated immunotherapy in breast cancer. The initial demonstration of multiple HLA-A2-binding peptides derived from the HER2/neu protein has led to multiple clinical vaccine trials. Initial studies using peptide and adjuvant have demonstrated safety with minimal toxicity (61,71–73), but induced cytotoxic T-cells that failed to lyse tumor cells (21). To augment CD4+ T-cell immunity, HER2-derived class II peptides (26,74), or the HER2 intracellular domain (75,76), have been used for vaccination. A recent study of vaccination of high-risk patients in the adjuvant setting showed a trend toward improved disease-free survival in patients who received a HER2 peptide-based vaccine (85.7% vs. 59.8% in unvaccinated patients).

hTERT

The catalytic subunit of telomerase, hTERT, is a widely expressed tumor antigen, present in more than 85% of all human cancers (22). Initial clinical trials of dendritic cells pulsed with hTERT-derived peptides or hTERT RNA resulted in measurable hTERT-specific immunity (78,79), but hTERT peptide vaccination with adjuvant generated T-cells that did not recognize endogenously-processed telomerase (80).

Overall, these antigen-specific therapies have been well tolerated, with minimal toxicity, but only sporadic disease responses have been observed. The majority of these vaccines have been tested in the advanced disease setting. The optimal method of delivery of tumor antigens is not yet known, although many approaches have been tried (Table 1). These include adoptive immunotherapy with ex vivo expanded T-cells (81), peptide-based vaccines, proteins, RNA, DNA, and viral vectors such as vaccinia and fowlpox, that also encode three costimulatory molecules [CD80/B7.1, ICAM-1, and LFA-3; designated TRICOM^{TM} (59)].

Cellular-Based Vaccines

Vaccines based on whole autologous or allogeneic tumor cells have been combined with strong adjuvants or cytokines, since tumor cells themselves generally stimulate poor antigen presentation (82). Both autologous tumor cells (83–85) and allogeneic cell lines (86–88) have been used in clinical trials in breast cancer, with isolated clinical responses reported. Whole tumor cells have also been fused with dendritic cells (89). In murine models, GM-CSF was the most potent cytokine adjuvant for vaccination (90), and GM-CSF-secreting autologous and allogeneic vaccines are currently being evaluated in clinical trials in breast cancer.

TARGETING IMMUNE REGULATION

The focus of tumor immunology is shifting from targeting specific antigens to targeting the regulation of immune responses that result in impaired host immunity and tolerance to tumor antigens (Fig. 2 and Table 2). By activating co-stimulatory molecules and inhibiting molecules that down regulate immunity, effective T-cell immunity can be generated. By combining these approaches of targeted antigenic

TABLE 2 Targets of Immune Regulation

Activating targets	Inhibitory targets
B7.1/CD80	Regulatory T cells
B7.2/CD86	FoxP3
CD40	CTLA-4
4-1BB	PD-L1/B7-H1
OX40	B7-H4
MICA, MICB	IDO
Toll-like receptors	TGF-β
TNF-alpha	IL-10
	FasL/CD95L

Abbreviations: TGF-β, transforming growth factor-β; TNF-alpha, tumor necrosis factor-alpha; CTLA-4, cytotoxic T-lymphocyte-associated antigen-4; IDO, indoleamine 2,3-dioxygenase.

vaccination with "regulating the regulators," it is hoped that specific anti-tumor T-cell-immunity can be generated.

Regulatory T Cells

One mechanism of immune regulation is the activity of regulatory T-cells. These CD4+CD25+FoxP3+ T-cells inhibit other cellular immune responses and the development of autoimmunity (91,92). Regulatory T-cells normally account for 5% to 10% of CD4+ lymphocytes in peripheral blood. In patients with breast cancer, however, regulatory T-cells are increased both in peripheral blood and in malignant effusions (93,94). In a study of patients with ovarian cancer, elevated levels of regulatory T-cells in the tumor and in ascites were associated with poor survival (95).

Targeted therapeutics that specifically inhibit regulatory T-cells have been developed and are being tested in clinical trials. Denileukin diftitox (Ontak), which is a fusion of the full-length of interleukin-2 and the active portion of diphtheria toxin, can deplete regulatory T-cells by directly binding to CD25 (interleukin-2 receptor). In combination with RNA-transfected dendritic cells, Ontak augments T-cell responses in patients with renal-cell carcinoma (96) and in those with ovarian carcinoma (97).

Cytotoxic T-Lymphocyte-Associated Antigen-4 Blockade

Cytotoxic T-lymphocyte-associated antigen (CTLA-4) is an inhibitory transmembrane molecule expressed on T-lymphocytes (Fig. 2). Activation of CTLA-4 strongly inhibits memory T-cell responses, as demonstrated by the development of lethal lymphoproliferative disease in CTLA-4 knockout mice (98,99). The observation that CTLA-4 blockade can augment anti-tumor immunity in mouse models, has prompted an intense effort to develop antibody therapeutics that target CTLA-4.

Early-phase clinical trials have used anti-CTLA-4 monoclonal antibodies in melanoma, and in ovarian, renal-cell, colon, and prostate cancers (101–106). CTLA-4 blockade has been associated with the development of significant Grade III/IV autoimmunity (dermatitis, colitis, hypophysitis) (106), but also with clinical responses in melanoma patients, including tumor necrosis (101–103). Notably, 9 of 29 patients with melanoma had either stable disease or extended periods without disease progression (23 to 36+ months) (102). Hodi et al. (101) used autologous vaccination to prime T-cells and subsequent administration of an antibody that blocks CTLA-4 (MDX-010) to boost memory T-cell responses. This vaccination strategy resulted in significant tumor necrosis in three of seven patients with melanoma. Although these studies have focused primarily on malignant melanoma, CA-125 responses have been reported in patients with ovarian cancer (107) and PSA responses have been reported in hormone-refractory prostate cancer patients (105), arguing that augmentation of memory T-cell responses can be clinically effective in adenocarcinomas. It is not yet known whether the development of autoimmunity can be separated from the antitumor effects of this potent immunotherapeutic target.

CLINICAL ISSUES IN VACCINATION

There are several challenges that affect the development of breast cancer immunotherapies. Molecular typing of breast cancer (108) and genomic identification of breast cancer antigens (109) have made it clear that there are specific biologic types of breast cancer with different levels and patterns of tumor antigen expression. The identification of multiple antigenic targets in breast cancer (Table 1) has required the development of immunologic assays for careful monitoring of antigen-specific immune responses. There is no global assay for assessing immunocompetence, but antigen-specific T-cell responses can now be quantitatively measured with the use of flow cytometry using recombinant tetrameric HLA molecules (110), and plate-based ELISA and Elispot assays for T-cell-dependent cytokine secretion. Whole-cell based vaccines and modulators of immune regulation are more difficult to assess. Delayed-type hypersensitivity to vaccine can be tested in skin-biopsy specimens, and tumor-biopsy specimens can be examined for evidence of infiltrating lymphocytes, but identification of target antigens in complex vaccines and after targeted anti-immunoregulation remains difficult. Ideally, genome-wide and proteome-wide approaches to monitor immune responses will prove useful (27,36).

Timing of Vaccination

The timing of prior chemotherapy may be critical to the successful development of tumor-specific immunity. Cytotoxic chemotherapy has several effects on immune responses [reviewed in (111)]. It can abrogate existing immune responses, deplete regulatory T-cells, and induce a minimal residual disease state, thereby enhancing the potential effectiveness of immunotherapies. Specific chemotherapeutic agents, such as doxorubicin, paclitaxel, 5-fluorouracil, and cisplatin, have effects on the local tumor microenvironment, enhancing apoptosis, antigen presentation, or sensitivity to cytotoxic T-lymphocyte-mediated killing (112,113). Cyclophosphamide, in particular, may decrease the function of CD4+CD25+ T-regulatory cells that inhibit immune responses (114). In addition, immunotherapy may enhance the efficacy of subsequent chemotherapies (115). These findings point to potential synergistic effects of chemotherapies and immunotherapies. Similarly, immunotherapies may be synergistic with other targeted therapeutics.

CONCLUSION

The development of cancer requires inhibition of effective immunity at multiple levels, from dysregulation of innate immune responses to active inhibition of adaptive immunity at the tumor microenvironment. As cancer progresses, so does the extent of immune dysregulation. Shifting the timing of vaccine delivery from the metastatic to the adjuvant setting (or earlier) should facilitate more effective anti-tumor immunity. To date, most vaccine strategies have focused on immune activation such as antigenic delivery, TLR activation by CpGs and adjuvant, and cytokine stimulation. However, the identification of immune regulatory pathways, such as B7-H1, B7-H4, CTLA-4, IDO, and regulatory T-cells has demonstrated that inhibition of immune regulation will be critical to establish effective anti-tumor immunity. The successful development of breast cancer vaccines will require combinatorial therapies that target both breast-cancer specific immune activation and inhibition of immune tolerance.

SUMMARY

The goal of cancer vaccines and immunotherapies is to train the immune system to recognize cancer cells and destroy them. Immune responses play a dynamic role in the development of cancers, from immunosurveillance to immune escape; from in situ immune dysregulation to metastatic spread. The systematic identification and targeting of molecules involved in the immune response has led to a wide variety of potential immunotherapeutic targets for the treatment of breast cancer. Extraordinary advances in molecular immunology have led to a detailed understanding of tumor antigens, antigen presentation, innate immunity, cytokine and chemokine pathways, and immunoregulation. Many of these vaccine therapies are already in clinical development. It is the rational and rapid translation of these scientific discoveries into effective therapies for patients with breast cancer that poses the greatest challenge, and opportunity, to realize the potential of tumor vaccine therapy for breast cancer.

ACKNOWLEDGMENTS

This work is supported by grants from the NIH, NCI (3 P30 CA006516-41S4 and U01 CA117374), and the AVON Foundation. The author thanks Dr. Ellis Reinherz and Dr. Glenn Dranoff for critical review, and Victoria Alexander for editorial assistance.

REFERENCES

1. Chaudhuri S, Cariappa A, Tang M, et al. Genetic susceptibility to breast cancer: HLA DQB*03032 and HLA DRB1*11 may represent protective alleles. Proc Natl Acad Sci USA 2000; 97:11451–11454.
2. Marincola FM, Jaffee EM, Hicklin DJ, et al. Escape of human solid tumors from T-cell recognition: molecular mechanisms and functional significance. Adv Immunol 2000; 74:181–273.
3. Campoli M, Chang CC, Oldford SA, et al. HLA antigen changes in malignant tumors of mammary epithelial origin: molecular mechanisms and clinical implications. Breast Dis 2004; 20:105–125.
4. Aaltomaa S, Lipponen P, Eskelinen M, et al. Lymphocyte infiltrates as a prognostic variable in female breast cancer. Eur J Cancer 1992; 28A:859–864.
5. Menard S, Tomasic G, Casalini P, et al. Lymphoid infiltration as a prognostic variable for early-onset breast carcinomas. Clin Cancer Res 1997; 3:817–819.
6. Jerome KR, Domenech N, Finn OJ. Tumor-specific cytotoxic T-cell clones from patients with breast and pancreatic adenocarcinoma recognize EBV-immortalized B cells

transfected with polymorphic epithelial mucin complementary DNA. J Immunol 1993; 151:1654–1662.

7. Disis ML, Calenoff E, McLaughlin G, et al. Existent T-cell and antibody immunity to HER-2/neu protein in patients with breast cancer. Cancer Res 1994; 54:16–20.

8. Bishop MR, Fowler DH, Marchigiani D, et al. Allogeneic lymphocytes induce tumor regression of advanced metastatic breast cancer. J Clin Oncol 2004; 22:3886–3892.

9. Lundqvist A, Childs R. Allogeneic hematopoietic cell transplantation as immunotherapy for solid tumors: current status and future directions. J Immunother 2005; 28:281–288.

10. Carella AM, Beltrami G, Corsetti MT, et al. Reduced intensity conditioning for allograft after cytoreductive autograft in metastatic breast cancer. Lancet 2005; 366:318–320.

11. Janeway CTP, Walport M, Shlomchik M. Immunobiology: The Immune System in Health and Disease. 6th ed. New York, NY: Garland Science Publishing, 2005.

12. Iwasaki A, Medzhitov R. Toll-like receptor control of the adaptive immune responses. Nat Immunol 2004; 5:987–995.

13. Vollmer J. Progress in drug development of immunostimulatory CpG oligodeoxynucleotide ligands for TLR9. Expert Opin Biol Ther 2005; 5:673–682.

14. Speiser DE, Lienard D, Rufer N, et al. Rapid and strong human CD8+ T cell responses to vaccination with peptide, IFA, and CpG oligodeoxynucleotide 7909. J Clin Invest 2005; 115:739–746.

15. Diefenbach A, Raulet DH. The innate immune response to tumors and its role in the induction of T-cell immunity. Immunol Rev 2002; 188:9–21.

16. Smyth MJ, Swann J, Cretney E, et al. NKG2D function protects the host from tumor initiation. J Exp Med 2005; 202:583–588.

17. Bauer S, Groh V, Wu J, et al. Activation of NK cells and T cells by NKG2D, a receptor for stress-inducible MICA. Science 1999; 285:727–729.

18. Groh V, Rhinehart R, Secrist H, et al. Broad tumor-associated expression and recognition by tumor-derived gamma delta T cells of MICA and MICB. Proc Natl Acad Sci USA 1999; 96:6879–6884.

19. Groh V, Wu J, Yee C, et al. Tumour-derived soluble MIC ligands impair expression of NKG2D and T-cell activation. Nature 2002; 419:734–738.

20. Singer G, Rebmann V, Chen YC, et al. HLA-G is a potential tumor marker in malignant ascites. Clin Cancer Res 2003; 9:4460–4464.

21. Zaks TZ, Rosenberg SA. Immunization with a peptide epitope (p369–377) from HER-2/neu leads to peptide-specific cytotoxic T lymphocytes that fail to recognize HER-2/neu+ tumors. Cancer Res 1998; 58:4902–4908.

22. Vonderheide RH, Hahn WC, Schultze JL, et al. The telomerase catalytic subunit is a widely expressed tumor-associated antigen recognized by cytotoxic T lymphocytes. Immunity 1999; 10:673–679.

23. Maecker B, Sherr DH, Vonderheide RH, et al. The shared tumor-associated antigen cytochrome P450 1B1 is recognized by specific cytotoxic T cells. Blood 2003; 102:3287–3294.

24. Kao H, Marto JA, Hoffmann TK, et al. Identification of cyclin B1 as a shared human epithelial tumor-associated antigen recognized by T cells. J Exp Med 2001; 194: 1313–1323.

25. Khong HT, Yang JC, Topalian SL, et al. Immunization of HLA-A*0201 and/or HLA-DPbeta1*04 patients with metastatic melanoma using epitopes from the NY-ESO-1 antigen. J Immunother 2004; 27:472–477.

26. Salazar LG, Fikes J, Southwood S, et al. Immunization of cancer patients with HER-2/neu-derived peptides demonstrating high-affinity binding to multiple class II alleles. Clin Cancer Res 2003; 9:5559–5565.

27. Anderson KS, LaBaer J. The sentinel within: exploiting the immune system for cancer biomarkers. J Proteome Res 2005; 4:1123–1133.

28. MacLean GD, Miles DW, Rubens RD, et al. Enhancing the effect of THERATOPE STn-KLH cancer vaccine in patients with metastatic breast cancer by pretreatment with low-dose intravenous cyclophosphamide. J Immunother Emphasis Tumor Immunol 1996; 19:309–316.

29. Sandmaier BM, Oparin DV, Holmberg LA, et al. Evidence of a cellular immune response against sialyl-Tn in breast and ovarian cancer patients after high-dose chemotherapy, stem cell rescue, and immunization with Theratope STn-KLH cancer vaccine. J Immunother 1999; 22:54–66.

30. Holmberg LA, Oparin DV, Gooley T, et al. Clinical outcome of breast and ovarian cancer patients treated with high-dose chemotherapy, autologous stem cell rescue and THERATOPE STn-KLH cancer vaccine. Bone Marrow Transplant 2000; 25: 1233–1241.

31. Musselli C, Livingston PO, Ragupathi G. Keyhole limpet hemocyanin conjugate vaccines against cancer: the Memorial Sloan Kettering experience. J Cancer Res Clin Oncol 127 Suppl 2001; 2:R20–R26.

32. Disis ML, Pupa SM, Gralow JR, et al. High-titer HER-2/neu protein-specific antibody can be detected in patients with early-stage breast cancer. J Clin Oncol 1997; 15:3363–3367.

33. Stockert E, Jager E, Chen YT, et al. A survey of the humoral immune response of cancer patients to a panel of human tumor antigens. J Exp Med 1998; 187:1349–1354.

34. Sioud M, Hansen MH. Profiling the immune response in patients with breast cancer by phage-displayed cDNA libraries. Eur J Immunol 2001; 31:716–725.

35. Sugita Y, Wada H, Fujita S, et al. NY-ESO-1 expression and immunogenicity in malignant and benign breast tumors. Cancer Res 2004; 64:2199–2204.

36. Wang X, Yu J, Sreekumar A, et al. Autoantibody signatures in prostate cancer. N Engl J Med 2005; 353:1224–1235.

37. Hodi FS, Schmollinger JC, Soiffer RJ, et al. ATP6S1 elicits potent humoral responses associated with immune-mediated tumor destruction. Proc Natl Acad Sci USA 2002; 99:6919–6924.

38. Gnjatic S, Atanackovic D, Jager E, et al. Survey of naturally occurring CD4+ T cell responses against NY-ESO-1 in cancer patients: correlation with antibody responses. Proc Natl Acad Sci USA 2003; 100:8862–8867.

39. Zou W. Immunosuppressive networks in the tumour environment and their therapeutic relevance. Nat Rev Cancer 2005; 5:263–274.

40. Zou W, Machelon V, Coulomb-L'Hermin A, et al. Stromal-derived factor-1 in human tumors recruits and alters the function of plasmacytoid precursor dendritic cells. Nat Med 2001; 7:1339–1346.

41. Rollins BJ. Inflammatory chemokines in cancer growth and progression. Eur J Cancer 2006; 42:760–767.

42. Greenwald RJ, Freeman GJ, Sharpe AH. The B7 family revisited. Annu Rev Immunol 2005; 23:515–548.

43. Muschen M, Moers C, Warskulat U, et al. CD95 ligand expression as a mechanism of immune escape in breast cancer. Immunology 2000; 99:69–77.

44. Brown JA, Dorfman DM, Ma FR, et al. Blockade of programmed death-1 ligands on dendritic cells enhances T cell activation and cytokine production. J Immunol 2003; 170:1257–1266.

45. Tringler B, Zhuo S, Pilkington G, et al. B7-h4 is highly expressed in ductal and lobular breast cancer. Clin Cancer Res 2005; 11:1842–1848.

46. Schuler G, Schuler-Thurner B, Steinman RM. The use of dendritic cells in cancer immunotherapy. Curr Opin Immunol 2003; 15:138–147.

47. Wilcox RA, Tamada K, Flies DB, et al. Ligation of CD137 receptor prevents and reverses established anergy of CD8+ cytolytic T lymphocytes in vivo. Blood 2004; 103:177–184.

48. Bansal-Pakala P, Jember AG, Croft M. Signaling through OX40 (CD134) breaks peripheral T-cell tolerance. Nat Med 2001; 7:907–912.

49. O'Neill DW, Adams S, Bhardwaj N. Manipulating dendritic cell biology for the active immunotherapy of cancer. Blood 2004; 104:2235–2246.

50. Gervais A, Leveque J, Bouet-Toussaint F, et al. Dendritic cells are defective in breast cancer patients: a potential role for polyamine in this immunodeficiency. Breast Cancer Res 2005; 7:R326–R335.

51. Munn DH, Sharma MD, Lee JR, et al. Potential regulatory function of human dendritic cells expressing indoleamine 2,3-dioxygenase. Science 2002; 297:1867–1870.

52. Mellor AL, Munn DH. IDO expression by dendritic cells: tolerance and tryptophan catabolism. Nat Rev Immunol 2004; 4:762–774.

53. Nair SK, Morse M, Boczkowski D, et al. Induction of tumor-specific cytotoxic T lymphocytes in cancer patients by autologous tumor RNA-transfected dendritic cells. Ann Surg 2002; 235:540–549.

54. Nestle FO, Alijagic S, Gilliet M, et al. Vaccination of melanoma patients with peptide- or tumor lysate-pulsed dendritic cells. Nat Med 1998; 4:328–332.

55. Avigan D, Vasir B, Gong J, et al. Fusion cell vaccination of patients with metastatic breast and renal cancer induces immunological and clinical responses. Clin Cancer Res 2004; 10:4699–4708.

56. Holtl L, Zelle-Rieser C, Gander H, et al. Immunotherapy of metastatic renal cell carcinoma with tumor lysate-pulsed autologous dendritic cells. Clin Cancer Res 2002; 8:3369–3376.

57. O'Rourke MG, Johnson M, Lanagan C, et al. Durable complete clinical responses in a phase I/II trial using an autologous melanoma cell/dendritic cell vaccine. Cancer Immunol Immunother 2003; 52:387–395.

58. Small E.J.SPF, Higano C, Neumanaitis J, Valone F, Herschberg RM. Immunotherapy (APC8015) for androgen independent prostate cancer (AIPC): Final survival data from a phase 3 randomized placebo-controlled trial, 2005 ASCO Prostate Cancer Symposium, 2005.

59. Morse MA, Clay TM, Hobeika AC, et al. Phase I study of immunization with dendritic cells modified with fowlpox encoding carcinoembryonic antigen and costimulatory molecules. Clin Cancer Res 2005; 11:3017–3024.

60. Morse MA, Nair SK, Mosca PJ, et al. Immunotherapy with autologous, human dendritic cells transfected with carcinoembryonic antigen mRNA. Cancer Invest 2003; 21:341–349.

61. Brossart P, Wirths S, Stuhler G, et al. Induction of cytotoxic T-lymphocyte responses in vivo after vaccinations with peptide-pulsed dendritic cells. Blood 2000; 96:3102–3108.

62. Wobser M, Keikavoussi P, Kunzmann V, et al. Complete remission of liver metastasis of pancreatic cancer under vaccination with a HLA-A2 restricted peptide derived from the universal tumor antigen survivin. Cancer Immunol Immunother 2006; 55:1294–1298.

63. Otto K, Andersen MH, Eggert A, et al. Lack of toxicity of therapy-induced T cell responses against the universal tumour antigen survivin. Vaccine 2005; 23:884–889.

64. Taylor-Papadimitriou J, Finn OJ. Biology, biochemistry and immunology of carcinoma-associated mucins. Immunol Today 1997; 18:105–107.

65. Goydos JS, Elder E, Whiteside TL, et al. A phase I trial of a synthetic mucin peptide vaccine. Induction of specific immune reactivity in patients with adenocarcinoma. J Surg Res 1996; 63:298–304.

66. Reddish M, MacLean GD, Koganty RR, et al. Anti-MUC1 class I restricted CTLs in metastatic breast cancer patients immunized with a synthetic MUC1 peptide. Int J Cancer 1998; 76:817–823.

67. Gilewski T, Adluri S, Ragupathi G, et al. Vaccination of high-risk breast cancer patients with mucin-1 (MUC1) keyhole limpet hemocyanin conjugate plus QS-21. Clin Cancer Res 2000; 6:1693–1701.

68. Karanikas V, Thynne G, Mitchell P, et al. Mannan Mucin-1 Peptide Immunization: Influence of Cyclophosphamide and the Route of Injection. J Immunother 2001; 24:172–183.

69. Snijdewint FG, von Mensdorff-Pouilly S, Karuntu-Wanamarta AH, et al. Antibody-dependent cell-mediated cytotoxicity can be induced by MUC1 peptide vaccination of breast cancer patients. Int J Cancer 2001; 93:97–106.

70. Karanikas V, Hwang LA, Pearson J, et al. Antibody and T cell responses of patients with adenocarcinoma immunized with mannan-MUC1 fusion protein. J Clin Invest 1997; 100:2783–2792.

71. Murray JL, Gillogly ME, Przepiorka D, et al. Toxicity, immunogenicity, and induction of E75-specific tumor-lytic CTLs by HER-2 peptide E75 (369–377) combined with granulocyte macrophage colony-stimulating factor in HLA-A2+ patients with metastatic breast and ovarian cancer. Clin Cancer Res 2002; 8:3407–3418.

72. Knutson KL, Schiffman K, Cheever MA, et al. Immunization of cancer patients with a HER-2/neu, HLA-A2 peptide, p369–377, results in short-lived peptide-specific immunity. Clin Cancer Res 2002; 8:1014–1018.

73. Disis ML, Gooley TA, Rinn K, et al. Generation of T-cell immunity to the HER-2/neu protein after active immunization with HER-2/neu peptide-based vaccines. J Clin Oncol 2002; 20:2624–2632.

74. Knutson KL, Schiffman K, Disis ML. Immunization with a HER-2/neu helper peptide vaccine generates HER-2/neu CD8 T-cell immunity in cancer patients. J Clin Invest 2001; 107:477–484.

75. Disis ML, Schiffman K, Guthrie K, et al. Effect of dose on immune response in patients vaccinated with an her-2/neu intracellular domain protein-based vaccine. J Clin Oncol 2004; 22:1916–1925.

76. Morse MA, Clay TM, Colling K, et al. HER2 dendritic cell vaccines. Clin Breast Cancer 3 Suppl 2003; 4:S164–S172.

77. Peoples GE, Gurney JM, Hueman MT, et al. Clinical trial results of a HER2/neu (E75) vaccine to prevent recurrence in high-risk breast cancer patients. J Clin Oncol 2005; 23:7536–7545.

78. Vonderheide RH, Domchek SM, Schultze JL, et al. Vaccination of cancer patients against telomerase induces functional antitumor CD8+ T lymphocytes. Clin Cancer Res 2004; 10:828–839.

79. Su Z, Dannull J, Yang BK, et al. Telomerase mRNA-transfected dendritic cells stimulate antigen-specific CD8+ and CD4+ T cell responses in patients with metastatic prostate cancer. J Immunol 2005; 174:3798–3807.

80. Parkhurst MR, Riley JP, Igarashi T, et al. Immunization of patients with the hTERT:540–548 peptide induces peptide-reactive T lymphocytes that do not recognize tumors endogenously expressing telomerase. Clin Cancer Res 2004; 10:4688–4698.

81. Ho WY, Blattman JN, Dossett ML, et al. Adoptive immunotherapy: engineering T cell responses as biologic weapons for tumor mass destruction. Cancer Cell 2003; 3:431–437.

82. Mach N, Dranoff G. Cytokine-secreting tumor cell vaccines. Curr Opin Immunol 2000; 12:571–575.

83. Ahlert T, Sauerbrei W, Bastert G, et al. Tumor-cell number and viability as quality and efficacy parameters of autologous virus-modified cancer vaccines in patients with breast or ovarian cancer. J Clin Oncol 1997; 15:1354–1366.

84. Wood G, Baynes R. Vaccination of Stage IV Breast Cancer Patients with Whole Autologous Malignant Cells and Granulocyte Mactrophage Colony Stimulating Factor. Proc Am Soc Clin Oncol; 1999 [abstr 168].

85. Dillman RO, Beutel LD, Barth NM, et al. Irradiated cells from autologous tumor cell lines as patient-specific vaccine therapy in 125 patients with metastatic cancer: induction of delayed-type hypersensitivity to autologous tumor is associated with improved survival. Cancer Biother Radiopharm 2002; 17:51–66.

86. Wiseman CL. Inflammatory breast cancer. 10-year follow-up of a trial of surgery, chemotherapy, and allogeneic tumor cell/BCG immunotherapy. Cancer Invest 1995; 13:267–271.

87. Schoof DD, Smith JW II, Disis ML, et al. Immunization of metastatic breast cancer patients with CD80-modified breast cancer cells and GM-CSF. Adv Exp Med Biol 1998; 451:511–518.

88. Jiang XP, Yang DC, Elliott RL, et al. Vaccination with a mixed vaccine of autogenous and allogeneic breast cancer cells and tumor associated antigens CA15–3, CEA and CA125–results in immune and clinical responses in breast cancer patients. Cancer Biother Radiopharm 2000; 15:495–505.

89. Avigan D. Fusions of breast cancer and dendritic cells as a novel cancer vaccine. Clin Breast Cancer 3 Suppl 2003; 4:S158–S163.

90. Dranoff G, Jaffee E, Lazenby A, et al. Vaccination with irradiated tumor cells engineered to secrete murine granulocyte-macrophage colony-stimulating factor stimulates potent, specific, and long-lasting anti-tumor immunity. Proc Natl Acad Sci U.S.A. 1993; 90:3539–3543.

91. Wang RF. Functional control of regulatory T cells and cancer immunotherapy. Semin Cancer Biol 2006; 16:106–114.

92. Khazaie K, von Boehmer H. The impact of CD4(+)CD25(+) Treg on tumor specific CD8(+) T cell cytotoxicity and cancer. Semin Cancer Biol 2006; 16:124–136.
93. Liyanage UK, Moore TT, Joo HG, et al. Prevalence of regulatory T cells is increased in peripheral blood and tumor microenvironment of patients with pancreas or breast adenocarcinoma. J Immunol 2002; 169:2756–2761.
94. DeLong P, Carroll RG, Henry AC, et al. Regulatory T cells and cytokines in malignant pleural effusions secondary to mesothelioma and carcinoma. Cancer Biol Ther 2005; 4:342–346.
95. Curiel TJ, Coukos G, Zou L, et al. Specific recruitment of regulatory T cells in ovarian carcinoma fosters immune privilege and predicts reduced survival. Nat Med 2004; 10:942–949.
96. Dannull J, Su Z, Rizzieri D, et al. Enhancement of vaccine-mediated antitumor immunity in cancer patients after depletion of regulatory T cells. J Clin Invest 2005; 115:3623–3633.
97. Barnett B, Kryczek I, Cheng P, et al. Regulatory T cells in ovarian cancer: biology and therapeutic potential. Am J Reprod Immunol 2005; 54:369–377.
98. Waterhouse P, Penninger JM, Timms E, et al. Lymphoproliferative disorders with early lethality in mice deficient in Ctla-4. Science 1995; 270:985–988.
99. Tivol EA, Borriello F, Schweitzer AN, et al. Loss of CTLA-4 leads to massive lympho-proliferation and fatal multiorgan tissue destruction, revealing a critical negative regu-latory role of CTLA-4. Immunity 1995; 3:541–547.
100. Leach DR, Krummel MF, Allison JP. Enhancement of antitumor immunity by CTLA-4 blockade. Science 1996; 271:1734–1736.
101. Hodi FS, Mihm MC, Soiffer RJ, et al. Biologic activity of cytotoxic T lymphocyte-associated antigen 4 antibody blockade in previously vaccinated metastatic melanoma and ovarian carcinoma patients. Proc Natl Acad Sci U.S.A. 2003; 100:4712–4717.
102. Ribas A, Camacho LH, Lopez-Berestein G, et al. Antitumor activity in melanoma and anti-self responses in a phase I trial with the anti-cytotoxic T lymphocyte-associated antigen 4 monoclonal antibody CP-675,206. J Clin Oncol 2005; 23: 8968–8977.
103. Phan GQ, Yang JC, Sherry RM, et al. Cancer regression and autoimmunity induced by cytotoxic T lymphocyte-associated antigen 4 blockade in patients with metastatic melanoma. Proc Natl Acad Sci U.S.A. 2003; 100:8372–8377.
104. Sanderson K, Scotland R, Lee P, et al. Autoimmunity in a phase I trial of a fully human anti-cytotoxic T-lymphocyte antigen-4 monoclonal antibody with multiple melanoma peptides and Montanide ISA 51 for patients with resected stages III and IV melanoma. J Clin Oncol 2005; 23:741–750.
105. Davis TA TS, Korman A, et al. MDX-010 (human anti-CTLA4): a phase 1 trial in hormone refractory prostate carcinoma (HRPC), Proc Am Soc Clin Oncol 2002; 21:2002 (abstr 74).
106. Attia P, Phan GQ, Maker AV, et al. Autoimmunity correlates with tumor regression in patients with metastatic melanoma treated with anti-cytotoxic T-lymphocyte antigen-4. J Clin Oncol 2005; 23:6043–6053.
107. Hodi FS, Seiden M, Butler M, et al. Cytotoxic T lymphocyte-associated antigen-4 (CTLA-4) antibody blockade in patients previously vaccinated with irradiated, autolo-gous tumor cells engineered to secrete granulocyte-macrophage colony stimulating factor (GM-CSF). J Clin Oncol 2004. ASCO Annual Meeting Proceedings 2004; 22(145):2536.
108. Perou CM, Sorlie T, Eisen MB, et al. Molecular portraits of human breast tumours. Nature 2000; 406:747–752.
109. Porter DA, Krop IE, Nasser S, et al. A SAGE (serial analysis of gene expression) view of breast tumor progression. Cancer Res 2001; 61:5697–5702.
110. Altman JD, Moss PA, Goulder PJ, et al. Phenotypic analysis of antigen-specific T lymphocytes. Science 1996; 274:94–96.
111. Emens LA, Jaffee EM. Leveraging the activity of tumor vaccines with cytotoxic chemotherapy. Cancer Res 2005; 65:8059–8064.

112. Yang S, Haluska FG. Treatment of melanoma with 5-fluorouracil or dacarbazine in vitro sensitizes cells to antigen-specific CTL lysis through perforin/granzyme- and Fas-mediated pathways. J Immunol 2004; 172:4599–4608.
113. Keane MM, Ettenberg SA, Nau MM, et al. Chemotherapy augments TRAIL-induced apoptosis in breast cell lines. Cancer Res 1999; 59:734–741.
114. Lutsiak ME, Semnani RT, De Pascalis R, et al. Inhibition of CD4(+)25+ T regulatory cell function implicated in enhanced immune response by low-dose cyclophosphamide. Blood 2005; 105:2862–2868.
115. Gribben JG, Ryan DP, Boyajian R, et al. Unexpected association between induction of immunity to the universal tumor antigen CYP1B1 and response to next therapy. Clin Cancer Res 2005; 11:4430–4436.

Index

Printed and bound by CPI Group (UK) Ltd, Croydon, CR0 4YY

17/10/2024

01775690-0008